Praise for *Better Baby Food* and *Better Food for Kids*

"Thank you so much for your advice. It has given me the push to implement many changes in [my son's] diet. Processed cheese is a thing of the past, juice is down to 4 ounces a day, and he is now eating 2 to 3 raw fruits a day. We are working on the veggies. Since cutting way down on juice and including water in his diet, he now eats with much more enthusiasm and is more willing to try new foods."
A few weeks later . . .
"Our son's diet is now more varied, with lots of fruit and only an occasional juice as a treat every few days. Quite a change from the juice-a-holic we had. The water is still a struggle, as is getting him to try new veggies, but we will persevere."
— Mother of a 4-year-old who is becoming less picky

"*Better Food for Kids* is one of my favorite cookbooks. I recommend it for all daycare/ home providers, parents and even seniors, as the recipes are so simple and great!"
— Mother

"We use *Better Baby Food* and *Better Food for Kids* and recommend them all the time."
— Mother

"Your book *Better Baby Food* is an excellent resource in our city library and is on our list of recommended books."
— Public Health Nutritionist

"I've purchased your books *Better Baby Food* and *Better Food for Kids* and found them to be excellent resources . . . I would love to see some changes to the menus in daycare centers. Judging from the reaction I've been getting from mothers and the staff in my son's daycare, I believe there is an immense need for education in feeding children 'better food' as early as possible."
— Mother of a preschooler

"A quick note to express my appreciation for your excellent book, *Better Baby Food*. I have an 8-year-old whom I breastfed for more than 2 years and an 8-month old whom I adopted at 4 months. I was concerned about giving him the best start, nutritionally speaking. I had questions about formula, the introduction of solid food, etc., that have been answered in just a quick review of the opening pages of your book. I had looked at other reference books, but they do not compare in terms of information or accessibility. Thank you for your excellent publication."
— Mother of two

"The second edition of this book is even better than the first. It is authoritative and easy to read, and contains great information and many useful recipes. Convenient sidebars emphasize the practical take-home messages."
— Robert Issenman, M.D.
Chief of Pediatric Gastroenterology and Nutrition, McMaster Children's Hospital, and Professor of Pediatrics, McMaster University

Better Baby Food

Second Edition

Your Essential Guide to Nutrition, Feeding
& Cooking for All Babies & Toddlers

Daina Kalnins, MSc, RD, **and Joanne Saab,** RD

Robert
ROSE

For complete cataloguing information, see page 326.

Disclaimer

This book is a general guide only and should never be a substitute for the skill, knowledge, and experience of a qualified medical professional dealing with the facts, circumstances, and symptoms of a particular case.

The nutritional, medical, and health information presented in this book is based on the research, training, and professional experience of the authors, and is true and complete to the best of their knowledge. However, this book is intended only as an informative guide for those wishing to know more about health, nutrition, and medicine; it is not intended to replace or countermand the advice given by the reader's personal physician. Because each person and situation is unique, the author and the publisher urge the reader to check with a qualified health-care professional before using any procedure where there is a question as to its appropriateness. A physician should be consulted before beginning any exercise program. The author and the publisher are not responsible for any adverse effects or consequences resulting from the use of the information in this book. It is the responsibility of the reader to consult a physician or other qualified health care professional regarding his or her personal care.

The recipes in this book have been carefully tested by our kitchen and our tasters. To the best of our knowledge, they are safe and nutritious for ordinary use and users. For those people with food or other allergies, or who have special food requirements or health issues, please read the suggested contents of each recipe carefully and determine whether or not they may create a problem for you. All recipes are used at the risk of the consumer.

We cannot be responsible for any hazards, loss or damage that may occur as a result of any recipe use.

For those with special needs, allergies, requirements or health problems, in the event of any doubt, please contact your medical adviser prior to the use of any recipe.

Editor: Sue Sumeraj
Proofreader: Sheila Wawanash
Indexer: Belle Wong
Design and Production: Kevin Cockburn/PageWave Graphics Inc.
Illustrations: Kveta

Cover: Walter B. McKenzie/Getty Images

Interior Food Photography: Colin Erricson
Food Styling: Kathryn Robertson
Prop Styling: Charlene Erricson

Interior Baby Photography (in order of appearance): Opposite page 96: © Studio Forza/Getty Images, Overleaf: © Jose Luis Pelaez Inc/Getty Images; Opposite page 97: © iStockphoto.com/Damir Cudic, Overleaf: © Masterfile; Opposite page 128: © iStockphoto.com/Adam Borkowski, Overleaf: © iStockphoto.com/loriel60; Opposite page 129: © iStockphoto.com/Heiko Bennewitz, Overleaf: © Masterfile; Opposite page 160: © VojtechVlk, 2008. Used under license from Shutterstock.com, Overleaf: © Szasz-Fabian Ilka Erika, 2008. Used under license from Shutterstock.com; Opposite page 161: Radoslav Stoilov, 2008. Used under license from Shutterstock.com, Overleaf: © iStockphoto.com/ Drew Hadley; Opposite page 224: © iStockphoto.com/Richard Hobson, Overleaf: © iStockphoto.com/Cherissa Roebuck; Opposite page 225: © iStockphoto.com/Kirill Zdorov, Overleaf: © iStockphoto.com/isabelle Limbach; Opposite page 256: © Masterfile, Overleaf: © George Doyle/Getty Images; Opposite page 257: © Blend Images/Alamy, Overleaf: © JUPITERIMAGES/BananaStock/Alamy; Opposite page 288: © Masterfile, Overleaf: © Sergei Chumakov, 2008. Used under license from Shutterstock.com; Opposite page 289: © SaferTim, 2008. Used under license from Shutterstock.com, Overleaf: © SW Productions/Getty Images

We acknowledge the financial support of the Government of Canada through the Book Publishing Industry Development Program (BPIDP) for our publishing activities.

Published by Robert Rose Inc.
120 Eglinton Avenue East, Suite 800, Toronto, Ontario, Canada M4P 1E2
Tel: (416) 322-6552 Fax: (416) 322-6936

Printed and bound in Canada

1 2 3 4 5 6 7 8 9 CPL 16 15 14 13 12 11 10 09 08

Contents

Acknowledgments

First we would like to thank the Hospital for Sick Children and Robert Rose Inc. for giving us the opportunity to write this book. It has been an amazing experience both on professional and personal levels. Thanks especially to Bob Dees and Marian Jarkovich at Robert Rose. To the editorial and design team at Robert Rose and PageWave Graphics, especially Sue Sumeraj, thank you for making our words and recipes come to life on paper.

Thank you to Margaret Howard, who worked with us and contributed nearly half the recipes for this book. Marg, it was such a pleasure working with you and we look forward to future collaborations.

For the first edition, a special thank you to Dr. Deborah O'Connor, Dr. Paul Pencharz and Debbie Stone, who took time out of their busy schedules to review the text portion of the book and provide insight and constructive comments to ensure our information was as accurate and up to date as possible with current research and opinion.

Also to all of our friends, family and co-workers, including Karen Kurilla, Lucy Dardarian, Christine Dunlop, Jess Haines, Denise Robichaud, Joyce Hawman, Joann Herridge, Inta Huns, Ilze Kalnins, Joanne Munro, Joanne Nijhuis and Connie Saab, who kindly contributed their favorite kid-friendly recipes.

A heartfelt thank you to our families, who helped test our recipes by chopping, cooking and even baking! You tasted our recipes when they turned out and even when they didn't. Most of all, thank you for always supporting us in whatever we do. Thanks especially to David, Blair, Natali, Matt, Denise, Barry and Joyce Hawman, Christine Micules and Joanne Munro.

We would also like to thank our co-workers in the department of clinical dietetics at Sick Kids, including Joan Brennan, Joann Herridge and Donna Secker, who provided us with information, reviewed our work and provided support. Also to Aneta Plaga, who helped ease the burden of typing when the deadline was looming near.

Throughout this project, many friends provided much appreciated advice and encouragement. Thank you Debbie O'Connor, Patrice Banton, Ted and Cathy Watson, Dr. Stan Zlotkin, Monica O'Reilly, Gord Munro and Abbe Klores.

Also, thank you to Linda Chow, who completed the nutritional analysis for over 200 recipes in this book. Thank you for being so patient as we tested and changed recipes. Your help was invaluable.

For the second edition, sincere thanks to Joan Brennan-Donnan, Jennifer Buccino, Megan Carricato, Sharon Dell, Gloria Green, Joanne Herridge, Nicole Inch, Kristen Lasky, Charlotte Miller, Debbie O'Connor, Donna Secker, Debbie Stone, Connie Stuart, Anna Tedesco-Bruce and Joyce Touw for your valuable contributions. Thanks again to Linda Chow, who completed the analysis on all recipes for this second edition. Your contribution was invaluable! Thanks also to Kristen Lasky and Savannah Stuart for their assistance.

Joanne would also like to thank Daina for making this book such a memorable project to work together on. Your support, and friendship, as well as your experience and expertise, are greatly valued. I think we make a great team, and look forward to working together again soon.

From Daina, a sincere thank you to Joanne Saab, a good friend, colleague and co-author. Throughout the long phone conversations, emails and meetings, you have demonstrated over and over again your knowledge, professionalism and commitment to this book. I have really enjoyed our partnership, and like you, look forward to future collaborations. Thanks also for your patience and understanding when Matt or Natali, or both, weren't quite so willing to let go of their mom's attention.

Introduction

In this second edition of *Better Baby Food*, we have talked more about many aspects of breastfeeding, including solutions to common questions and concerns; we've updated the formula section to include some of the new formulas available on the market; and we've provided more information on some important components of a healthy, balanced diet, such as fiber and omega 3 fatty acids. We responded to comments we received from readers of the first edition of *Better Baby Food* and have reduced the amount of sugar and salt in many of the recipes. We have also added 50 exciting new recipes for families to try.

Some important changes include less restriction on foods in the first year of life. For the majority of infants, food restrictions are unnecessary after 6 months of age; however, current literature still recommends introducing one new food at a time.

Other changes have occurred in the lives of the authors. Daina's young children are now older — her daughter turned 9 in 2008, and her little boy is now 7 years old. Both were breastfed and are great eaters today. They enjoy variety and always do the "lick test" when new foods are presented (see page 61 for more on the lick test).

Joanne has twin girls who are now 5 years old. Both were breastfed, and Joanne does admit to the challenge of breastfeeding multiples. People are constantly amazed by the variety of foods Joanne's children eat, and while they may not always like the new foods they try, they are willing to try almost anything, which is fantastic!

Nutritional Analysis

The nutrient databases used for recipe analysis were the Canadian Nutrient File 1998 and the USDA National Nutrient Database for Standard Reference. The Recipe Analyzer from the Dietitians of Canada was also used in combination with the nutrient databases.

The nutrient analyses were based on:

- imperial measures and weights (except for food typically packaged and used in metric);
- the smaller amount where there is a range;
- the first ingredient listed where there is a choice;
- the exclusion of "optional" ingredients; and
- the exclusion of ingredients with non-specified or "to taste" amounts.

Nutritional Advice in Brief

Here, in no particular order, we offer our top 10 recommendations for parents of infants and toddlers. Each provides references for additional information within the book.

1 Breastfeeding is recommended for infants (see pages 9–31). Formula-feeding is an adequate nutritional alternative (see pages 32–41), but does not provide the many immunological (and other) benefits of breastfeeding.

2 Be sure to supervise children when new solid foods are introduced into their diet (see pages 42–65). Learn what measures to take to prevent choking (see pages 67, 76–77).

3 Parents need to be educated on principles of good nutrition if they want to provide the most nutritious food choices for their children. They should understand the basic elements of food — such as protein, fat, carbohydrates, vitamins and minerals — and the role played by each (see pages 93–104).

4 Children should understand from an early age the importance of good nutrition and its effects on their growth and well-being (see pages 61, 69, 94, 95). This will help to promote good eating habits later in life.

5 Commercially prepared foods can provide adequate nutrition, but homemade foods and fresh foods (see pages 48–52) should make up the majority of a child's diet — and that of the family as a whole. (This is why we felt it was important to include a wide variety of nutritious, tasty recipes in this book).

6 Ensure that your child's diet contains an adequate supply of iron-rich foods. Inadequate iron intake can affect their behavior, learning ability and general well-being (see page 57). Young children are particularly at risk of iron deficiency (see pages 101–102).

7 As much as possible, ensure that your child has ready access to a supply of cut-up fresh fruit and vegetables (see pages 59–60, 67). When these foods are at hand, they are more likely to be eaten as snacks. As well, increased fruit and vegetable consumption helps to boost fiber intake, which helps with digestion and reduces constipation.

8 Encourage your child by example to eat nutritious foods and to be physically active. Childhood obesity is on the rise. It is up to parents to help prevent this epidemic (see pages 115–120).

9 Choose whole grains more often than processed grains.

10 Include a variety of fats in cooking and in the diet.

CHAPTER 1

Breast Milk

Mothers face many challenges in caring for a newborn. But preparing healthy, nutritionally balanced meals need not be one of them.

With breast milk, nature has provided the perfect food for your baby. It is very easy to digest and is designed to meet just about all of a healthy infant's nutritional requirements for the first 4 to 6 months of life. The only real exception is vitamin D, which may need to be given as a supplement, particularly in sun-deprived northern locations (see box, page 22). Also, infants who are born extremely premature, weighing less than 2 kg (4 lbs), must receive breast milk that is fortified with extra calories and nutrients.

Breast milk is an unequalled source of nutrition for a baby. Whether it's delivered directly from the breast to the baby's mouth or via a bottle for women who are unable to feed from the breast, breast milk is the preferred choice as the sole source of nutrition for a baby's first 6 months of life. Breastfeeding offers a number of significant health benefits to both mother and child.

Benefits for baby

Breastfeeding offers many health benefits for the baby. In some cases, the longer exclusive breastfeeding continues, the more these health benefits are observed. The benefits to the baby from breastfeeding, as compared to formula feeding, may include, but are not limited to:

Can breast milk help reduce the risk of allergies?

Recent research has shown that for infants with a high risk of allergies (for example, when one or both parents, or a sibling, has an allergy), prolonging breastfeeding for a minimum of 4 to 6 months can decrease the child's risk of developing allergy. Even for families with no history of allergy, exclusive breastfeeding can provide some protection against allergies from infancy through the preschool years. Studies in both families with a history of allergy and those with no history of allergy show that the longer the duration of breastfeeding (with some protection even with as little as 3 months of breastfeeding), the less likely an infant is to develop atopy, which includes asthma, food and respiratory allergy or wheezing. Some studies show that the incidence of these is about 50% lower in breastfed children. Other studies have not found this positive effect; nevertheless, breastfeeding remains the recommended feeding method for babies. Even very small amounts of breast milk, such as the colostrum in the first few days, provide protection for an infant.

- a decreased risk of developing allergies;
- an improved fatty acid profile in the blood, which can prevent heart disease in later years;
- enhanced immunity, which means lower rates of ear infections, lower respiratory tract infections and diarrhea (gastroenteritis);
- some protection against cancer;
- better bone health;
- protection against inflammatory bowel disease, such as Crohn's disease and ulcerative colitis;
- possible protection against celiac disease; and
- possible protection from obesity.

Benefits for mom

Women who breastfeed not only experience the close bonding and psychological well-being that this form of feeding provides, but may also experience less stress. The hormones, such as oxytocin and prolactin, that are released during breastfeeding can reduce a mother's anxiety level and provide a calming effect during the first few weeks of feeding. Some researchers believe breastfeeding may reduce postpartum depression.

Other possible health benefits for mom include:

- protection against the development of diabetes and heart disease, because of the effect breastfeeding has on the metabolism of nutrients such as carbohydrate and fat;
- a reduced risk of osteoporosis later in life; and
- a decreased risk of breast, ovarian and endometrial cancers (the longer a woman breastfeeds, the more she will be protected against these cancers in later years).

While women who breastfeed may not lose weight dramatically after delivery, they usually do have an easier time losing weight than woman who choose to feed their babies formula. One reason is that in the first few months, a woman's body requires an additional 500 calories a day to produce breast milk. Another is that the fat stores that accumulate during pregnancy are used to provide energy

---

Prevention of SIDS

There is some evidence to indicate that babies who are breastfed have a lower risk of sudden infant death syndrome (SIDS). The frequent feedings and lower incidence of infection in breastfed infants may play a protective role.

for a breastfeeding mom to produce milk. Within 6 to 12 months after delivery, a breastfeeding mom may lose weight more readily than one who formula-feeds her baby. However, attention has to be paid to the appropriate energy intake; if more calories are consumed than are required, weight loss will not occur with either feeding method.

Breastfeeding, by way of the hormone oxytocin, causes the uterus to contract and return to its normal pre-pregnancy size more quickly than in women who choose not to breastfeed. When the uterus contracts more quickly, there is less bleeding after delivery, which can help prevent the loss of iron. The contractions of the uterus, which sometimes occur during breastfeeding, are called afterpains. While these contractions can sometimes be uncomfortable or even painful, they do not typically last longer than 6 to 7 days after delivery. If your afterpains are very uncomfortable and interfere with breastfeeding, you should contact your health care provider, who may prescribe medication to ease the pain.

In addition to the health benefits, breastfeeding is very convenient, as it can be done anytime, anywhere. Breast milk is always fresh, costs nothing and does not require preparation or sterilization techniques that are dependent on a clean water supply.

Breastfeeding positions

There are four main positions women find comfortable for breastfeeding, but there are many other ways you could hold your baby. Experiment to find out what works best for you. In whatever position you choose, you should feel relaxed and your baby should have easy access to your breast. As your baby gets older, you will have figured out what works best for you.

Cross cradle position

This is a good learning position, allowing you good control of your baby's head. Sit with your baby totally on his side and close to you, well supported on pillows, so his chest, abdomen and knees are facing and touching you. If you are feeding on your left breast, you will use your right arm to support your baby's body and your right hand to support

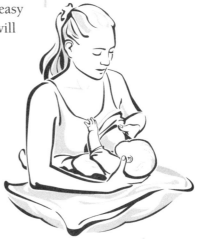

your baby's head. How you support the head is important because babies generally fuss if you hold them around the top of their heads. Open your hand up wide and hold your baby's head low down at the base of the head, with your thumb on one side of the head and your fingers on the other side. Your left hand supports the left breast.

Football position

This is also a good learning position, preferable for many mothers after a C-section. The upright football position keeps your baby more awake. Put a pillow vertically behind your back to move you forward in the chair. This allows more room for your baby's legs behind you.

Hold your baby at your side, supported on pillows. If you're breastfeeding on your right breast, you would seat yourself as far to the left side of the chair as possible. Use your right arm to support your baby at your side, with your right hand supporting the baby's head at the base of the head. Your left hand will support the breast.

Side-lying position

This position is often used during the first feeds and at night and when you want to rest as your baby feeds beside you. It is best if you and your baby are able to latch well before trying the side-lying position, because it is a little harder to have both hands accessible in this position. To feed on the left breast, lie on your left side with your back well supported. You might find it easier in this position to have your head and shoulders well supported on a pillow so that you can see your baby. Lay the baby on the bed on his right side facing you, with his chest against your chest. A pillow or roll behind him will also keep him positioned on his side. Your right arm will support your baby's body and your right hand will support the baby's head, bringing your baby toward your breast. Some mothers are more comfortable with the baby supported in the crook of the arm.

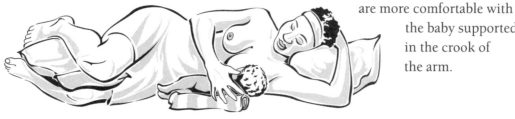

Cradle position

This is a common position for older babies who can easily latch. You can use it initially if it works for you. It is a little harder to control the head in this position. You are sitting with your baby well supported on pillows on your lap. Turn your baby totally on her side and close to you so her chest, abdomen and knees face and touch you. If you are feeding on the left breast, your left arm supports her head, with her head being supported by the forearm but not over the bend in your arm. Her nose should be opposite the nipple to begin. You should not feel you need to move the breast sideways for your nipple to reach her mouth. Your right hand supports the breast.

Not enough moms are breastfeeding!

Eighty-five percent of women in Canada and 75% of women in the United States initiate breastfeeding after the birth of their babies. By the time the baby is 3 months old, however, only about 40% of women in Canada and the U.S. are exclusively breastfeeding their infant (with about 50% providing some breast milk and some formula). By 6 months, only 19% of Canadian women and 13% of American women exclusively breastfeed (39% of Canadian women and 35% of American women offer some breast milk). By 1 year, only 16% of American women continue to offer some breast milk.

Women give many reasons for stopping: they believe they do not have enough milk; they have to return to work; they are very fatigued; the child weans himself. Some women do not even start breastfeeding because they find it unappealing; they believe bottle-feeding to be easier; or they or their child have a medical condition at the time of birth. While certain situations that hinder breastfeeding are unavoidable, clearly a great deal of education on the benefits of

When you shouldn't breastfeed

While breast milk is generally the best food for newborns, there are some cases where breastfeeding is not recommended. One example, although extremely rare (less than 1 in 60,000 births), is in cases of galactosemia, a condition in which infants are born unable to metabolize breast milk. More common examples are when the breast milk may pose a danger to the baby because of the mother's health or lifestyle — for example, if she is HIV positive, has untreated active tuberculosis, or is using illegal drugs.

breastfeeding needs to take place if more women are going to initiate and continue breastfeeding.

The influence of mom's diet on baby

During your pregnancy, your baby had a "taste" of the kinds of food you like, because the food you ate "flavored" your amniotic fluid. The same is true of your breast milk: your food choices affect the flavor of the milk you provide for your baby. Exciting new research confirms that babies taste foods early on — even before solids or complementary foods are introduced; therefore, your diet likely influences your baby's future food preferences. Don't avoid your favorite spices or unusual foods while you are pregnant or breastfeeding. In the future, your baby may be more likely to try different foods that you enjoy, as opposed to simple bland choices, if you have given him a taste of what is to come!

What about foods that are commonly associated with food allergies, such as fish, eggs, peanuts and whole milk? Should breastfeeding moms avoid these foods to help prevent food allergy for her infant? Current advice is that there is no reason to avoid any foods while breastfeeding. If an infant has a known allergy to a certain food, however, then it is recommended that the breastfeeding mother avoid that food. For more on breastfeeding and allergies, see page 9.

Breastfeeding as a form of contraception

Exclusive breastfeeding throughout the day and night can have a contraceptive effect during the first 6 months, because breastfeeding suppresses the release of luteinizing hormone, thereby preventing ovulation. However, breastfeeding should not be relied upon as a complete contraception method — a lot depends on breastfeeding patterns and the health of the mother. As the frequency of breastfeeding decreases, or the amount of time between feeds increases, the chances of ovulation increase. Breastfeeding women who wish to prevent pregnancy should discuss other methods of contraception with their physician, especially if they are giving any formula to the baby.

Mom's nutrition needs during breastfeeding

The production of breast milk requires energy, or calories. A breastfeeding mom needs about 500 extra calories per day for the first 6 months, and about 400 extra calories per day in the following 6 months. (If you have twins, you will need an extra 1,000 calories per day for the production of milk!) But remember, energy needs also depend on your weight. If you were over your ideal body weight before going into pregnancy, and gained more weight than you should have during pregnancy, chances are you were eating too much before becoming pregnant and during pregnancy. Now is a good time to evaluate how much you are eating; add more calories only if you really need them. Listen to your body: eat when you are hungry and stop when you are full.

What nutrients do moms need more of while breastfeeding?

While you are breastfeeding, you need more vitamin A, vitamin E and vitamin C than you did when you were pregnant (see the box at right for some sources of these nutrients). Your need for the B vitamins, which include thiamin, riboflavin and niacin, is about the same as when you were pregnant. (See page 16 for information on vitamin D.) While folate needs are a little less for women who are breastfeeding than for those who are pregnant, it is still important to ensure adequate intake of this vitamin. A supplement of folic acid (400 µg/day) is often recommended for breastfeeding women.

In terms of minerals, your calcium needs remain the same as they were during pregnancy and pre-pregnancy, and you actually need less iron than you required during pregnancy and before you became pregnant. However, women who are anemic after pregnancy (determined by a blood test) may require additional iron until they are no longer anemic. It's best to check with your doctor.

As for fiber, you need about 29 grams per day, about the same amount you needed during pregnancy. If you are not eating 29 grams a day, increase your intake of fiber gradually, by a couple of grams a day; if you increase it quickly over a short period, you may experience bloating. See pages 96–98 for information on the benefits of fiber and a list of foods that contain fiber.

Nutrient sources

Here are some good sources of the nutrients that are important to breastfeeding moms:

- **Vitamin A:** carrots, sweet potatoes, apricots, pumpkins, mangos, milk, cheese, liver
- **Vitamin B:** cereals, meats, legumes
- **Vitamin C:** kiwifruit, oranges, grapefruit, cantaloupes, mangos, strawberries, broccoli, tomatoes, red and green bell peppers
- **Vitamin D:** fatty fish (such as salmon, herring and sardines), fortified margarine and milk, some types of mushrooms, sunlight (spending time in the sun is one of the best ways to ensure that your vitamin D is in good supply)
- **Vitamin E:** wheat germ, corn oil, olive oil, almonds, soy oil
- **Folate:** dark green vegetables, such as spinach, romaine lettuce and broccoli, fortified whole grains

tip

A balance of omega 3 and omega 6 fatty acids in the diet helps to keep inflammation processes in check and to keep blood cholesterol levels within a healthy range.

DHA and your breast milk

Talk of DHA (docosahexanoic acid), one of the omega 3 fatty acids, is everywhere in the news because of its tremendous health benefits. Sources of DHA are fatty fish, such as salmon, trout, herring and sardines. Other omega 3 fatty acids, found in sources such as flaxseeds, flaxseed oil, canola oil and soy oil, also provide important health benefits. But omega 3 fatty acids are not just good for *your* health, they are also good for your breast milk, and thus your baby's health. While breast milk is itself a source of DHA, studies have shown that your diet can influence the DHA content of your milk.

Among other benefits, DHA helps your baby's brain and vision develop. Some studies suggest that the infants of breastfeeding women who have a high intake of omega 3 fatty acids score better on cognitive tests.

Should I try supplements?

Omega 3 supplements are available, but women should check with their family physician to see if they should be taking this type of supplement, based on current recommendations.

Moms and vitamin D

Recent studies indicate that many people, especially those who live in northern climates and those with limited exposure to sunlight, do not get enough vitamin D, as reflected by low levels of this vitamin in their blood. Women with darker skin have an increased risk of deficiency, as darker skin has a diminished ability to produce vitamin D with sun exposure. Wearing sunscreen prevents the body from producing vitamin D. The Canadian Paediatric Society suggests that infants and children should be exposed to just less than 15 minutes of sun per day in the right season (i.e., not winter) to get a good supply of vitamin D.

tip

Recommendations for vitamin D during pregnancy and lactation can also be found on the websites of national health advisory groups, such as Health Canada or the U.S. Food and Drug Administration (see the Resources, page 323).

Mothers can also improve their vitamin D intake, and thus the vitamin D content of their breast milk, by consuming foods rich in vitamin D (see box, page 15) or by taking vitamin D as a supplement. Unfortunately, no one knows how much vitamin D to recommend as a supplement for a pregnant or breastfeeding woman, to keep her baby's vitamin D levels in an appropriate range. It is hoped that ongoing research will soon answer this question. Until more is known about increased vitamin D intake, pregnant or breastfeeding women should avoid taking very high doses of vitamin D (more than 2,000 IU a day).

While the current DRI (Dietary Reference Intake) for pregnant and lactating women is 200 IU (international units) per day, some researchers suggest that this recommendation is too low, especially for women with limited sun exposure (for most of the winter in Canada, for example, the sunlight is not strong enough for the body's own production of vitamin D). Studies looking at the safety and effectiveness of daily doses of 1,000 IU to 2,000 IU (or more) are under way (these amounts do not necessarily increase the vitamin D concentration in breast milk to a level that the milk could serve as a substitute for an infant vitamin D supplement), but you are advised to check with your physician before starting any supplements. Until this research is sorted out, it is recommended that exclusively breastfed infants receive a vitamin D supplement of 400 IU per day. The recommended supplemental form of vitamin D is cholecalciferol, or vitamin D_3.

> ### Benefits of vitamin D
> Not only does vitamin D help you maintain healthy bones by enhancing calcium absorption, but recent evidence links a decrease in vitamin D intake to many diseases, including diabetes, cancers and heart disease.

The basics of breast milk

Breast milk develops in stages, with each providing an important component of the baby's nutrition.

Colostrum

This is the milk produced by moms in the first few days of a newborn infant's life. Colostrum is colorless, often thick and sticky, and contains high amounts of anti-infective properties called immunoglobulins. It also helps babies pass their first stool, which is called meconium. Often only very small amounts of colostrum are produced in those first few days of life, which can be frustrating for mothers who expect a greater volume of milk. However, it is important for new moms to continue to breastfeed. The volume will typically increase by Day 3 or 4, as this first stage gives way to the production of mature milk.

tip
Many prescription and over-the-counter drugs are compatible with breastfeeding. In most cases, the baby receives less than 1% of the maternal dose through breast milk. To find out which medications are safe, talk to your doctor or call the Hospital for Sick Children's "Motherisk" hotline at 416-813-6780 or, toll-free, at 1-877-327-4636. www. motherisk.org

Daina's diary

When my first baby, Natali, was born, I was overwhelmed with the many feelings first-time moms experience. Fortunately, breastfeeding seemed easy, pain-free and enjoyable. Natali, however, had loose, explosive stools and seemed hungry all the time, never quite appearing satisfied. When she failed to gain enough weight in the first few weeks, I realized that she was not receiving enough hindmilk to satisfy her energy needs. I let her feed longer, and soon her gassiness and explosive stools subsided, and she gained weight beautifully!

Mature milk

This milk consists of two different components: foremilk, which is the milk a baby receives at the beginning of any feeding; and hindmilk, which is produced during each feed as the pressure in a mother's breasts decreases.

- Foremilk has a high water and sugar content, and quenches a baby's thirst. It is produced between feeds in response to previous suckling.
- Hindmilk, by contrast, is rich in fat and calories, and is produced during each feed as the pressure in the breast decreases. To ensure the infant receives this calorically dense milk, mothers should breastfeed until the baby pulls away or begins to nibble at the breast or when the infant falls asleep at the breast and doesn't start to feed again if milk is squeezed into its mouth. (See "How much is enough," page 24, for more information on feeding techniques.) Signs that a baby is not receiving sufficient hindmilk include frequent feeding, inadequate weight gain, lots of gas and explosive production of green stools instead of the yellow, seedy-textured type. (See chart, page 25.)

Breastfeeding for two: When you have twins

It is definitely possible to successfully breastfeed twins, because breast milk production is based on a supply-and-demand system. That is, the more milk your babies demand, the more your body makes to replace what they have removed. Prior to delivery, you should speak with a lactation consultant or someone experienced with breastfeeding twins. You may also want to get regular breastfeeding support in your community while you are trying to initiate breastfeeding. As with breastfeeding singletons, when feeding twins you have different options for feeding positions and timing. Speak to your lactation consultant for advice.

Potential issues with breastfeeding, and their solutions

Some of the issues women experience when trying to breastfeed their newborns include engorgement (breast fullness), blocked milk ducts and mastitis. Fortunately, solutions exist for each of these potential issues.

Engorgement (breast fullness)

A woman's breasts start to feel different in the first 2 to 4 days after delivery. They become harder, heavier and more tender as breast milk is produced. Women also sometimes feel pain or discomfort under their arms, because milk-producing tissue is found there as well. The way to relieve the feeling of engorgement is to feed frequently and/or express milk. As more milk is released, the breasts eventually feel softer and are not as tender. Don't worry: breast milk is still being made. It just takes time to get used to the changes in your breasts as milk production increases.

Tips on preventing sore nipples

- Position your baby comfortably and correctly on the breast (see "Breast-feeding positions" on pages 11–13).
- Wash your nipples once a day with warm water.
- Apply breast milk to each nipple after breastfeeding.
- Air-dry nipples, if possible, between feedings.
- Use a 100% cotton bra and reapply dry cotton nursing pads often (avoid plastic-backed pads).
- Avoid creams and ointments unless they are recommended by a breastfeeding specialist — they may only aggravate your skin.
- To take your baby off the breast, insert your finger gently between the baby's lips and gums to break the suction. Remove the nipple before removing your finger from the baby's mouth.

Joanne's diary

While it is possible to exclusively breastfeed multiples, it is not without its challenges. I was very committed to breastfeeding my twin girls when they came home from the hospital. I was fortunate in that the girls were born full-term, but they were small and had individual problems getting a good latch. As a first-time mom, I too was learning the art of breastfeeding, and the fact that I had twins seemed to make this more challenging.

I think the most important thing a new mom can do is ask for help. I asked to see the hospital's lactation consultant, who helped the babies get a proper latch. I also rented an electric pump and pumped after each feeding for 10 to 15 minutes for the first month or so to get my supply up so that I would be able to breastfeed two babies. After a few weeks of feeding the babies one at a time, I visited a lactation consultant in my community to help me get them on the breast at the same time. (Note to first-time moms of multiples: twins will likely need to feed individually first before you will be able to feed them at the same time, which will help reduce the amount of time you spend breastfeeding). I had to work very hard over the next months to provide my twins with breast milk.

Blocked milk ducts

Milk can plug up a milk duct, resulting in blocked ducts, if not enough milk was emptied or if there was increased pressure on the duct. A small lump may form, and the area may become red and tender. You will not have fever with plugged ducts.

To resolve plugged ducts within 24 to 48 hours, try the following:

- feed frequently;
- wear a supportive, well-fitting wireless bra;
- choose a different feeding position and ensure a good latch;
- massage breasts gently while feeding;
- apply warm compresses before and after feeding;
- take a warm shower and massage the breast;
- line up the baby's nose or chin over the plugged duct to help draw the milk out.

If your ducts become plugged frequently, you may want to ask a lactation consultant to assess the latch. Always speak to your physician if you have concerns.

Mastitis

Mastitis is an inflammation in the breast tissue due to infection. Women who have mastitis may notice a red, hot, painful area on the breast. Red streaking may also appear. They may feel unwell and fatigued, and may have chills and a fever. Treatment includes antibiotics, prescribed by a physician. Getting plenty of rest, eating well and applying warm (or cool) compresses to the affected breast will all help you recover. You can continue to express milk or breastfeed from the affected breast. If breastfeeding is too painful, feed from the unaffected breast. You can express the milk from the affected breast and feed it to your baby at another time.

Is it safe to breastfeed while I'm on antibiotics?

You can continue breastfeeding while taking almost any antibiotic. If you are unsure whether your antibiotic, or any other prescribed or over-the-counter medication, is safe, check with Motherisk at the Hospital for Sick Children (see the Resources, page 322) or your public health office.

Supplies for breastfeeding

While you don't need to buy cans of formula or several bottles and nipples if you are exclusively breastfeeding, there are some items that can make breastfeeding more comfortable or that a lactation consultant may recommend in certain situations:

1. a comfortable, wireless nursing bra;
2. washable cotton nursing pads;
3. storage bottles or bags for breast milk;
4. nipple shields (if recommended);
5. a good-quality, hospital-grade double electric breast pump (recommended if mothers need to pump for extended periods of time or choose to pump their milk for bottle feeding).

Breast milk to go

In an ideal world, mothers would always be available to breastfeed their babies. But the realities of life often make this impossible. For such occasions, it is important to have a supply of milk that has been expressed from the breast and is available for whenever the baby is hungry.

Choosing a breast pump

While it's possible to express breast milk manually, the task is considerably easier with a breast pump. There are many different types of breast pumps available, ranging from simple hand-operated models (costing between $20 and $80, depending on quality) to electric or battery-powered pumps designed for home use (between $90 and $300). The most powerful and efficient of all are professional- or hospital-grade electric pumps, which are prohibitively expensive to purchase but can be rented from some hospitals, pharmacies or medical supply companies at a nominal cost. Your birth hospital should be able to provide details. You can also contact Hollister Ltd. (a breastfeeding equipment manufacturer) or Medela Inc. to locate a supplier of breast pumps available for rental in your community. (For contact information, see the Resources, page 322.) Finally, for Internet-enabled moms, it is now possible to shop for breast pumps online.

tip

Infants who are born extremely premature can be breastfed, although the breast milk will generally initially need to be fortified with extra calories and nutrients until the baby reaches a certain weight.

Before you buy, however, compare the cost of purchasing a home-use pump against that of renting a professional-grade device. Depending on how often you expect to use a pump, one option may be significantly less expensive than the other.

Preparing and using a breast pump

Before pumping breast milk, be sure to wash your hands thoroughly with soap and water. Breast milk is relatively free of bacteria, but care must be taken not to contaminate the breast milk with bacteria from hands or dirty equipment. Breast pump kits should also be washed well with hot soapy water and air-dried. Follow the manufacturer's instructions for sterilizing the pump, which is usually done on a daily basis. Mothers should pump each breast for 10 to 15 minutes or until milk stops flowing. Pumping should be done as often as a mother would breastfeed her infant — every 2 or 3 hours for newborns, with longer periods between feedings for older infants.

Storing expressed milk

After using the breast pump, expressed milk should be stored in the refrigerator or freezer in sterile glass or hard plastic containers. Another option is to use plastic freezer bags that have been specially designed for freezing breast milk. (You can also use ordinary freezer bags, although these should be double-bagged to avoid punctures.) Once milk is collected in sterile containers, it should be labeled clearly with the date and time of expression so that the milk can be consumed by the baby in the order it was pumped. Frozen breast milk should be stored in small (2- to 4-oz/60 to 125 mL) portions, since these will defrost quickly and less will be wasted if baby doesn't drink the entire amount of thawed milk. When freezing breast milk, be sure to leave some space at the top of the storage container as the milk will

tip

Once thawed, frozen breast milk should be refrigerated and consumed within 24 hours. Do not freeze again.

Breast milk express

8 steps to success

1. Wash hands and equipment thoroughly.
2. If you are at work or away from your baby, find a quiet place to pump. An article of clothing or a blanket that smells like baby may help let down the milk.
3. Pump — approximately 10 to 15 minutes per breast until empty.
4. Collect milk in sterilized containers. Label clearly with date and time.
5. Freeze or refrigerate for later use.
6. Defrost frozen milk overnight in refrigerator or run under warm running water. Do not microwave or place breast milk in hot water. Test temperature before using.
7. Feed baby.
8. Discard any breast milk that remains after feeding.

expand during freezing. Fresh breast milk can be stored for up to 48 hours in the refrigerator, and up to 6 months in the freezer if frozen using the proper techniques.

Defrosting frozen breast milk

Defrosting should be done overnight in a refrigerator, where it will take approximately 8 to 12 hours to thaw completely. For parents in a hurry, frozen milk can be placed under warm running water or in a dish of warm water. Do not use boiling water, since this can destroy the milk's immunological (infection-fighting) properties. Breast milk should never be heated in a microwave, which changes the composition of breast milk and can cause "hot spots" that could burn the baby's mouth.

How often and how long should you breastfeed?

Newborn infants should feed on cue about 8 to 12 times per day until satisfied. They will usually breastfeed for 10 to 15 minutes per breast at each feeding, although this time typically decreases as the baby gets older and learns to feed more efficiently. If a newborn infant, in the first few weeks of life, is not demanding to be fed at least every 4 hours, he should be awakened to feed. Crying is

tip

If you alternate breasts between feedings, it's often helpful to attach a safety pin to the corresponding bra strap to remind you which breast was used.

a late sign that an infant is hungry. Other signs or "cues" that an infant is ready to feed include increased fussiness or agitation, tongue or lip movements, fists in mouth, or opening his mouth when the skin around his mouth, cheeks or lips is touched.

How much is enough?
Newborns

The best way to know if a newborn infant is receiving enough breast milk is by counting the number of wet diapers produced in a day. Weight gain is another. A newborn infant should have 6 to 8 wet diapers a day after the first week of life. During the first days of life wet diapers may be fewer. For example, on Days 1 to 3 of life, infants may only have 3 wet diapers in a day. Wet diapers should increase in frequency and volume each day.

On Day 4 and 5, there should be 4 to 5 wet diapers. These diapers should be quite heavy and wet. Babies should also have about 3 to 5 stools per day. Babies should breastfeed on cue (or demand), about 8 to 12 times per day (that is, every $1\frac{1}{2}$ to 2 hours). There may be a longer period during the night if the baby feeds frequently during the day.

Length of time spent at the breast is also a good indicator that your baby is receiving enough breast milk. Babies spend about 10 to 15 minutes per breast and should not routinely be falling asleep at the breast without feeding. While the baby feeds, there should be a rhythmic suckling and you should hear the baby swallowing. After feeding, breasts should feel softer.

To ensure adequate weight gain, be sure to have your baby properly weighed (not on a home scale) after the first week (Day 7).

Older infants

Between the ages of 1 to 4 months, babies will feed less frequently than newborns — in most cases, between

Eating and sleeping

Most parents are grateful for newborn infants who like to sleep. But sleepy babies are often hard to feed for more than 5 or 10 minutes before they nod off. To encourage longer feeding and adequate nutrition, newborns can be kept awake by tickling their toes or undressing them slightly.

When to get help

4 signs that you need assistance with breastfeeding your baby

1. Baby has fewer than 2 soft stools per day in the first month.
2. Baby has dark urine and produces fewer than 3 wet diapers on Days 1 to 3, and fewer than 6 wet diapers by Day 5 or 6.
3. Baby is unusually sleepy and difficult to wake for feedings.
4. Baby is feeding less often than 8 times per 24 hours.

6 to 8 times a day (or every 3 to 4 hours). They may also begin to sleep through the night (or longer) without feeding. Throughout this period, the infant should continue to produce 6 or more heavy, soaked diapers per day. Stool frequency varies between babies, but may be 3 to 5 daily. Weight gain provides a good indicator that the older infant is getting enough nutrition from breastfeeding. Ask to see your baby's growth chart at his or her next doctor's appointment.

What goes in, what comes out

Determining whether your newborn is getting enough breast milk

DAYS AFTER BIRTH	NUMBER OF FEEDS	STOOLS	WET DIAPERS
1 to 2	Number of feeds will increase each day. Should feed 8 to 12 times/day	Dark green or black meconium. May only have 1 sticky stool	1 to 3 wet diapers, increasing in fullness each day *Note:* Occasional brick-red staining is normal in Days 1 to 3.
3 to 4	8 to 12 times per day, every 2 to 3 hours	Day 3 stool may still be black Day 4 stool will be lighter (yellowish) in color	3 or 4 soaked diapers
5 to 6	8 to 12 times per day	Minimum of 2 to 3 bowel movements per day. Stools will be odorless, a few tablespoons in volume and yellow/seedy in color and texture	6 or more, heavy soaked diapers. Will continue to have this many diapers for many months

Monitoring growth in the fully breastfed baby

In 2006, the World Health Organization (WHO) produced growth charts that reflect the normal growth pattern of the exclusively breastfed infant. These growth charts differ from the ones that are usually used (the Centers for Disease Control and Prevention charts) because the other charts reflect the growth of infants who have been fed formula alone or both formula and breast milk. Breastfed infants grow more quickly in the first 2 to 3 months of life, and more slowly in the later months, than formula-fed infants. When the CDC charts are used, some exclusively breastfed babies appear not to be growing well, and their mothers may be told to give the babies formula when in fact they are gaining adequate weight on breast milk alone. Using the WHO growth charts, fewer babies appear to be "falling off the chart," or gaining at a slower rate. Plotting exclusively breastfed babies on the WHO charts is therefore recommended.

Poor weight gain and the breastfed baby

By 4 to 5 months, breastfeeding should be well established. If an exclusively breastfed baby is growing poorly at 4 or 5 months of age, as demonstrated by his growth curve on the WHO growth charts, then a full evaluation by a physician and a breastfeeding expert is required. One explanation for the poor growth could be that inadequate breast milk is being provided because of a poor latch or decreased milk supply. Other children may be demanding more of their mother's attention, resulting in fewer feeds for the baby than in the first few months of life. Mom may be taking on more responsibilities and feeding her baby less often, especially if the baby is

How to Read WHO Growth Charts

The baby's actual height and weight at his corresponding age are plotted on the chart. The line along which height and weight are plotted indicates the percentile for that height and weight. Weight should be at about the same percentile as height.

The 50th percentile indicates the average height and weight of a breastfed baby at that age. If a child's height and weight are plotted on a higher percentile (for example, the 97th), it does not necessarily mean that there is a problem. Nor is there necessarily something wrong if a child's height and weight are plotted on a lower percentile (for example, the 3rd). This usually just means that they have larger or smaller parents. It is growth over time — the growth pattern — that is most important.

Feeding can be assessed by tracking growth and weight gain. If there are any significant deviations from the growth curve over time, your family doctor or pediatrician will discuss this with you. If you are worried about the size of your baby, growth charts can help determine whether you have cause for concern, provided that growth over time has been charted. The growth pattern is more important than single measurements.

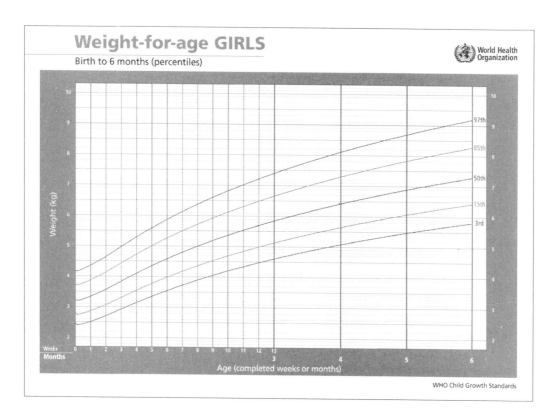

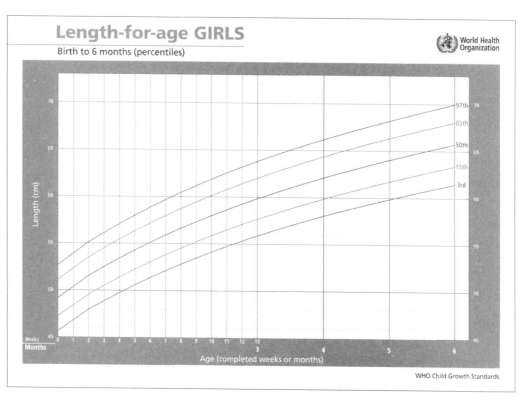

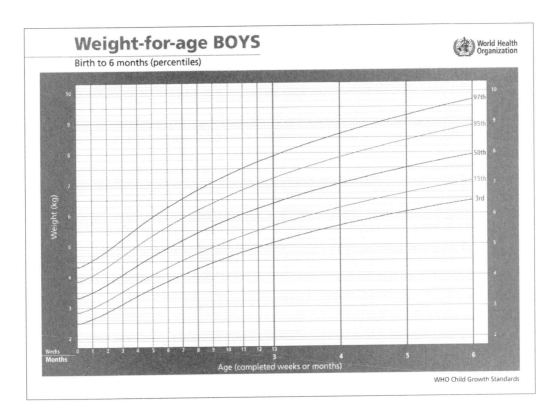

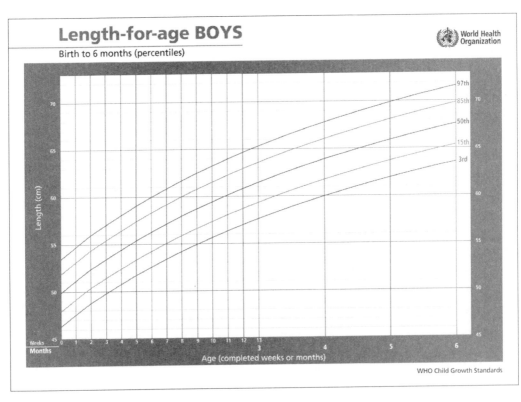

sleeping longer at night. Other lifestyle choices can also affect breastfeeding.

If a mother wishes to continue exclusively breastfeeding at this stage, rather than offering complementary food, she must continue to provide an adequate supply of breast milk as the sole source of nutrition. Inadequate nutrition can affect an infant's growth and brain development. An assessment by a breastfeeding expert or lactation consultant is recommended, to assess the latch, feeding pattern and milk volume. Breast milk production can be increased by increasing the number of breastfeeds, by breast compression and/or with medications.

Additional feeding — bottle-feeding expressed breast milk or formula 1 to 2 times a day — may be warranted for infants who are not growing adequately. While exclusively breastfeeding until the baby is 6 months old is recommended, complementary feeding must be considered if the mother's lifestyle choices do not allow for adequate feeding. The growth and development of the infant is critical, and inadequate feeding can affect a baby for life.

When to wean your infant

There are many factors to consider when deciding when to wean an infant off the breast, including a mother's decision to return to the workforce (although many mothers are able to continue breastfeeding at work) and/or the baby's preference for finger foods or sip cups after these have been introduced to the diet. It is normal for mothers to continue breastfeeding until the infant is transitioned to whole milk at 12 months or even longer. If an infant is weaned off the breast prior to the introduction of whole milk, both the American and Canadian pediatric societies recommend the use of an iron-fortified, cow's-milk-based infant formula as your best alternative to breastfeeding. (See Chapter 2, page 32.)

tip
While exclusive breastfeeding to 6 months is the accepted advice from international health authorities, some experts still suggest that more studies are needed to ensure that all nutrients (for example, iron) are being met through breast milk alone up to this age. Keeping informed about the latest advice is always recommended. Check out your national health advisories for up-to-date information and speak with your family doctor.

Top 10 Breastfeeding Questions

1 My baby was sick at birth, and we were not able to breastfeed for his first 2 weeks of life. Can I still try to breastfeed even though he's been bottle-feeding?

The most important gift of immunity a mother can give her baby is her breast milk. If she cannot breastfeed because of infant or maternal illness, she can still establish a milk supply by using a hospital-recommended electric breast pump on the same schedule that the baby is feeding, about every 3 hours on average. As long as she is producing breast milk and the baby is receiving breast milk, both are enjoying the many health benefits that breastfeeding provides. The birthing hospital nurses or community health nurses should be able to provide resources, such as lactation consultants, to assist mom with latching a baby who has not been at the breast. Even though your baby has been bottle-fed for 2 weeks, it is still possible that he will be able to latch. If he has difficulty latching, ask to see a breastfeeding expert.

2 Are there any foods I should avoid while I am breastfeeding?

There is no need to avoid specific foods while you are breastfeeding. Some women believe foods that give them gas, such as cabbage or onions, can make their baby gassy as well. There is no evidence to support this. The more variety in the foods you eat while breastfeeding, the more variety your baby is tasting. This may actually help prevent your baby from becoming a picky eater later on. Keep in mind that while up to 25% of babies may develop colic or irritability in the first few months of life, this is not necessarily associated with foods the mother is eating while breastfeeding.

Women who are pregnant or breastfeeding should, however, limit their intake of caffeine (no more than 1 to 2 cups of coffee a day) and certain herbal teas (safe ones — at 2 to 3 cups per day — include citrus peel, orange peel, ginger, lemon balm and rose hip, but check with your physician first).

3 Can I have a glass of wine if I am breastfeeding?

It is best to save that treat for when your breastfeeding is established, at about 4 to 6 weeks, when you have a better idea of your baby's usual feeding times. Alcohol does appear in breast milk, and can decrease milk supply if consumed in large quantities. If you want to enjoy some wine (about 5 ounces/150 mL) or beer (about 12 ounces/341 mL) with your meal, it's best to do so either after you breastfeed or at least 2 hours before the next feeding, so that the alcohol will not be present in your breast milk. Keep in mind that women who are lighter in weight may have a lower tolerance. If your baby is hungry while you are having your wine, it would be best to give him or her bottled breast milk.

4 I am not sure if I have enough milk for my baby, and my breasts really hurt when she is feeding. Where can I go for help with breastfeeding issues?

Lactation consultants are trained professionals (they may be nurses or other health professionals) who can help with just about any breastfeeding issue. Check with your birthing hospital or your public health department to find the LC support clinic nearest you. See the Resources, page 322, for more information.

5 The breastfeeding position I was taught does not seem very comfortable. Are there any alternative positions I can try?

Absolutely. Breastfeeding positions include cradle, cross cradle, football and side-lying (see "Breastfeeding positions" on pages 11–13). As long as your baby is removing milk, you can experiment with each of these positions until you learn what is comfortable for you. Together, you will find the position that works best for both of you.

6 My nipples are very sore when I breastfeed. What can I do to decrease the pain?

Sore nipples can really prevent a woman from enjoying breastfeeding. While it is normal to have some degree of tenderness in the first week or so, the pain should not persist. It is important to know why you are feeling pain. The most common cause is a poor latch. Other reasons include incorrect positioning, incorrect sucking, a plugged nipple pore, a yeast infection or andvasospasm (where the nipple changes color after feeding as the temperature changes from the warmth of the baby's mouth to cool air). All of these can be "treated" with the appropriate advice from an experienced lactation consultant (see the Resources on page 322). For tips on preventing sore nipples, see page 19.

7 Will skipping a breastfeed or prolonging the time between pumping increase my milk supply?

Many mothers believe that skipping a feeding or prolonging the time between pumping will build their milk supply. In fact, the opposite is true. Skipping feeds sends a message to the mother's body that it has produced enough milk and does not need to produce more.

8 My pumped breast milk is often a different color on different days. Is there something wrong?

The color, consistency and odor of breast milk can vary depending on many things, including the foods you eat. If you are freezing your breast milk, different foods found in your refrigerator or freezer can also affect the odor of your breast milk.

9 Is it all right to give my breastfed baby a bottle? I've heard that it can lead to something called "nipple confusion."

The mechanisms of breastfeeding and bottle-feeding are quite different. If a baby is offered a bottle too soon — that is, before breastfeeding is well established — it is possible for a baby to develop "nipple confusion." This happens when a baby is unable to learn techniques of both breast- and bottle-feeding. This can result in inefficient sucking at the breast. By delaying the introduction of a bottle until breastfeeding is well established (about 4 weeks), nipple confusion can be avoided.

Alternatively, some babies have a hard time going from breast to bottle or cup when breastfeeding has been well established. What can you do if your baby refuses a bottle or cup? One good suggestion is to use expressed breast milk as your milk of choice for the bottle- or cup-feeding. That way, your baby will still smell your milk. For older infants who are able to handle the fast flow, try removing the stopper from a sippy cup. If your baby is 6 months or older, it is sometimes necessary to spoon the milk into his mouth. Even though having an older baby who refuses milk from anything but the breast is stressful, rest assured that he will also be getting fluid from mashed or puréed/strained foods, which are about 85% to 90% water. Babies will eventually drink from a bottle or cup.

10 I am breastfeeding and taking many vitamin and herbal supplements. Could this be harmful to my baby?

While there are many medications and supplements that can be taken while breastfeeding, there are some that should not be used. Herbal supplements, for example, should be avoided or used with caution while breastfeeding. Vitamins can also pass through to breast milk. So while a single multivitamin taken every day is beneficial to many mothers, this may not be the case if a number of vitamins are taken at once. This is especially true for single-vitamin preparations. Your doctor, pharmacist or dietitian can guide you about specific supplements.

For more infant-related Q & As, see Chapter 2, pages 40-41.

Infant Formula

While breast milk is generally accepted to be the best food for newborns (as discussed in Chapter 1), there may be some circumstances in which a mother will, having considered the alternatives, choose not to breastfeed. Here the most acceptable alternative is to give the baby a cow's-milk-based infant formula until she is 12 months old and begins to drink conventional whole milk.

With so many different types of formula available in the marketplace today, new parents may find it difficult to know which is the most appropriate choice for their child. The good news is that the composition of infant formula is subject to strict regulations, so you can be confident that just about any choice will provide nutrition that is similarly balanced.

Formula fundamentals

While all types of infant formula are intended to provide good nutrition, they differ according to the food source on which they are based. These are described below.

Is that formula fortified?

While most formulas will state quite clearly on their packaging whether or not they are iron-fortified, some may not. If you are unsure, read the nutritional analysis on the label. Iron-fortified formulas must contain 1 mg iron per 100 kcal (about 6.8 mg per 1 L). Non-fortified formulas are still required to contain at least 0.15 mg iron per 100 kcal.

Cow's-milk-based formula (*examples: Enfamil with Iron, Similac*). This is the most common type of infant formula on the market — and the best choice for healthy term (that is, not premature) infants who have no family history of allergy. These formulas come in both low-iron and iron-fortified varieties. The low-iron type is designed to mimic the iron content of breast milk. However, for non-breastfed infants who will be consuming formula exclusively until they are 9 to 12 months old (when they have transitioned to whole milk and other foods), most health authorities recommend using iron-fortified formula. This is based on the fact that between the ages of 4 and 6 months, formula-fed infants will have depleted their own body's iron stores and will require additional iron from the foods they eat. Although low-iron formulas do contain small amounts of iron, the quantity may be insufficient to prevent deficiency in infants over 6 months of age.

Infant formula with omega 3 and omega 6 fatty acids (*examples: Enfamil A+, Similac Advance, Good Start with Omega 3 and Omega 6, Isomil with Omega 3 and 6*). The latest trend in infant formula is to add omega 3 fatty acids. These formulas come in cow's-milk-based and soy-based varieties. They have added DHA (docosahexanoic acid) and ARA (arachidonic acid), two fatty acids found in breast milk that support normal brain, eye and nerve development. There is a lack of evidence at this time to support the claim that full-term, healthy children will have better visual acuity or mental test scores because they consumed formula containing DHA and ARA; however, there is reasonable evidence to support these claims when these formulas are given to premature infants. It is important to remember that breast milk contains DHA and ARA, so by choosing to breastfeed you will be supplying these nutrients to your infant naturally.

Soy-based formulas (*examples: Enfamil Soy, Isomil, Alsoy*). Parents choose soy-based formulas for a number of reasons —- many having to do with their own dietary preferences. For example, they may be strict vegetarians (vegans). They may have an allergy (or intolerance) to dairy, and they may interpret symptoms such as loose stools, vomiting and colic as evidence of a similar allergy in their newborn. In fact, there are few cases where the use of a soy-based formula is medically necessary. These include cases of galactosemia, a disorder in which infants are unable to digest the carbohydrate galactose.

Does iron cause constipation?

Like many parents, you may have heard that iron-fortified formulas can cause constipation in newborns, and are therefore cautious about using this type of product. Well, don't worry. Research into this claim has not been able to demonstrate that iron-fortified formulas are any more constipating than their low-iron counterparts.

tip

Unlike those derived from cow's milk, all soy-based formulas available for purchase in the U.S. and Canada are iron-fortified.

Still, it has become common practice to prescribe soy formula for children with cow's milk protein allergy. While soy formula may be appropriate for children with IgE-mediated allergy, it may not be tolerated by children with non-IgE-mediated cow's milk intolerance, also known as cow's milk colitis. Speak to your doctor about the type of cow's milk allergy your child may have. See page 83 for more information. Where cow's milk allergy is a real concern, an alternative may be a hypoallergenic formula (such as Nutramigen), in which the protein is extensively broken down. (See below for details.)

Although soy formulas are not recommended as the first choice for healthy term infants who are not being breastfed, the American Academy of Pediatrics suggests that soy-protein-based formulas are safe and effective alternatives to breast milk or cow's-milk-based formulas, to provide appropriate nutrition for normal growth and development.

Protein hydrolysate formulas, casein-based (*example: Nutramigen*). This type of formula is considered to be hypoallergenic, which, as noted earlier, is a better choice for non-breastfed infants who have a confirmed allergy to cow's milk protein. (Of course, as we have also mentioned previously, breast milk poses the least risk for children at high risk of developing allergy.) Here the protein is broken down into very small units called peptides and free amino acids. Although less palatable to some infants, this type of formula is generally well-accepted by those whose sense of taste is not well developed. This type of formula is also very expensive.

Protein hydrolysate formulas, whey-based (*examples: Nestle Good Start, Enfamil Gentlease A+*). This type of formula contains proteins that have been slightly broken down to form smaller incomplete proteins. The proteins are still quite large, however, so this formula is not appropriate for children with a confirmed allergy to cow's milk protein. It is uncertain whether the formula is suitable for those children at high risk of milk allergy (that is, where a parent or sibling is allergic). The formula offers the benefits of being similar in taste and having a cost comparable to that of standard cow's-milk-based formula.

Lactose-free formulas *(examples: Enfamil Lactose Free, Similac Sensitive Lactose Free)*. Lactose-free formulas are based on cow's milk, but have had the lactose removed and replaced with corn syrup solids. They are intended for infants who are unable to digest lactose, a carbohydrate (sugar) found in cow's milk. These infants, described as having primary lactose intolerance, are actually quite rare. More common are children who develop a temporary version of this condition, called secondary lactose intolerance, which typically accompanies an episode of diarrhea. Lactose-free formulas can also be useful in these cases, providing nutrition until the diarrhea subsides and the ability to digest lactose returns.

Follow-up formulas *(examples: Nestle Follow-Up, Nestle Follow-Up Soy, Enfapro A+)*. These formulas are intended for older infants between the ages of 6 to 12 months. They are a better choice than whole cow's milk for children at an age where they can benefit from different proportions of nutrients, including calories, iron and essential fatty acids. These formulas also have a lower renal solute load than whole cow's milk (see page 38 for details), and are therefore easier on a baby's kidneys. This type of product can be based on cow's milk or soy; both varieties are iron-fortified. While follow-up formulas claim to offer benefits over traditional infant formulas, this has not been proved. Parents can comfortably use the same "starter" formula from birth until 12 months of age.

tip

Lactose-free formulas are not appropriate for infants with galactosemia, a disorder in which infants cannot digest the sugar galactose, since these formulas contain residual galactose.

Iron-fortified formula

Iron-deficiency anemia is the most common childhood nutritional deficiency in North America (and the rest of the world). You will hear us discuss iron deficiency over and over in this book. A full-term baby is typically born with adequate iron stores to last about 6 months, but it may be difficult for moms to remember when to switch to an infant formula that contains extra iron. For that reason, we suggest that, if you choose to formula-feed, you use an infant formula fortified with iron from the get-go.

It may be difficult for premature infants who weigh less than 2.2 lbs (1,000 g) to meet their iron needs with breast milk or formula alone. Talk to your doctor about whether your premature infant requires an iron supplement.

Added-rice formulas *(example: Enfamil Thickened A+ for babies who spit up)*. For otherwise healthy infants who occasionally spit up, this product combines rice starch and a conventional cow's-milk-based formula. The starch is intended to help the formula remain settled in the child's stomach. If your child spits up persistently, you should see your family physician or pediatrician for further recommendations.

Specialty formulas *(examples: Alimentum, Neocate Infant, Pregestimil)*. Specialty formulas are available for those infants who have problems with digestion and/or absorption of carbohydrates, protein, fat, or other nutrients. These formulas are generally used in a hospital setting under the supervision of a dietitian and doctor. They are the most expensive formulas available. If your child is on a specialty formula, and you have questions, contact your dietitian or pediatrician for more information.

Powder, liquid or ready-to-use?

Formulas are typically sold as concentrates (powdered or liquid) that must be mixed with water before using, or in pre-mixed form. While their nutritional content remains the same for any given type of formula, they are significantly different in terms of cost and convenience.

How can I speak with a registered dietitian?

In Canada, you can call your local public health unit and ask to speak with the registered dietitian who deals with prenatal and infant nutrition. Alternatively, you can go to www.dietitians.ca to find a local dietitian who can meet with you personally. This service may not be covered by your provincial health insurance. In the United States, you can visit www.eatright.org to find a registered dietitian in your community.

Form and substance

Determining which form of infant formula is best for you

FORM	PROS	CONS
Powdered concentrate	Cost (see next page) Keeps for 1 month after opening	Risk of measuring error
Liquid concentrate	Easy to measure Easy to mix	Must be used within 48 hours of opening
Ready-to-use	No mixing Convenient Not reliant on water supply	Cost (see next page)

Counting the cost
How different types of formula compare

FORMULA TYPE	RELATIVE COST		
	POWDER	LIQUID	READY-TO-USE
Cow's-milk-based	Low	Moderate	Very high
Lactose-free CMB	Moderate	Moderate	N/A
Soy-based	Moderate	Moderate to high	Very high
Follow-up	Low	Moderate	N/A
Specialty	Very high	N/A	N/A

Powdered concentrate is the least expensive type of formula (see chart, above). It must be measured and mixed with clean water. (Use sterilized water for children under 4 months.) Once opened, a tin can be stored for up to 1 month before discarding.

Liquid concentrate is easier to measure and mix than the powdered variety, and is typically 30% to 40% more expensive. It's shelf life is also considerably shorter: once opened, a container of unmixed formula must be used within 24 hours. (Formula that has been mixed with water must be used up or thrown out within 24 hours.)

Ready-to-use formula offers the greatest convenience, since it requires no mixing and does not depend on having a clean water supply (which can be useful when traveling). Convenience has a cost, however, since this is by far the most expensive way to buy formula — up to four times as costly as powdered concentrate. While all types of formula are available in powdered form (and most types as liquid), ready-to-use formats are typically offered only for cow's-milk- and soy-based formulas.

So which format to choose? Ultimately, that will depend on your budget, time constraints and personal preference.

Milk by any other name

So how does formula compare with breast milk? How does it compare with whole cow's milk? As noted earlier and as shown in the chart below, formula manufacturers attempt to provide the same nutritional balance as breast milk. Comparing breast milk with cow's-milk-based formula, we see that the distribution of calories from carbohydrates and fat are roughly the same, although proteins are slightly higher in formula.

In the case of whole cow's milk, however, we see a dramatically higher protein content than is found in either formula or breast milk. This is why whole milk is not recommended for infants before the age of 9 months. The excess protein (and salt) in cow's milk creates what is called a high renal solute load, which means that these nutrients can be difficult for an infant's kidneys to process.

By avoiding cow's milk during the first 9 to 12 months, infants give their kidneys a chance to develop to the point where they are able to handle this additional protein. If consumed at a younger age — say, before 6 months — cow's milk can cause a variety of problems, which can include bleeding in the digestive tract.

Cow's milk is also very low in iron, which is another reason to avoid giving it to infants before the age of 12 months. If is introduced earlier — that is, before the infant is consuming a variety of foods (including iron-fortified rice cereal and meat) — she could be at risk of developing iron-deficiency anemia. (This condition is discussed in greater detail in Chapter 7; see pages 101–102.)

Liquid assets

Comparing the nutrient composition of milk and formula

	BREAST MILK	COW'S-MILK-BASED FORMULA	WHOLE COW'S MILK
Protein	6%	8% to 9%	20%
Fat	50%	45% to 50%	50%
Carbohydrates	40% to 45%	41% to 43%	30%

Preparing and using formula

1 **Sterilize.** Before preparing formula, it is important to sterilize all bottles, nipples and caps (particularly important for infants younger than 4 months old). To do this, all equipment should be boiled for 5 minutes.

2 **Boil the water.** Most domestic water supplies contain at least some bacteria that may be harmful to an infant — again, particularly when the baby's age is less than 4 months. To ensure that the water is sterile, it should be boiled for 2 minutes, then allowed to cool until lukewarm, before preparing the formula according to the package instructions.

3 **Use it or lose it.** Once prepared, formula can be stored in the refrigerator for up to 24 hours, after which any unused formula should be discarded.

For more information on infant feeding, see Chapter 1.

How much formula is enough?

Unlike breastfeeding, where it is not possible for mothers to know exactly how much a baby is drinking, it is possible to measure an infant's formula intake. The volume of formula consumed will increase with age and will vary depending on size and activity. The following chart gives an example of estimated intake.

AGE	FEEDS/DAY	QUANTITY/FEED*
Birth to 1 week	6 to 10	2 to 3 oz (60 to 90 mL)
1 week to 1 month	6 to 8	3 to 4 oz (90 to 120 mL)
1 to 3 months	5 to 6	4 to 6 oz (120 to 180 mL)
3 to 7 months	4 to 5	6 to 7 oz (180 to 210 mL)
7 to 12 months	3 to 4	7 to 8 oz (210 to 240 mL)

* Values are approximate; actual intake will vary with infant's size and activity level.

Top 10 Formula Questions

❶ Which formula is best? There are so many to choose from.

In cases where the mother decides not to breastfeed, virtually all pediatricians and dietitians recommend a cow's-milk-based, iron-fortified formula as the next best choice for healthy, full-term babies with no family history of allergy. Nutritionally, it does not matter if it is powder, liquid concentrate or ready-to-use. These choices must be made based on affordability and lifestyle. See pages 36–37 for more information.

❷ Will giving my 7-week-old son cereal at bedtime help him sleep through the night?

Research has not shown that the early introduction of cereals at bedtime will help babies sleep through the night. Babies generally begin to sleep through the night (8 consecutive hours) sometime after the age of 2 to 3 months, regardless of whether they are fed cereal at night.

❸ Do I need to spend the extra money for infant formula with added omega 3 and omega 6 fatty acids?

Omega 3 fatty acids have been much touted in the media, with the claims that they improve visual acuity and mental test scores. While it is unclear whether these claims hold true for full-term infants, there is evidence to suggest that preterm infants (less than 33 weeks or 4 lbs/1,800 grams) can benefit from these formulas.

❹ My child has an allergy to cow's milk. What kind of formula can I use?

For many children with cow's milk allergy, a soy-based formula is a reasonable alternative. However, if your child has an intolerance to cow's milk called colitis (often diagnosed because of blood in the stools; see pages 83–85 for more information), then soy-based formula may not be appropriate and you may need to use a protein hydrolysate formula such as Nutramigen.

Speak with your doctor for specific information about your child's situation.

❺ Do I need to switch to a follow-up formula when my child is 6 months old?

No, you do not need to switch from a starter formula to a follow-up formula. There are no significant nutritional differences between starter formulas and follow-up formulas. Follow-up formulas are superior to homogenized cow's milk, providing a better balance of calories, iron and essential fatty acids, and are a better choice than cow's milk for families who had planned on introducing cow's milk before 12 months of age. Starter formulas can be used until an infant is 12 months old, or longer; follow-up formulas can be used from 6 to 12 months.

❻ Is it still safe to use powdered formulas? I have heard they can be contaminated with the bacteria _Enterobacter sakazakii_.

Infants who were born prematurely, who are ill or who have a degree of immune suppression should not receive powdered formulas. Powdered infant formulas are not sterile, and the bacteria ES can grow, potentially causing meningitis and infections of the intestine. If you choose to give your baby powdered formula, heat the water to 158°F (70°C), which will maintain the nutrient integrity of the formula and help destroy the bacteria.

❼ Are soy-based formulas safe?

Yes, they are safe, but they should not be the first choice for infants. If lactose intolerance is suspected, a better choice would be lactose-free cow's-milk-based formulas. Soy-based formulas are appropriate for vegan mothers who have decided not to breastfeed. The end products of soy digestion do appear in the blood of infants, but it is not known what, if any, effect these end products have on the infants' health. See pages 33–34 for more information on soy.

8 How long can an opened can of concentrated formula remain in my refrigerator?

An opened can of liquid concentrate can be stored in the refrigerator for up to 24 hours. Once it is prepared with water and distributed into bottles, it should be consumed within 24 hours or discarded.

9 When can I start using cow's milk instead of formulas?

Although dairy products can be introduced sometime after the age of 6 months, breast milk or formula is still recommended as the primary fluid for babies until the age of 12 months, to ensure that their nutritional needs are being met. (See question about follow-up formulas, above, for more information.)

10 My 2-month-old daughter spits up a lot. I have heard that adding infant rice cereal to her formula may help. Is this true?

Many pediatricians do suggest adding a small amount of rice cereal to a bottle of formula or expressed breast milk (1 to 2 tbsp/15 to 25 mL per $\frac{1}{2}$ cup/125 mL) to help with spitting up. However, research has not proven that the addition of rice cereal will always be effective. If spitting up is a problem for your infant, seek further advice from your doctor or pediatrician.

CHAPTER 3

Introducing Solids (6 to 8 months)

A diet of breast milk alone is recommended for babies in the first 6 months of life. "Immune-rich" breast milk protects the infant's gut, supplying appropriate nutrition for the growth and health of the digestive and immune systems. If a woman chooses not to breastfeed or to provide breast milk, then infant formula should be the sole source of nutrition for the first 6 months.

When to begin

There is ongoing research on when is the best time to introduce solids, and the reports are sometimes contradictory. That is why the recommendations on when to begin solids change over the years. At this time, it is recommended to delay the introduction of solid foods until the infant is about 6 months old (this is true for both breastfed and formula-fed infants). By this age, the digestive tract is mature enough to digest complex proteins, fats and carbohydrates. In addition, at 6 months most infants are able to sit and to swallow non-liquid foods. Younger babies have what is called an extrusion reflex, which can prevent them from swallowing — and possibly choking on — solids; this reflex disappears between 4 and 6 months.

Don't wait too long

While many parents recognize the importance of not starting solids too soon, they may not realize that it's also possible to start too late. Research has shown that if a child is not introduced to solids before 9 months, he or she may have difficulty accepting textures later.

A 6-month-old also has the motor skills necessary to accept non-liquid foods, such as the ability to close his lips over a spoon when it is removed from his mouth. By 4 to 6 months a baby will typically be able to grasp a spoon, as well as other objects. He will be able to express hunger by opening his mouth and sitting forward when food is presented to him. Conversely, he will be able to show disinterest in food (or fullness) by leaning back in his high chair, pushing food away with his hands or turning his face away from what is being offered. The ability to chew solid foods begins to develop between 7 and 9 months.

It is important to remember that solids must be introduced gradually. During the initial transition period, breast milk or formula will continue to be your baby's primary source of nutrition. Gradually give him more food and let him guide you about when he is hungry and when he has had enough. Use the chart on page 49 as a guideline on how much food to offer, but certainly not as a rule about how much your child needs. Every baby is different.

Be patient!

While you are the one offering your baby a variety of foods, it is up to him to decide whether he will eat them. Let him guide you. As you introduce a new food, offer it to him on a spoon. Touch the spoon to his lips. If he is not interested or appears not to like the food, do not force the issue. Try the food again another day. The same food may need to be presented many times (research says up to 15 times!) before your infant will accept it.

Foods to avoid

Health authorities used to recommend avoiding foods that can cause allergic reactions, such as eggs (egg whites), fish and nuts, until a child reaches 1 or 2 years of age. The theory was that avoidance of these foods in the early development stages would potentially prevent a child from developing allergies to them. However, authorities have reviewed the results of studies and now recommend including these foods in the diet after 6 months of age. There is one exception to this recommendation: if a breastfed baby younger than 4 months is diagnosed with atopic dermatitis, it may be advisable to avoid foods that contain peanuts when introducing solids.

Spice it up!

Don't be afraid to add spices to your infant's food. There's no reason babies can't enjoy the wonderful flavors spices provide, and adding spices now may help your child enjoy a greater variety of foods later on!

Indications your child is ready to start solids

1. He can sit up in a high chair.
2. He can hold his head up.
3. He opens his mouth wide when offered food on a spoon.
4. He turns his head away from food when he is full or disinterested.
5. He uses his lips to remove food from the spoon.
6. He can control his tongue so that it does not push food back out of his mouth.
7. He looks at you with interest when you are eating.

Growth spurts

Growth spurts are common at the ages of 2 to 3 weeks, 4 to 6 weeks and 3 to 4 months. Your child may want to breastfeed more often during a growth spurt, but this is not an indication that he is ready to start solid foods.

Don't believe everything you hear

There is no good evidence to suggest that solids will help an infant sleep through the night. Don't let this popular wisdom tempt you into offering solids earlier than recommended.

If you have a family history of allergy, it is still best to get your family physician's or pediatrician's advice on what is right for your baby. Remember, every baby is different, and strict rules about feeding should be weighed against what is best for the individual baby.

Types of solid foods

Transition foods provide infants with the opportunity to learn how to eat. They will learn to move food around their mouth, move food to the back of the tongue and initiate a swallow. When they swallow, they will learn they must hold their breath for a moment. All of this requires time and lots of practice. Allow your child to explore food, and let him get messy.

In the early days, solid food is more for development than for nutrition. Gradually, your baby will start to eat enough food to satisfy his hunger, and the food will provide a nutritional complement to his liquid diet. As you introduce more solids, your child's intake of breast milk or formula will decrease accordingly.

Let's take a look at the types of solid foods, in general order of introduction.

Iron-fortified single-ingredient foods

Health authorities generally recommend that the first solid food be a single-ingredient food that contains iron. The single-ingredient composition is important, as this makes it easy to identify the source of any allergic reaction. As for the iron, a baby's iron stores begin to deplete by around the age of 6 months and must be supplemented from the diet. This is particularly true for infants who are exclusively breastfed or whose infant formula is not iron-fortified. Iron-deficiency anemia is the most common nutritional deficiency in North America (see pages 101–102).

Good choices include iron-fortified rice, barley, wheat or oat cereal, and strained meats, such as beef, chicken, turkey, lamb, pork or fish. Mashed cooked egg yolks, tofu and legumes (such as beans or lentils) are also reasonable choices. Remember, the iron from meat sources is better absorbed than the iron from non-meat sources.

Infant cereal should be mixed to a thin texture, like applesauce or slightly thicker, and fed to the baby with an infant-sized spoon. An infant beginning solids will eat about 2 to 4 teaspoons (10 to 20 mL) once or twice daily; this volume will gradually increase. There is no set amount that your baby needs. Use the chart on page 49 as a guide, but let your child determine whether he is interested in the food and when he is full.

Give each new food to your baby for a number of days before introducing the next so it is easy to determine the source of an allergic reaction should one occur. An allergic reaction could be rash, hives, vomiting, diarrhea or difficulty breathing. Stop feeding your baby the offending food if you think he may be allergic, then speak with your doctor about whether or not he needs further allergy testing or screening. If your baby is having trouble breathing, call 911. See pages 81–88 for more information on food allergies.

Can I feed my baby homemade cereal?

Homemade cereals may not contain enough iron for a growing baby. Consider mixing a commercial iron-fortified cereal with your homemade version to ensure an adequate iron intake. If you choose to provide your child with only homemade cereal varieties, ask your pediatrician or dietitian about an iron supplement.

---

tip

New foods should be introduced one at a time with a couple of days in between each new food offered. This enables parents to identify which foods are not tolerated well by their infant.

Zinc

In addition to iron, zinc is another important mineral that must be supplemented after 6 months of exclusive breastfeeding, as the zinc content of breast milk declines with time (for more on zinc, see page 103). Researchers have recently suggested that meat might be the best first food, as it contains both iron and zinc.

tip

When introducing solids, stool color and frequency may change. The amount produced will sometimes decrease and have a more pungent smell — particularly in the case of breastfed babies.

When to offer solids

Find a time of day when your child is most interested in solids. The morning, when your baby is alert and is not overtired, is generally a good time to start. Offer the solids after a breastfeed or bottle, but with enough time in between so that your child is hungry and eager to eat.

Signs of allergy

Signs of food allergy include rash, vomiting, diarrhea and breathing problems. Call 911 if your baby is having trouble breathing.

Vegetables and fruit

Between the ages of 6 and 7 months, your baby should be ready to start eating strained vegetables and fruit. Not only do these foods add taste, texture, color and variety to an infant's expanding diet, they are also good sources of vitamins A and C. As with the grains, introduce a new food every few days, satisfying yourself that it is well tolerated, before moving on to the next.

If you choose to use commercially prepared baby fruits, be sure to avoid fruit "desserts," which contain added sugar your baby doesn't need. While commercial jarred varieties of fruits or vegetables are acceptable sources of nutrition, it is less expensive to make your own, and it's not all that time-consuming. Some fruits, such as a ripe banana or pear, can simply be mashed with a fork. For more ideas, check out the recipes for mashed or puréed/strained fruits and vegetables (pages 148–153).

Keep choosing fresh fruits and veggies for your baby as he grows. Serve platters of cut-up fruits and veggies as snacks every day — good for children, and for you.

Nitrates and vegetables

Some types of strained vegetables and fruits — including spinach, beets, turnips, carrots, green beans, mixed vegetables and bananas — contain nitrates, and should therefore not be given to infants younger than 4 months (and solids should not be introduced at this age). In sufficient concentrations, nitrate can cause these children to develop methemoglobinemia, a condition in which blood cells do not transport oxygen efficiently. After the age of 6 months, however, vegetables and fruits do not pose a risk, since infants are then able to handle nitrates in their diet.

Fruits or vegetables first?

Should you start your baby with fruits or vegetables? Some authorities believe that it is better to have an infant become accustomed to vegetables before introducing sweet-tasting fruits. But this is not always true. In fact, some infants who start exclusively with vegetables may continue to prefer vegetables over fruit! Like adults, infants have their own likes and dislikes. Try a variety of fruits and vegetables, perhaps alternating the introduction of one fruit with one vegetable. Nutritionally, it makes no difference, since breast milk or formula supplies most of the infant's nutrients at this stage.

Start with a few tablespoons of either a puréed vegetable or fruit, served twice a day. All vegetables and fruits are good choices, including strained sweet potato, peas, squash, pears, apples and mangos.

Avoid fruit juice

You may be wondering when it is okay to offer fruit juice. Although babies are able to digest fruit juice around the same time they can start eating fruits, there is no need for juice in an infant's diet. When your child is thirsty, offer milk (breast or formula) or, after 9 months, water from a sippy cup instead.

Grains

After single-ingredient iron-fortified cereals such as rice, oats, barley and wheat have been introduced, you can try mixed-grain cereals. When purchasing mixed cereal varieties that contain fruit, be aware that many of these products also contain added sugar, which your baby doesn't need.

Meats and alternatives

Between the ages of 6 to 9 months, babies can be introduced to meats and meat alternatives, including puréed or mashed beef, lamb, pork, fish, chicken, turkey,

Did you know?

Not only are fruits a great source of many vitamins (such as vitamin C, an important antioxidant) and phytochemicals, as well as fiber, but they may also help to protect infants from developing asthma. In one study, infants who were fed fresh fruits in infancy were less likely to develop asthma after 1 year of age.

Be enthusiastic!

Sure, you may have an aversion to certain types of vegetables. But your baby doesn't. So try to avoid letting your personal tastes interfere with what veggies and fruit you choose to serve. Believe it or not, your reaction (including words and/or facial expressions) can have a profound effect upon an infant's willingness to try and enjoy new foods.

Bottles are for liquids only

Some parents believe that adding a little infant cereal to their baby's bottle is the best way to introduce the texture of solid foods. This is not recommended, since adding cereal to liquid actually dilutes the texture of the food and can interfere with the development of an infant's feeding skills.

If your child does not tolerate or does not want plain cow's milk, one option is to continue offering breast milk or formula until he is more accepting of cow's milk. You can also try mixing the breast milk or formula with cow's milk. Start with one-quarter milk, then increase to half, then to three-quarters, then to full-strength milk. While soy, rice and nut milks can be suitable substitutes, they do not contain a sufficient amount of energy or calcium to be included as a regular part of a toddler's diet.

cooked egg yolks, legumes and tofu. These foods provide additional flavor and variety, as well as a good source of supplemental protein. And, of course, strained meat is an excellent source of iron. You can begin by offering about 1 to 3 tablespoons (15 to 45 mL) per day.

If you choose to use commercially prepared products, start with strained meats with broth. If your child tolerates these well, you can move on to mixtures of vegetables and meat, which contain less meat and therefore less iron and fewer calories. Check the label to see which ingredient is listed first; that will be primarily what's in the jar.

Of course, as an alternative to buying prepared plain meats with broth, you can always make your own! See page 199 for a recipe.

Milk products and milk

Once you have introduced some iron-containing foods and tried fruits and veggies, you can begin to offer your baby milk products. Milk products provide fat, protein and calcium. Start by giving your infant 1 to 2 tablespoons (15 to 25 mL) per day.

Good choices include plain yogurt, cottage cheese or grated hard cheeses. Cow's milk should be offered only after 12 months. Breast milk or iron-fortified formula are recommended until that time. "Follow-up" formulas, intended for infants over 6 months, are also preferable to cow's milk before 12 months, although they do not offer any meaningful nutritional benefits over traditional "starter" formula.

Store-bought or homemade?

Are homemade baby foods better than the store-bought variety? Certainly, commercially prepared foods are more convenient, although homemade baby foods are very easy to prepare. There is no significant nutritional difference between commercially prepared and homemade baby foods. Children grow and develop equally well on both.

What about milk allergies?

Research shows that as many as 2% to 3% of infants have an allergy to cow's milk, although most grow out of it by the time they are 3 years old. Higher-risk babies — specifically, those whose parents and/or siblings have a milk allergy — should be checked by a physician before they are placed on a milk-free diet. (See pages 83–85 for more details.)

Introduction to solids

FOODS	BIRTH TO 6 MONTHS	6 TO 9 MONTHS	9 TO 12 MONTHS
Breast milk	Nursing on demand* *Exclusively breastfed infants should receive a vitamin D supplement	Nursing on demand	Nursing on demand
Iron-fortified formula	Bottle feeding on demand (about 8 to 4 feeds per day). Boil all water for formula	Bottle feeding on demand (about 5 to 3 feeds per day)	Bottle feeding of formula or whole cow's milk (about 4 to 3 feeds per day)
Iron-fortified single-ingredient food	NONE	Iron-fortified infant cereal (2 to 4 tbsp/25 to 60 mL twice daily)	Continue with a variety of cereals
Other grain products	NONE	Other whole grains, such as dry toast or unsalted crackers	Other plain cereals, bread, rice, pasta (8 to 10 tbsp/120 to 150 mL per day)
Meat and alternatives	NONE	Mashed or strained meat, fish or poultry, mashed silken tofu, well-cooked legumes (beans, lentils, chickpeas) or egg yolks (1 to 3 tbsp/ 15 to 45 mL per day)	Minced or diced cooked meat, fish, chicken, tofu, beans or egg yolks (3 to 4 tbsp/45 to 60 mL per day)
Vegetables	NONE	Puréed or mashed cooked vegetables of all colors (yellow, green and orange); progress to soft mashed consistency (4 to 6 tbsp/60 to 90 mL per day)	Mashed or diced cooked vegetables (6 to 10 tbsp/90 to 150 mL per day)
Fruit	NONE	Puréed or mashed cooked fruits or very ripe mashed fruit (e.g., banana or avocado) (6 to 7 tbsp/90 to 105 mL per day)	Soft peeled, seeded and diced fresh or canned fruit (packed in water or juice) (7 to 10 tbsp/105 to 150 mL per day)
Milk products	NONE	Plain yogurt (≥3.25% MF), cottage cheese or grated hard cheese (1 to 2 tbsp/15 to 30 mL per day)	Continue with yogurt, cottage cheese and diced/grated cheeses (2 to 4 tbsp/25 to 60 mL per day)
Texture	Liquid	Thickened cereal; finely mashed, soft solids	Soft minced or diced table foods
Other advice		Avoid honey, added sugar and salt	Avoid honey, added sugar and salt

Note: Check with your physician about when to start nut products, including nut butters. See pages 86–87 for information on nut allergies.

However, if you make your own baby food, you can offer your baby a greater variety of flavors. Homemade foods also tend to have more texture than their commercial counterparts. And because you control what ingredients go in, you know the food contains no additives. Although sugar, salt and modified starch are not routinely used in commercial baby foods, you should always check the label to make sure. (Desserts and toddler foods still contain sugar and modified starch.)

Note that commercial frozen baby food is anywhere from three to five times more expensive than the jarred varieties, yet you can make your own frozen baby food for a fraction of the cost! When the ingredients are only a vegetable or fruit and water, you can see why it is much more cost-effective to make your own! There is also much less waste with home-prepared food, as individual portions can be thawed and eaten one at a time.

Making your own baby food

So you have decided to make your own baby food. Hooray! When it comes to home-prepared foods, the potential variety is limitless: you can use any fruit,

Types of additives

- **Sugar** is sometimes used in baby desserts as a sweetener.
- **Salt** is another common additive, although often more so in homemade baby foods than in commercial varieties. Why? Simply because parents tend to season foods to suit their own taste buds, often forgetting that infant palates have not been similarly conditioned to need the flavor of salt. So if you decide to make your own baby food, leave the salt out of the recipe. What tastes bland to you may not taste bland to your infant.
- **Modified starch**, typically based on corn or tapioca, is sometimes added to commercial baby foods. These compounds act as stabilizers to provide a desired consistency, texture and shelf life, primarily in desserts and junior foods. Research has demonstrated that modified starch is not harmful, and is fairly well digested by infants.

vegetable or meat. Asparagus or avocado purées may be difficult to find on grocery store shelves but can be prepared in your kitchen with ease.

For a selection of flavorful and nutritious first solid food recipes — including fruits, vegetables and meat — see pages 148–153 and page 199. These recipes can be made ahead of time and frozen in ice-cube trays, which divide the food into portion sizes that are ideal for a young infant. Baby foods are safe in the freezer for up to 3 months, by which time your baby may be on to textured solids or mashed or diced table foods. Thaw frozen baby food overnight in the refrigerator, or defrost in a container of warm water.

Preparing homemade fruits or vegetables

Many ripe fresh fruits, including banana, avocado, mango, pear and melon, do not need to be cooked before they are puréed or mashed. For those that do, here are the steps to follow:

1. Peel, seed and slice the fruit or vegetable. Place in a small saucepan and cover with water.
2. Bring to a boil and cook until tender. Drain, reserving cooking liquid.
3. Purée the fruit or vegetable until smooth, or mash with potato masher for a lumpier consistency. You may need to add water or cooking liquid to achieve the desired consistency.
4. Place in ice-cube trays and freeze. Once frozen, transfer individual cubes to freezer bags.

Preparing homemade meats

1. Place a piece of meat in a small saucepan. Cover with water and bring to a boil. You can add a stalk of celery or a carrot to flavor the broth, if desired.
2. Reduce heat and simmer until meat is very tender and starts to fall off the bone. Drain, reserving broth, and discard celery or carrot, if used. Remove skin and bones from meat.

What you will need
- A food processor or handheld blender
- A wire sieve
- A potato masher
- Ice-cube trays
- Freezer bags

tip

Make baby food with whatever vegetables you are cooking for dinner that night. Cook extra veggies, purée or mash what you don't eat, then freeze it. Presto! Minimal extra work involved.

tip

An average-sized ice-cube tray will hold about 2 tablespoons (25 mL) per unit, or about 1 1/2 cups (375 mL) of baby food per tray.

tip

Homemade baby food can be frozen and used for up to 3 months. Thaw overnight in the refrigerator, or defrost in a container of warm water.

3 Transfer meat to a food processor and purée until smooth, adding cooking broth or water as needed to achieve desired consistency. Meats may also need to be put through a wire strainer once puréed to achieve a smooth texture.

4 Place in ice-cube trays and freeze. Once frozen, transfer individual cubes to freezer bags.

Baby organics

Is organic baby food a better choice than non-organic? What does organic mean?

Organic food differs from conventional food in the way it is grown, processed and handled. To protect the soil, water and the environment, organic farmers do not use conventional pesticides and fertilizers. So that consumers will know when they are buying a food that has been grown organically, government agencies have set national standards and have developed strict labeling rules. But organic foods are not the only ones that are safe to consume. Government agencies also have strict regulations on the amount and type of pesticides and fertilizers that can be used for non-organic farming.

The decision about whether to purchase organic or non-organic foods is ultimately one that everyone must make on their own. Here are some factors to consider.

Cow's milk

In the United States, the FDA allows cows to be treated with a growth hormone to increase milk production, but cow's milk is free of antibiotics. If a cow is being treated with antibiotics for an infection, the milk from that cow is discarded. All milk is tested before being sent to a plant for processing.

Regulations on organic food

The United States Department of Agriculture (USDA) has developed national standards for food that is labeled organic, and strict labeling rules. The "USDA Organic" seal tells you that the food is at least 95% organic.

In Canada, the Canadian Food Inspection Agency (CFIA) is the lone certifying body for organic food. To be assigned the official "Canada Organic" logo, food must be made up of at least 95% organic material.

Local food

Buying local food, organic or not, is always the better choice. You will not only support your local farmers, but you'll benefit from fresher foods. In addition, buying local helps the environment, because it cuts down on the fuel emissions that result from transporting foods over long distances.

Safety

Whether or not a food is organic, food safety concerns always apply. Wash all fresh fruits and vegetables under cold running water to remove undesirable contaminants, and handle meat, poultry and fish in a safe manner (see page 78).

In Canada, conventional cow's milk is free of both growth hormone and antibiotics. Health Canada does not permit the use of bovine growth hormone for dairy cows (effective since 1999).

While these are the regulations in North America, laws differ in other countries. Check with the health regulatory agency in your country for more information on the regulations on milk production and processing.

Nutrients

While some studies show that organic foods are higher in vitamin C and some minerals than conventional foods, the difference is not significant enough to affect the daily contribution of these nutrients to the diet, and therefore to overall health. In addition, it is difficult to make comparisons between organic and non-organic foods because factors such as soil conditions, type of seeds, temperature and light all affect the quality of the products.

Pollutants

The amount of pesticides and pollutants used varies depending on the soil conditions where the food is grown. While there are restrictions on the amount of pesticides and other chemicals that can be used in non-organic farming, non-organic foods usually do have more pesticide residues than organic foods. At this time, the degree to which foods contribute to an individual's exposure to environmental pollutants, and the effects these pollutants may have, is not known.

Cost

In general, organic food — including organic baby food — continues to be more expensive than conventionally grown food, but this is changing as the demand for organic food increases. Whether you use organic or non-organic food, it is always more cost-effective to make your own baby food.

Here come the teeth

Teething can begin as early as 3 months or as late as 1 year, but usually begins at around 6 to 8 months and lasts for about 2 years. The first teeth cut are usually the incisor (or front) lower, then upper teeth.

The pain of teething — and the irritability that can accompany it — varies from one child to the next. In some cases, the discomfort can affect a child's appetite, but typically for no longer than a day or two. Some relief can be obtained by giving your baby cool teething rings or bagels or crusts of bread. Be wary of using teething gels, however. These products are essentially surface anesthetics that numb the contact area. While intended for the gums only, these gels are often applied inadvertently to the tongue, which may cause a child to choke or be insensitive to hot foods. Check with your GP or pediatrician before using these products. (For more information on teething and tooth care, see pages 62–63.)

Top 10 First Solids Questions

1 When is my child old enough to start solids?

The current recommendation from the World Health Organization, the American Academy of Pediatrics and Health Canada is to start solids at 6 months of age. Starting too early can disrupt the protective factors provided by exclusive breastfeeding, and is unnecessary for the formula-fed infant. See pages 42–43 for more details.

2 My 6-month-old daughter hates the taste of rice cereal. What can I do?

Commercial infant rice cereal is often the first food given to babies, since rice is very unlikely to cause an allergic reaction and it is a great source of dietary iron. If your child appears to dislike the taste of rice cereal, try changing the temperature at which you serve it, or change the consistency by adding more or less liquid. Also, for a change in flavor, try preparing the cereal with breast milk or formula.

3 My 7-month-old son doesn't seem to like any of the strained fruits and vegetables I am offering him. What should I do?

The first reaction of some babies to an unfamiliar food is to spit it back out. It is important to persist, however; keep offering the food for a few days to see if he will eventually accept it. Once a food has been tried for a few days without success, move on to another food. Also, try not to let your personal tastes (or, more importantly, distastes) affect the manner in which you present the food. No matter how unappetizing you may find them personally, always offer new foods with enthusiasm. (See page 47 for more details.)

4 Why should new foods be offered at intervals of at least 3 days?

Solids should be introduced one at a time with about 3 days between each new food so that if an allergy or intolerance is to occur, it will be easy to identify which food is the cause.

5 My husband and I both had food allergies as young children and I am worried about starting solids for my 6-month-old infant. What should I do?

Introducing single foods, one at a time every 3 days or so, will help you identify any allergy if it occurs. Exclusive breastfeeding for at least 3 to 4 months may prevent the development of cow's milk allergy. Delaying the introduction of common sources of food allergy (e.g., cow's milk, eggs and nuts) is no longer recommended (including for children who are at high risk for developing allergy), as this has not been proven to prevent food allergies but may only delay the identification of them. Speak with your family doctor for advice. See pages 81–88 for more information on food allergies.

6 Should I make my own baby food, or are commercial foods okay?

If you have the time and desire to make your own baby food, then by all means do so. It provides a great opportunity to try some different fruits, vegetables and meats. But if you don't have the time or inclination, don't worry — commercially prepared baby foods are perfectly acceptable and offer comparably good nutrition. Just be sure to read the labels on store-bought baby foods. Some older toddler desserts may include unnecessary sugar. Beginner foods should not contain salt, preservatives or color.

7 My 7-month-old son is teething. What can I give him to soothe the pain?

Teething can be a difficult time for both infant and parents. Acceptable methods for managing pain include a cooled plastic teething ring or biscuit or bagel pieces. (See page 53.) It is best to check with your family doctor for advice.

⑧ How long can homemade baby foods be frozen?

Homemade baby foods can be frozen for up to 3 months. This should be plenty of time, as most infants will progress to mashed or diced table foods within this period.

⑨ If I'm using jarred baby foods, how long does an open jar keep?

First of all, when using jarred baby food, always be sure to spoon the food into a separate bowl; otherwise, the food will need to be thrown out immediately after use. If the baby has not eaten directly from the jar, the food should keep in the refrigerator for up to 48 hours. Also, remember that food should never be heated in the glass jars in the microwave.

⑩ Can I make my own homemade infant cereal?

There are many recipes available (particularly on the Internet) for homemade infant cereal. While it is possible to make your own, homemade varieties are lower in iron than their commercial counterparts, so they may not provide enough iron for the exclusively breastfed infant and may place him at risk for iron deficiency.

CHAPTER 4

Time for Table Food (8 to 12 months)

By the age of 8 months, many infants are able to progress from mashed or puréed/strained foods to more solid or textured foods: pieces of bread, small slices of ripe peaches or pears, cooked green beans. For parents and infants alike, this is a time of ongoing discovery, occasional frustration and eventual reward.

Ready for textures?

There is no specific time to make the transition to more textured food since, as we have stated previously (and no doubt will again), each child is different. Very often a parent will know when the child is ready — either intuitively or from previous experience. Sometimes the emergence of teeth is taken as an indication of readiness, although this does not always matter. As a rule, however, if an infant is able to eat small slices of soft food without gagging or choking, and clearly enjoys these types of foods, then she is ready. But if you have doubts, seek the advice of your pediatrician.

Ultimately, the decision must be one with which you are comfortable. If you are not ready to offer textured foods, then wait until you are. An infant will sense your anxiety, and a few extra weeks of mashed or puréed/strained foods will not make any difference.

Take cover!

Making the transition to textures can be (okay, is almost always) a messy business. It is at this stage that infants learn to handle food themselves, with the result that much of it will end up someplace other than in their mouths. So invest in a good bib — one with a water-resistant backing and a soft, easy-to-clean front. If you prefer, you can use a harder plastic bib with a "trap" in front to catch food. Either way, the bib should dry quickly after cleaning, so it is ready to use for the next meal. Or have a few handy so that a clean one is always available.

Making the transition

The introduction of more textured foods to your baby's diet should be a gradual one. You can continue to offer some mashed or puréed/strained foods and introduce one textured food at a time. There is no need to stop giving all mashed or puréed/strained foods at once. Indeed, many infants really enjoy their mashed or puréed/strained foods and, by continuing to provide them, you will also have a more precise idea of how much food your child is eating.

Throughout the transition, your child's intake of breast milk or formula will continue to decrease, as solids replace this source of calories. Expect the number of breastfeedings to drop to about 4 or 5 per day, while bottles or cups of formula may decrease from 4 to 6 bottles (each 6 to 8 oz/175 to 250 mL) to about 2 or 3 per day.

Dairy debut

At 12 months, whole cow's milk can begin to replace formula-feeding or breastfeeding if the mother chooses. It is best to gradually introduce cow's milk by replacing half a bottle to one bottle a day of formula or breast milk with whole cow's milk. This gradual phase-in period may make it easier for the baby to adjust to the change in the types of carbohydrate and protein she is consuming.

By 1 year of age, a child should be taking in a good supply of iron-rich foods, such as meats, tofu and iron-rich cereals, to keep up with her body's high demand for iron during this period of rapid growth. If her intake of foods high in iron is limited, and her mother is not providing breast milk, then it may be wise to continue giving her an iron-fortified formula until iron-rich foods are a more significant part of her diet. (Check out the table on food sources rich in iron on page 101.)

Iron-clad nutrition after 6 months

Iron plays a very important role in a child's development, and studies have shown that iron deficiency can affect a child's learning ability early on in life. Low iron can also leave a child pale, irritable and tired. This can result in decreased appetite, which only compounds the problem.

For the exclusively breastfed infant, the natural supply of iron with which she is born is usually exhausted by 6 months. However, mothers who have a low iron intake during pregnancy may affect their infant's iron stores; therefore, it is especially important that a good food source of iron be provided at 6 months. Iron-fortified formulas contain adequate amounts of iron, as does breast milk. After 6 months, as solid foods are introduced, the amount of iron absorbed from breast milk can decrease, so it is particularly important that these solid foods include good sources of iron.

Because of its relatively low iron content, liquid cow's milk is not advised until an infant is 12 months of age; however, the latest research suggests that other milk protein products, such as cheese, yogurt or ice cream, can be offered after 6 months of age, along with other complementary foods. If your family has a strong history of allergy, check with your family physician or pediatrician for a recommendation based on current guidelines. Of course, if your child has a confirmed milk protein allergy, all milk and milk products should be avoided.

Cup-feeding versus bottle-feeding

Health authorities recommend weaning from the bottle between 12 and 18 months, but parents often choose to delay bottle-weaning until much later, allowing their child to keep using a bottle to 24 months and beyond. A recent Canadian study revealed that children between 12 and 38 months who were allowed to continue drinking from a bottle were more likely to become iron-depleted than children who drank from a cup. The reason? Bottle drinkers tended to drink more milk, which resulted in eating less food, which would have provided them with more iron. So keep trying with that cup!

Why is iron so important?
Iron is a mineral that is part of hemoglobin, a protein in blood. It helps carry oxygen to cells in the body so that vital cell functions can take place. Iron also helps build tissue in the nervous system so that signals can be shared effectively. In addition, many brain chemicals, which help to send signals within the brain, need iron to function.

Choosing starter foods

There are three things to keep in mind when selecting more textured foods to introduce into your baby's diet.

Softness. Foods should be soft enough to be easily mashed in an infant's mouth. These may include certain fruits and vegetables (see specific recommendations below), pieces of cheese, meat or fresh bread. Other foods to try include grains such as quinoa, brown rice and couscous.

Size. Pieces of food should be small enough to eat without choking (see sidebar) — typically no larger than $1/4$ to $1/2$ inch (5 mm to 1 cm) in size. Pasta (another good starter food) should be cut into similarly short lengths.

Variety. Based on the experience you've had feeding your baby mashed or puréed/strained foods, you will have already discovered that your infant has her preferences — vegetables over fruit, for example, or meats over cereals. This is only natural since, as with adults, infants cannot be expected to like all foods equally. Still, it is important to offer your baby a wide variety of textured foods. This helps to build familiarity with a range of tastes and textures. More importantly, it ensures a balanced diet that includes all food groups (see page 108).

Good choices for starter foods include the following.

Soft fruits. These can include ripe bananas, pears or peaches — fresh in season, otherwise canned in juice (avoid the variety packed in heavy syrup, which is excessively sweet and provides a lot of empty calories). Prepare the fruit by slicing, then cutting it into pieces approximately $\frac{1}{4}$ to $\frac{1}{2}$ inch (5 mm to 1 cm) in diameter. Other soft-fruit choices include fresh mango (peeled and cut into pieces as above), seedless grapes (cut into quarters), apricots, plums and pitted cherries (cut into quarters). Other choices include papayas, strawberries, melons (honeydew, cantaloupe) and avocado.

Vegetables. Cooked until soft, then cooled, vegetables offer a great variety of flavors and textures for your child to enjoy. Good choices include wax or green beans, spinach, carrots, peppers, zucchini and potatoes. Fresh tomatoes (try plum or cherry tomatoes cut in quarters) are also good. Serve vegetables without salt or butter so your child can enjoy

Don't choke up

At 8 to 12 months, infants are generally able to manage small pieces of soft food without difficulty. Occasionally, however, they can swallow food without mashing it with their tongue or palate, which causes them to choke. The signs of choking can include persistent coughing, gagging, wheezing and sputtering. As alarming as these sounds are, they also mean that the food is not totally blocking the airway — a much more dangerous situation in which the child turns red or blue and makes no sounds at all. (See page 76 for information on infant cardiopulmonary resuscitation [CPR] — a skill that all parents and caregivers should master.) Where choking sounds are heard (e.g., coughing or gagging), some physicians recommend that you allow the child to cough the food particle out herself. Other remedies include turning the child upside down to let gravity get food out, or if necessary, giving a few light hits on the back.

Ultimately, the best defense against choking is to provide safe foods (see page 77 for a list of foods to avoid) and to monitor your infant constantly during mealtimes.

Water instead of juice

While fruit juices are often given to young children, they are nutritionally unnecessary for a child whose diet includes fresh fruit. In fact, water is better for quenching thirst and it does not leave residual sugars on the teeth. So get your infant into the water habit early. If you do serve juice, do so only infrequently and limit it to 4 oz (125 mL) per day.

tip

To save time, cook fresh vegetables in the microwave oven. In a microwave-safe bowl, add 2 tbsp (25 mL) water to 1 cup (250 mL) vegetables (such as green or wax beans or broccoli); cover with a microwave-safe lid (not plastic wrap) and cook on High for 3 minutes or until soft. Allow to cool 5 minutes before serving.

the undisguised taste of each. For best flavor, use fresh produce. Less flavorful but faster to prepare, frozen and (low-sodium) canned vegetables are acceptable substitutes, and they provide comparable nutritional value. Rinse canned vegetables under cold water to remove salt.

Soft cheeses. Try mild or medium Cheddar cheese, grated or thinly sliced and cut into small pieces. (Some infants prefer the stronger cheese, however, so experiment!)

Meats. These foods are an important source of iron and protein for growing infants and children, but are often the most difficult to get children to eat when starting textures. A good place to start is with chicken, including tender pieces of thigh, leg or breast meat. (Mixing it with some low-salt gravy or vegetable broth can help to soften the texture.) Other meat choices include soft beef (from shepherd's pie or stew, for example) or fish without the bones, such as salmon, sole and tuna. Serve canned tuna in its own water or light broth, or mixed with a little mayonnaise. Try plain or herbed soft tofu. See the meat recipes in this book for suggested preparation methods.

Why babies love to shop

A trip to the grocery store, with all its interesting sights and smells, can be great fun for infants and parents alike. Just keep in mind that babies sitting in shopping carts can have a surprisingly long reach — and they will try to grab things that are familiar or are of interest to them.

Pasta and grains. Soft pasta is often an infant favorite. Look for whole wheat pasta, or varieties made with chickpeas and legumes, for added fiber, protein and omega 3 fatty acids. Try "pastina" (child-size pieces of pasta), macaroni, fusilli, spaghetti, linguine or penne; serve plain or with a sauce. Be sure to cut long-strand pasta, such as spaghetti or linguine, to prevent your child from gagging or choking. Other grain foods include small pieces of soft bread. Some cereals are also good for their size and consistency.

In all cases, start by giving your infant small amounts of each new food. Keep watch as she chews and mashes the food. At this age, you should NEVER leave your infant without supervision while she's feeding.

Dealing with fussy eaters

When young children are at the stage of trying new foods (as well as their parents' patience!), there will be times when they seem not to be hungry, and refuse their usual favorite foods. This is quite common and should not be a cause for concern. Just as a child's growth and weight gain do not always increase smoothly, appetite may also be inconsistent. Also, with all the little things they eat throughout the day, children who refuse a main meal could be getting more food than their parents realize.

Consider, for example, the sample menu shown on page 62. Here a 1-year-old might appear to receive insufficient amounts (bites) of food, yet in fact gets 850 calories — or over 80% of her energy needs — from various foods nibbled on throughout the day. (Only 50% of iron needs would be met, however, so you'd eventually need to add iron-rich foods.)

If your child refuses to eat, continue to offer one or two main items per meal along with milk at the end of the meal. Allow your child to nibble on foods such as whole-grain bread and cheese or pieces of fruit, so that she gets some form of nutritious energy.

Try preparing new foods in different ways. For example, you could prepare fish with different herbs or different-colored vegetables. Show your child that you are enjoying the food you are offering her. Give her time to eat. Do not hurry your little one's appetite. On the other hand, don't let mealtime go on too long — 20 to 30 minutes is a reasonable limit. Express your delight over the food she does eat. Do not threaten or bribe her with activities or other foods.

Try, try again

Studies show that it sometimes takes 10 to 15 tries before a child decides to eat a new food. So don't give up! Repeat exposures to new foods can encourage young eaters. Do not try to hide veggies — keep offering the vegetable in its recognizable form. This will likely make it easier for your child to accept a variety of vegetables. Don't forget to be the role model: eat your veggies and demonstrate that you are enjoying them.

Daina's recommendation: The "lick test"

Even if you provide young children with lots of food variety, there comes a time when they will be exposed to a food they have never seen and may not be willing to try. That's where the lick test comes in. I have always encouraged my daughter and son to at least lick a new food to taste it, even if it does not look like something they think they would like. More often than not, after the lick, they agree to a serving of the food. If this does not happen the first time, I just try again later, encouraging another taste. Don't be discouraged: kids may not like something the first, second, third or even tenth time you give it to them, but they may like it later. Recent research proves this! The more often you expose a young child to a new food, the better the chances that she will eventually accept it.

Bits and bites

Sample menu of a picky (but still well-nourished!) 1-year-old eater

BREAKFAST			LUNCH			SUPPER		
1 oz	cheese	30 g	1 tbsp	tomato pasta sauce	15 mL	¼	slice whole-grain bread	¼
¼	banana	¼	2 tbsp	pasta	25 mL	1	mini yogurt (2 oz/60 mL)	1
½	egg	½	¼ cup	fresh strawberries	50 mL	¼	apple	¼
SNACK			**SNACK**			2 cups	whole milk (4 servings, each ½ cup/ 125 mL, taken throughout the day)	500 mL
6	small bite-size whole-grain crackers	6	2	arrowroot cookies	2			
¼	banana	¼	¼ cup	low-sugar whole-grain cereal (1 tbsp/ 15 mL, taken 4 times)	50 mL			

Introducing utensils

Between the ages of 8 and 12 months, infants will be able to feed themselves with their hands, but can start to learn to use utensils such as plastic spoons or forks. This will be a messy business, so be prepared. Start by letting your infant watch how you eat with your spoon and fork, then allow her to try using utensils with foods such as cereals or yogurt. Chances are it will seem like only a small amount of food ends up in your child's mouth (at first, anyway), but eventually she will succeed and will feel proud of the accomplishment. Be sure to encourage this new skill enthusiastically.

Teething and tooth care

Teething can begin from as early as 3 months to as late as 10 to 14 months. The first teeth cut are usually the incisors (front teeth), which come in around 6 to 8 months. As with most aspects of child development, teething can be more difficult for some infants than others, and can affect their sleeping, general mood and appetite. In many cases, however, teething is used as a catch-all explanation for

---

Eating out with baby

When having a meal at a restaurant, you may find that your infant demonstrates interest in your plate. By all means let the baby try those foods that are soft enough. Don't offer salty, high-fat foods. Allow your child to try small bits of salad, pieces of chicken breast or boneless fish, pasta or soup (be careful to cool it down first). At this young age, it is best to have your child sample from the food you choose, instead of getting the kids-choice menu items, which in many restaurants are high in fat and salt and offer little protein and iron.

any of these symptoms when the cause may lie elsewhere. If the symptoms persist, check with your pediatrician or general practitioner, who will be able to tell you if teething is the problem or if there is some other cause. An infant's irritability is often blamed on teething pain, but there is no evidence that teething causes any real pain. Cooled teething rings can be offered, but medications are not usually recommended.

What about cleaning your infant's teeth? The time to start is when the teeth first appear. You can begin by using a damp cloth to wipe away plaque. Or you can brush the teeth with a soft baby toothbrush, using a small (less than pea size) amount of fluoride-free toothpaste once a day. Be sure to wipe or brush the teeth gently, since the gums may be tender, and occasionally you may see some blood. It is a good idea for your child to see you brushing your teeth as well. By 12 months, brushing teeth should be well established, even if the child is not fond of the practice.

tip

Don't give your child a bottle of juice or milk right before falling asleep. The sugar in either beverage can pool around the teeth and cause decay. Try a bottle of water instead.

What about fluoride?

If your water supply does not contain fluoride (or contains concentrations of less than 0.3 parts per million), fluoride supplementation may be required when your child's first tooth appears. Why? Fluoride is necessary for proper tooth development. Check with your dentist or pediatrician to see if a supplement is needed. The first trip to the dentist should be when the first teeth erupt, according to both the American and the Canadian dental societies. However, if your pediatrician goes over proper tooth care with you, you can wait to seek out a dentist until your child is $2\frac{1}{2}$ to 3 years of age.

Top 10 Table Food Questions

1 How do I know when it is safe to feed my child more textures?

You won't really know until you try — with small, soft pieces of food. (Your pediatrician or family doctor can also guide you as to whether your child is ready.) The presence or absence of teeth need not make a difference, since many toothless infants do very well with mashing soft food between their palates (top and bottom of mouth) and tongue.

2 What can I do to minimize my child's risk of choking?

Children under the age of 4 years are at the highest risk of choking, and about 75% of choking incidents involve food. But choking can be prevented by ensuring that your child's food is sufficiently soft and is cut into small (no larger than ½-inch/1 cm pieces). Always stay with your child and supervise feeding. Keep infants seated at meal and snack times and do not allow them to run around with food in their mouths. (See page 77 for information on foods that present a danger of choking.)

3 What are the signs of allergy to a new food?

Allergic reactions usually manifest themselves in changes to the skin (such as hives or a rash) but may also lead to vomiting or diarrhea. If you suspect an allergy to a certain type of food, eliminate that food from your child's diet for a few weeks. Call your family doctor or pediatrician for advice. (See pages 81–88 for more information on allergic reactions to food.)

4 When eating in a restaurant, what foods can I safely offer my 10-month-old, who is just starting on textures?

Soft fruits and vegetables or pastas, as well as soft meats, should be fine. Avoid offering foods that are high in fat or sugar. Higher-fat foods tend to remain in the stomach longer, and this sometimes causes stomach upsets.

5 Should I give my 8-month-old daughter "junior foods" before offering her table foods?

Commercially prepared "junior foods" are essentially smooth purées with small pieces of food added. They are meant to advance the older infant to more solid textures. Some infants may find it difficult to make the transition from smooth purées to those containing small pieces of solid food. But you do not need to use junior foods. Mashing fruits, vegetables or other foods to a thicker consistency is also perfectly acceptable. For example, spaghetti and meat sauce can be puréed in a food processor to a smooth consistency so that pieces of pasta are just visible.

6 Should I be switching my child to whole milk or should I offer 2% or 1% milk instead? I am worried about fat and cholesterol.

Whole milk is recommended for infants who are older than 12 months. You do not have to worry about cholesterol at this age. The fat in whole milk is an important source of energy for a growing child. However, for infants whose weight is greater than it should be for their length (or height) — or if there is a history of high cholesterol in the family — it may be worth considering 2% milk. Check with your family doctor or pediatrician for advice.

7 Should I be giving my 10-month-old infant vitamin or mineral supplements? I want to make sure that he is getting the right amounts.

If your child's diet includes balanced amounts from all the four food groups (see page 108 for more information), then he probably does not need a supplement. However, since some North American children do not get enough iron (even those who are apparently well-fed), you should be sure that he is receiving a sufficient quantity of this mineral through foods such as iron-fortified infant cereal, tofu and meat. For example, the recommended daily iron intake for infants between 8 and 12 months can be supplied by about 8 to 10 tbsp (120 to 150 mL) cereal and 4 to 6 tbsp (60 to 90 mL) meat in a day. (See page 102 for a table of iron requirements.) If you suspect that your child is lacking in one or more specific nutrients, discuss this with your family doctor or pediatrician before offering a supplement. See pages 103–104 for more information about the role of specific vitamins and minerals.

8 My child eats much less on some days than on others. Should I be force-feeding her or trying to increase the number of snacks offered?

Because a child's growth rate is not always consistent, she may often demonstrate a general lack of interest in food. Other (less frequent) causes can include teething, lack of sleep, snacks too close to mealtime, low iron reserve or illness. Although poor appetite can be worrying for a parent, don't worry — your child will not starve herself. Chances are she will eat better the next day. If she doesn't, or if her growth or weight gain is below normal, consult with your doctor. Try to avoid tempting your low-appetite child with choice after choice at any given meal. Offer one or two choices and, if they are refused, offer them again at snack time.

9 My baby's high chair was given to me by a friend who bought it for her child a number of years ago. I am concerned about it still being safe for my child to use. What are the important features to look for?

A good high chair should have a cushioned, supportive seat; strong, supporting straps; and a foot rest. Other helpful features include wheels (for easy mobility), and a removable tray that can be easily cleaned. (If not cleaned properly, the tray area is a perfect breeding ground for bacteria; wash it thoroughly after each meal, using a clean cloth and soap or a mild detergent, then wipe off with water alone.)

10 Can I give foods that contain whole eggs to my 14-month-old?

Yes, eggs, including the egg whites, can be introduced after 6 months of age, when other solids are being introduced, based on the new guidelines on introduction of solid foods. If you have a strong family history of allergy, however, you may want to check with your family doctor or pediatrician for advice.

The Toddler Years (12 to 24 months)

Somewhere between the ages of 12 and 24 months, it suddenly becomes clear that your baby is no longer the helpless creature he once was. As speech develops — usually starting with the ability to say "no!" — children are less inclined to accept whatever they are fed. They are able to communicate their preferences of foods more clearly, and to say when they are hungry using words more often than gestures. At this stage, the task of planning meals and feeding your toddler can be quite the challenge. But it can also be fun and rewarding, especially if good eating habits have already been established.

Love that fat!

Fat-phobic parents may hesitate to give their baby whole milk (which contains between 3% and 4% fat). But the added fat and calories are actually good for most young children, which is why whole milk is generally recommended over 2%, 1% or skim milk until 24 months.

Goodbye formula, hello milk

As long as your child's weight is good, infant formula is usually no longer required after the age of 1 year. (You can continue breastfeeding, however.) Formulas may still be recommended for those with minimal iron intake or those with poor weight gain. If you are unsure about whether to switch from formula to whole (cow's) milk, ask your family doctor or pediatrician for advice.

If you wish, you can supplement whole milk with iron-fortified formula. (Remember that iron remains an important nutrient at this age, since it is essential for growth.) These have more iron and other minerals than whole milk but, nutritionally speaking, are unnecessary for any child older than 1 year whose diet is varied and includes recommended foods from the various food groups (see page 108).

Bigger and better

As your child's ability to chew and swallow improves, he can manage a greater range of foods.

Fruit can now be given in larger pieces, although softer varieties — such as bananas, peaches, pears and mangos — are still recommended. While you can let your child experiment with bite sizes (holding larger pieces or a whole fruit), only do so under close supervision. In cases where a whole fruit could possibly lodge in a small airway (such as grapes or berries), continue to cut the fruit into smaller pieces. Ultimately, let your common sense prevail. Each child develops differently, and you will know what is best suited for your toddler.

Vegetables should still be cooked until soft in most cases — although you may wish to try introducing your child to thin slices of fresh cucumber or green peppers. Raw carrots and other hard vegetables can be served grated. Children also enjoy peas and corn, but you should keep a close watch, since it is easy to swallow these vegetables without chewing. Baked potatoes are a good choice, as are (surprisingly) french fries. While higher in fat than baked, french fries still contain many important nutrients and, if properly prepared, are not the empty-calorie food that many people believe them to be.

Meats are often more readily accepted as a child gets older and finds them easier to chew — especially when he watches the rest of the family eat these foods. Allow your child to sample what the family is having. For more variety of flavor, try preparing meats with herbs and different (mild) spices. Other good choices for protein and iron include chicken, fish, eggs and tofu. (For interesting ideas on how to prepare meat, chicken, fish and tofu, try the recipes in this book.)

tip
For a healthier version of french fries, lightly brush potato slices or wedges with vegetable oil and bake them until lightly browned.

Timing is everything

Wherever possible, try to maintain a reasonable time schedule for meals and snacks. If a child is too tired or hungry, he will not enjoy his meals — and neither will you. Try to ensure that your child gets at least some amount of food around mealtime, and allow him to have his proper rest. Even if you are away from home, you can provide a light portable meal or more substantial snack (see chart, below). Remember that children like to have a routine, even if they are not in their usual setting. A child's schedule is important, so allow for it during the course of your busy day.

Nutritious meals in a hurry

As babies grow into toddlers, preparing meals for them often becomes increasingly time-consuming. Here are some helpful and practical tips for fast and nutritious meals.

It is often difficult for many parents to plan their children's meals in advance. But you can still ensure that that they get a nutritious diet by serving a variety of dishes that represent all the main food groups (see page 108), including bread or cereals, vegetables and fruit, milk or milk products, and meat or alternatives. For example, a balanced meal could consist of: bread, rice or pasta; a fresh or frozen vegetable; fresh or frozen

Baby food to go

Portable meals and snacks for your toddler

1. Whole-grain bread with cheese pieces
2. Low-sugar, whole-grain cereal mixed with whole-grain crackers
3. Sliced nitrate-free turkey or ham (found at organic meat markets and some delis) with a fresh whole-grain roll
4. Homemade soup
5. Pita bread cut in small pie-shaped pieces, served with vegetable dip
6. Sliced green, yellow or red bell peppers
7. Cut-up pears or peaches, berries, sliced banana, apple slices
8. Grated carrots and shredded cheese

fruit; and cheese, tofu, or canned tuna with mayonnaise, or leftover chicken or fish. Milk may be given during or after the meal.

Some good "combination meals" include macaroni and cheese, or tuna noodle casserole (which contains grains, fish and milk) — preferably homemade. For either of these dishes you can add extra cheese, as well as broccoli or some other vegetable, for a complete meal. You can also try quinoa with tofu and peas.

Soups are also good choices, since you can complement them with a grain such as quinoa or wheat berries, or bread and cheese, and add tofu for extra protein. Homemade oatmeal or chocolate chip cookies are simple but nutritious desserts. Ice cream served in a small cone is also a welcome treat, and is ideally suited for little hands.

Stocking your pantry

When you have a toddler to feed, be sure to keep some staples on hand (see list, page 71). Before purchasing packaged foods, read the labels carefully — many contain too much salt (see page 105) and other additives (see page 88). While commercially prepared meals can be quite nutritious, try to find the time to make a home-cooked meal more often. You'll find it personally satisfying and, as you'll discover with the recipes in this book, easier than you might think.

Wouldn't it be great if you could have a home-cooked meal just waiting for you to heat it up when you're short on time? You can! When you have the time, make large amounts and freeze portions for later. Meals that can be made in large quantities and frozen include pasta sauce, soups (to make soup a meal, add tofu or grains such as wheat berries or quinoa), pot pies, meatballs, chili, meatloaf (uncooked) and casseroles. Try Chicken Pot Pie (page 230), Shepherd's Pie (page 229), Easy Meatloaf (page 228), Fish, Tomato and Spinach Casserole (page 239), Easy Meatballs (page 226) and Vegetarian Chili (page 251).

tip

Giving your toddler nutritious meals is important, but don't forget to feed yourself as well! Your eating habits not only affect your own health, but also serve as an example to your child.

tip

Infants between 7 and 12 months need only 370 mg of sodium a day; children between 1 and 3 years need only 1,000 mg of sodium a day (1 tsp/5 mL table salt = 2,300 mg sodium).

Fast and easy
Quick menus for hungry toddlers

	DAY 1 (12 TO 24 MONTHS)	DAY 2 (12 TO 24 MONTHS)	DAY 3 (18 TO 24 MONTHS)
Breakfast	1 slice whole-grain toast with ½ tsp (2 mL) butter 1 oz (30 g) Cheddar cheese ¼ banana ½ cup (125 mL) whole milk	½ cup (125 mL) iron-rich oatmeal ½ cup (125 mL) whole milk ¼ orange	½ cup (125 mL) Baby's Fruit Smoothie (page 128) 1 slice whole-grain toast with 1 tsp (5 mL) peanut butter
Snack	1 Great Oatmeal Cookie (page 296) ½ cup (125 mL) whole milk	½ apple ¾ cup (175 mL) whole milk	¼ cup (50 mL) blueberries (fresh or frozen, thawed) ½ cup (125 mL) whole milk
Lunch	¼ cup (50 mL) Spinach Soup (page 162) 2 Meatballs and Mushrooms (page 227) ½ slice whole-grain bread with ½ tsp (2 mL) butter ½ cup (125 mL) whole milk	¼ cup (50 mL) green beans with ½ tsp (2 mL) butter 2 Simple Salmon Cakes (page 235) ½ cup (125 mL) whole milk	½ grilled cheese sandwich prepared with whole-grain bread 4 baby carrots, cooked and sliced lengthwise ½ cup (125 mL) whole milk ¼ to ½ cup (50 to 125 mL) diced fruit
Snack	2 unsalted whole-grain crackers 1 oz (30 g) Cheddar cheese ¼ cup (50 mL) whole milk	½ banana 1 Great Oatmeal Cookie (page 296) ½ cup (125 mL) water	¼ pita bread with 2 tbsp (25 mL) Hummus (page 277) ½ cup (125 mL) water
Supper	¼ cup (50 mL) broccoli ¼ cup (50 mL) Macaroni and Cheese (page 191) ½ cup (125 mL) whole milk ¼ cup (50 mL) strawberries	¼ chicken breast ½ cup (125 mL) quinoa with peas ¼ cup (50 mL) cooked carrots ½ whole-grain bagel with ½ tsp (2 mL) butter ½ cup (125 mL) whole milk	½ cup (125 mL) Fish, Tomato and Spinach Casserole (page 239) ½ to 1 seedless mandarin orange, sectioned 1 cup (250 mL) whole milk
Snack	¾ cup (175 mL) whole milk	½ cup (125 mL) whole milk	¼ cup (50 mL) plain yogurt with diced fruit
	Calories: 1356 Protein: 65.2 g Iron: 6.1 mg	Calories: 1250 Protein: 62 g Iron: 7.0 mg	Calories: 1200 Protein: 67 g Iron: 7.0 mg

Essential ingredients

Fresh, frozen and canned foods to keep on hand

- Eggs
- Milk
- Cheese
- Unsweetened or lightly sweetened yogurt, to which you can add mashed fresh berries, ripe pears, peaches or bananas
- Fresh fruits, such as oranges, apples, bananas, kiwifruit, melons, mangos, avocados
- Fresh or frozen berries
- Canned fruit, packed in water or its own juice
- Fresh or frozen vegetables, such as carrots, cucumbers, beans, peas, soybeans, broccoli, cauliflower, tomatoes
- Canned vegetable soup (low-sodium), to which you can add chickpeas, quinoa, whole wheat pasta or rice
- Homemade vegetable broth
- Dried or canned legumes, such as chickpeas, lentils, black beans (rinse canned varieties to reduce salt)
- Fresh or frozen fish
- Canned tuna, salmon (packed in water) and sardines
- Fresh or frozen chicken (boneless skinless breasts or thighs)
- Other lean cuts of meat
- Nut butter
- Whole-grain breakfast cereal (low-sugar, low-sodium, high-fiber)
- Whole-grain bread, rolls, bagels, pitas, wraps (freeze for later use)
- Whole-grain crackers (low-sodium)
- Whole-grain or enriched pasta (look for varieties made from lentils or chickpeas, which have more protein and fiber)
- Brown or mixed rice, quinoa, wheat berries, oats
- Olive oil, canola oil, sunflower oil
- Light mayo
- Fresh or frozen herbs

Not much cooking or baking in your house?

Even having a few recipes on hand can help make suppertime easier to manage, especially when you have limited time. Try out a couple of new recipes a week, and work up to about 10 that your family really enjoys. Then keep your kitchen stocked with the ingredients you need to prepare them.

tip

Mash a ripe avocado and use it in place of mayonnaise.

Eating with (and like) grown-ups

Between 12 to 24 months, children continue to build upon the rudimentary self-feeding skills they acquired at the age of 8 to 12 months. In addition, they begin to understand the social aspects of eating with parents and other family members.

Spoons and forks

Developing the skill of using utensils is important for toddlers, since it reinforces their independence. Security and affirmation are extremely important at this stage. So be positive — clapping your hands, smiling and showing approval — as your child gets better at using a spoon and fork. If you are worried about the amount of food he is actually eating, then try starting with spooning food yourself, and let him finish the last two-thirds of the meal. Soup may be more difficult for a toddler to manage on his own, so you may want to guide him with this food. Continue to let him pick up food with his fingers as well.

Toddlers can use their own cutlery, or they may want to try the grown-up version. The smaller forks and spoons made for children are generally easier to use, however. You can also start serving food on plates (if you have not already done so) instead of putting food on the tray. Toddlers learn quickly that this is where food should be. Try to teach them early on that the plate is not a toy, but meant for food. It can be done! Patience is important.

Taking the cup

By the time your child reaches the toddler stage, you may have already allowed him to take sips from your glass. But this is the time to introduce a cup of his own. Spill-proof ("sippy") cups are ideal at this age,

Sani-tray

Feeding trays are often cleaned too quickly and/or not thoroughly enough — especially if the meal has been a prolonged or frustrating one. This can be dangerous, since bacteria like nothing better than a moist area coated with various food residues. So get scrubbing. Use a clean cloth with mild soap, and rinse thoroughly with water.

Healthy snacks

Give your child fresh fruits and veggies as snacks at least twice a day, every day. Here are some ideas for platters:

- Strawberries, kiwis and pineapple
- Tomatoes, cucumbers, feta cheese, hummus, olives (without the pits) and pita bread
- Carrots, celery, cucumber and dips (either salad dressings or hummus)
- Avocados, tomatoes and cucumbers
- Lentil or quinoa salad, with whole-grain pita bread or unsalted crackers
- Whole wheat pasta with sauce (meat- or legume-based)

since they encourage independence and, for bottle-fed children, help to make the transition from bottle to cup.

A family that eats together

Meals are important events to share with your child. Try to interact with him for at least part of the meal. Allow him to feed you as well. As you are preparing the food and during the cleanup, talk to your child and explain what you are doing. Describe food that is hot and let him see where hot foods are prepared (the oven or stove). Allow him to touch hot food, so that he understands what this means. You can teach him to blow on food to cool it down.

What a mess!

As children become more independent in feeding themselves — but before their skills are fully developed — they are capable of creating a substantial mess. So there's no better time to start teaching them the importance of cleaning up. Always clean your child's hands and face after a meal, or let him do this himself (with a little help from you). Let him see you clean up the tray and high chair. Have a supply of clean cloths on hand to ensure a fresh cloth is used after each meal. You will certainly notice an unpleasant smell from the plastic tray if it is not cleaned properly. The same holds true for bibs. Invest in several bibs so that one is always clean and ready to use.

tip

If done gradually and with gentle persuasion, you can encourage your child to switch from his favorite night-time bottle to a "sippy" cup. Just remember that, whether it's a bottle or a cup, teeth should always be brushed once it is finished.

When your child won't eat veggies

If your child simply refuses to eat vegetables, keep trying. Research shows that it can take six or more tries before a child accepts a new vegetable or fruit. Here are some other suggestions:

- Make sure the vegetable is fresh, or cooked just right.
- Try dipping the vegetable in a light dip, such as yogurt or balsamic vinaigrette.
- Eat the vegetable yourself and demonstrate by your facial expression and satisfied "yum" that it is good.

Top 10 Toddler Years Questions

1 I don't always have time to prepare homemade meals. Are there nutritious alternatives?

Certain frozen dinners can be very nutritious, and are good choices when you don't have the time to prepare your own. Read the labels carefully, though, to ensure that they do not contain too much salt or other additives. We encourage you to try to prepare some of the recipes in this book, however. They're really fast and simple.

2 My child has a cold, and I've heard that milk can cause an increase in mucus. Should I avoid milk products?

Simply put, no. There is no research that confirms that milk causes an increase in mucus, so you can safely continue to give your child milk and milk products while he is sick. (Milk contains fat, which can adhere to an already mucusy throat and cause a sensation, albeit a false one, of increased mucus.) The important thing to consider is that milk is an essential source of Vitamin D and calcium (both important for bone growth), as well as protein and energy.

3 My child refuses to eat vegetables. What can I do?

While many children dislike one or two vegetables, it is unusual to dislike them all. The important thing is that you don't become discouraged if your child refuses a vegetable once. Introduce it again using a different preparation method, or at a different temperature and with a different food. Experiment with herbs or spices, or sauces or dressings (in small amounts), to enhance flavor. Focus on those vegetables that are popular with most children, such as corn, peas, carrots, beans and sweet potatoes. Soups are another good way to get your child to eat vegetables. (See the soup recipes in this book for ideas.)

4 How often should my daughter have snacks?

Snacks are a very important part of your child's diet, and should be offered at least 2 to 3 times a day. This will prevent her from getting too hungry and tired before mealtimes, and will allow you some flexibility in your schedule.

5 I usually give my daughter Cheerios and digestive cookies because they are so convenient. What other healthy snacks can you suggest?

For an alternative to your current snacks, try fresh fruit, cut into small bite-size pieces, or vegetables such as slices of green or red bell peppers; these can be kept a container in the refrigerator and enjoyed at any time. Thawed frozen fruit is another great fast food option. Other nutritious snacks include shredded cheese, pieces of a bagel, pita or other kind of bread, low-salt whole-grain crackers and homemade cookies. (See pages 68, 72 and 272–300 for more snack ideas.)

6 My husband tends to feed our daughter more quickly than I do, with the result that she eats less, and anticipates playtime less patiently. I often want to feed her myself, because I know that she will feed better for me, but realize that my husband has to feed her as well. What can we do to remedy this?

It is important for both of you to be consistent in your approach to feeding. Have your husband eat with your child, preferably for the same amount of time that you do. Make sure you both interact with your child at mealtimes, and that you are not using that time to read the paper, answer phone calls or read the mail. Above all, discuss the importance of consistency with your husband, and allow some time for change to take place. But remember also that there are many reasons why a child may be eating less (such as teething, fatigue or illness).

7 I have heard that some children tolerate goat's milk better than cow's milk. Is this true?

No. Not if they have an allergy to cow's milk. Children with an allergy to cow's milk protein should not be given goat's milk as an alternative, since they will most likely react to the protein in goat's milk as well. Claims of better tolerance to goat's milk are not supported by any research. Goat's milk is similar to cow's milk in that it is a good source of many important nutrients, including calcium and vitamin D. One difference between the two is in the types of protein each contains. Goat's milk may be deficient in folic acid (which is important for the production of red blood cells). If you choose goat's milk, make sure that it has folic acid added.

8 We drink soda pop in our house, and my 18-month-old son keeps asking to try some. Is it okay to give him a few sips?

Soda pop provides little in the way of beneficial nutrients except for calories and, in some cases, a bit of vitamin C. In addition, some of these drinks contain significant amounts of caffeine. As such, they are not really suitable for toddlers. Of course, a few sips here or there will not damage his health. A better alternative is to mix 1 part fruit juice with 3 parts unflavored sparkling water (such as Perrier). This is a refreshing, tasty drink that is good for your toddler — and the whole family.

9 Is it safe for my child to eat canned tuna?

It is safe for children to eat up to 2 servings per week of canned light tuna. Health authorities, however, recommend that canned albacore (white) tuna be limited to 1 serving per week for children between the ages of 1 and 4 years. Fish can be an important part of a well-balanced diet. See pages 79–81 for more details.

10 My child is an extremely picky eater. To be sure she is meeting her nutrient needs, should I be trying those oral milk supplements (with the added vitamins and minerals) that are aimed for children in their toddler years?

It is usually not advised to give energy-boosted oral supplements to young children. A child may fill up on these supplements at the expense of other foods. The transition to table foods is a time to provide new tastes and textures; it's not a good idea to simply substitute another liquid to satisfy your young child's food intake. While many parents feel anxious about whether their child is eating enough, remember that child-sized servings are much smaller than adult ones. Also, kids do not grow as fast in their second year of life as they did in the first, and it is normal for their appetite to vary. See page 62 for an example of what a "picky" eater might eat in 1 day, while still satisfying most of her needs.

Growth is the best way to measure whether energy needs are being met. Children who have poor weight gain and are falling off their regular growth curve may benefit from these supplements. Speak with your family doctor or pediatrician if you are concerned about your child's growth.

CHAPTER 6

Adverse Reactions to Food

Many foods that are safe for adults can be dangerous for young children. For example, a food's consistency may be such that it is hard to chew and/or swallow, thereby presenting a choking hazard. A food may be contaminated with bacteria, or it may contain compounds that cause an allergic reaction. Foods may cause digestive problems such as diarrhea or constipation. In each of these cases, it is important that parents understand the risks and remedies involved.

CPR certified?

If your child, or someone else's child, were to choke in your presence, would you know how to handle the situation? With training in infant cardiopulmonary resuscitation (CPR) you would be prepared. Infant CPR training can be organized through your local community center or the Red Cross. (Keep in mind that infant CPR is very different from adult CPR.) You may be able to get someone qualified to come to your home, where they can teach a group of friends and family.

Choking hazards

Anyone who has been around infants knows that they love to put things in their mouths. This makes them very susceptible to choking. Also, when eating, some infants swallow food without mashing it with their tongue or palate, which causes them to gag or to choke. Parents need to do all they can to minimize the risk of choking for their children.

Children should always be supervised while eating. Do not allow toddlers to walk or run with food in their mouths. Eating in the car is also considered unsafe for young children: If they choke in the car, you may not be able to pull over to the curb safely to help them. In addition, unexpected motion in a car (such as a sudden stop) can cause choking.

For infants, a "propped bottle" (that is, where no one is holding the bottle) is potentially hazardous, since the flow of milk can exceed their ability to drink it, thereby causing them to choke.

Many foods are considered unsafe for toddlers because of their shape. These include hard, small, round or sticky foods that have the potential to block their small airways. Some of these foods are listed in the table below.

Hard to swallow
Foods to avoid for children under 4 years old

- Chewing gum
- Cough drops
- Fish with bones
- Whole grape tomatoes
- Hard candies
- Sunflower seeds
- Popcorn
- Raisins (whole)
- Peanuts/nuts
- Snacks with toothpicks/skewers
- Whole carrots
- Whole grapes
- Whole wieners or hot dogs

Post this list on your refrigerator for all family members and friends to read.

Tips to reduce the risk of choking
- First and most importantly, *always supervise young children while they are eating.*
- Avoid foods listed in "Hard to swallow" (above).
- Become educated in CPR for infants and young children.
- Grate raw carrots and hard fruits, such as apples.
- Cook carrots (including baby carrots) until tender and slice lengthwise.
- Quarter or chop grapes and grape tomatoes.
- Slice hot dogs in lengthwise strips.
- Remove pits and seeds from fruit.
- Chop raisins or dates.
- Spread peanut butter or other nut butters thinly on crackers or toast (young children may not be able to handle thickly spread peanut butter with bread).

Food-borne illness

Infants are at an increased risk of "food poisoning" because of their immature digestive and immune systems. Food-borne illnesses are caused by eating foods contaminated with bacteria, viruses, parasites, or bacterial or chemical toxins. Parents can help minimize the risk of these illnesses by taking the following precautions.

Safe food-handling practices

1. Always wash your hands well before handling foods, and keep work surfaces and utensils clean.
2. Avoid cross-contamination between raw and cooked foods. Do not handle raw meats and raw fruits and vegetables at the same time. Wash your hands after handling raw meat, and wash surfaces, cutting boards and utensils thoroughly with soap and water after they come in contact with raw meats, before using them for other foods.
3. Cook meats, fish, poultry and eggs to the proper internal temperature (see table, page 79). Check with a food thermometer. Adequate cooking and reheating of foods will destroy any microorganisms that may infect foods.
4. Always keep hot foods hot (over 140°F/60°C) and cold foods cold (under 39°F/4°C). Bacteria multiply quickly in the warm temperatures in between.
5. Store foods properly, at the correct temperature. Refrigerate leftovers as soon as possible.
6. Thaw foods in the refrigerator, not on the counter at room temperature.
7. Read the "best before" date when purchasing items. Do not buy cracked, dirty or unrefrigerated eggs. Do not purchase canned foods if the can is dented or the top of the can is bulging.
8. Do not give honey, or food products that contain honey, to infants less than 12 months old. Honey may contain spores of the bacterium *Clostridium botulinum*, which can cause infant botulism.
9. Do not give foods that contain raw eggs (uncooked cookie dough, homemade Caesar salad dressing, homemade mayonnaise) to young children. Raw eggs may contain salmonella, which can cause a type of food poisoning called salmonellosis.
10. Do not give your child raw meats or poultry, raw fish or sushi, or unpasteurized milk or juice/cider products.

Other culprits to be aware of

Food poisoning is commonly caused by improperly prepared home-canned foods, improperly stored fruit juice or vegetable juice, or improperly stored baked potatoes. Also, do not eat any food from a dented, leaking or bulging can. Remember, even if your food does not have an off smell, it could still be contaminated with harmful bacteria.

Honey and infant botulism

Did you know that honey should not be given to infants under 1 year of age, due to the risk of infant botulism? Honey may contain the spores of a bacterium known as *Clostridium botulinum*, which can cause botulism. Adults and older children are not typically susceptible to the bacteria because their mature digestive systems are able to eliminate it before it can do any harm. Young babies, however, cannot handle the bacteria and, if ingested, the bacteria may produce a toxin that can affect an infant's ability to move, eat and breathe. Symptoms typically appear within 18 to 36 hours of consuming the affected food and may include constipation, a flat facial expression, muscle weakness, difficulty swallowing or breathing problems.

In North America, it is very rare that an infant becomes ill with botulism: fewer than 100 cases are reported in the U.S. each year. Most babies with infant botulism recover fully with appropriate medical treatment. The best treatment is prevention, so avoid giving your child honey before her first birthday.

Minding mercury

Mercury is an element that occurs naturally in the environment; however, it is also a by-product of industry and can be released into the air as a pollutant. When mercury pollution falls from the air and enters our rivers, lakes and oceans, it turns into methylmercury. Fish absorb methylmercury as they feed in polluted

---

Safe internal food temperatures

Beef
Ground beef . . . 160°F–165°F (71°C–73°C)
Medium . . . . 160°F (71°C)
Well-done . . . . 170°F (76°C)

Pork. . . . . 160°F–170°F (71°C–76°C)

Poultry . . . . 165°F–180°F (73°C–82°C)

Fish . . . . 165°F (73°C)

Egg dishes . . . . 160°F (71°C)

Buy pasteurized corn syrup

Corn syrup is also sometimes mentioned in connection with infant botulism; always read the label when purchasing corn syrup to make sure it has been pasteurized (in Canada, all corn syrup must be pasteurized and therefore poses no risk).

waters. Fish that swim and eat at the bottom of the ocean accumulate more mercury than other types of fish.

Pregnant and nursing women, as well as young children, should limit intake of these fish, because consumption of fish with high levels of methylmercury has been linked to the development of cerebral palsy and microcephaly (an abnormally small head). Consumption of these fish should also be limited in the general population.

Don't avoid fish altogether!

A recent study found that women who ate fish with low mercury levels twice a week had babies that did better on cognitive tests than babies whose mothers ate less fish. The message? Fish is an important and healthy part of the diet, contributing protein and essential fats, including the omega 3 fatty acids eicosapentaenoic acid (EPA) and docosahexaenoic acid (DHA). But choose the type and quantity of fish carefully.

How much fish is safe, and what types should be avoided?
FDA/EPA statement
The U.S. Food and Drug Administration (FDA), in conjunction with the Environmental Protection Agency (EPA), announced a joint statement on methylmercury in fish in March 2004. They recommend that women who are planning to become pregnant, are pregnant or are breastfeeding should "reduce their exposure to the harmful effects of mercury" by following these guidelines:

1. Avoid shark, swordfish, king mackerel and tilefish, which all contain high levels of mercury.
2. Eat up to 12 oz (375 g) per week (two average meals) of fish and shellfish that are low in mercury to receive the beneficial health effects of fish. Examples of fish low in mercury include canned light tuna, salmon, pollock, sole, shrimp, haddock, catfish and mahi mahi.
3. Limit intake of canned albacore (white) tuna to one meal, or 6 oz (175 g), per week, because canned albacore tuna has higher levels of mercury than canned light tuna. Eat fish lower in mercury for the balance of the week.
4. Check with your local authorities about the safety of fish caught in local waters. This includes fish caught by friends and family in local rivers and lakes. If no information is available, the FDA and EPA suggest consuming a maximum of 6 oz (175 g) of the fish in question, and not consuming any more fish that week.

The FDA/EPA statement suggests that you "follow these same recommendations when feeding fish and shellfish to your young child, but serve smaller portions."

Health Canada recommendations
Canada's Food Guide currently recommends that Canadians eat at least 2 servings of fish per week, choosing fish and shellfish that are high in omega 3 fatty acids but low in mercury, such as salmon, pollock, Atlantic mackerel, rainbow trout, anchovies, capelin, char, hake, herring, mullet, smelt, lake whitefish, blue crabs, shrimp, clams, mussels and oysters.

Predatory fish — including fresh and frozen tuna, shark, swordfish, marlin, orange roughy and escolar — may be high in mercury, and young children should limit their intake of these fish to $2\frac{1}{2}$ oz (75 g) per month. This recommendation does not apply to canned tuna, one of the most common types of fish consumed by Canadians. Canned tuna comes in two varieties: albacore (white) tuna and light tuna (also known as skipjack, yellowfin or tongol). Canned light tuna is relatively low in mercury, and young children can consume up to 5 oz (150 g), or 2 servings, per week. Albacore tuna consumed in high quantities may contain more mercury than is considered acceptable, and should be limited in children between the ages of 1 and 4 years to 1 serving, or $2\frac{1}{2}$ oz (75 g), per week.

> ## Dietitians' recommendations
> Both the American Dietetic Association and the Dietitians of Canada believe that fish contributes to a well-balanced diet. We should not forget all the benefits of eating fish when we are talking about mercury concerns. Fish contains omega 3 fatty acids, which contribute to heart health. Research also suggests that omega 3 fatty acids improve visual and neural acuity in unborn babies. Fish is an excellent high-quality protein, is low in saturated fat and has other essential nutrients, such as zinc and iron, that can contribute to a healthy diet.

Food allergies
Food allergy, or "hypersensitivity," is defined as an immune-system response to a food protein that the body identifies as foreign. As such, it is different from a food intolerance (such as lactose intolerance), which is an adverse reaction to a food that results in symptoms, but is not caused by a reaction of the immune system.

Children under 5 years are especially susceptible to food allergies because of their immature digestive system. So why do allergies occur in some and not in others? There is no straightforward answer. In past years, some thought that avoidance of certain foods in the first year of life would be protective, but this was not supported by studies. Some experts now believe that a young child's immune system can be "educated" by introducing foods that commonly cause allergies. In this way, some feel that allergies can be prevented (therefore, there is no need to avoid certain foods in the first year of life).

Most commonly, symptoms of food allergy involve the skin, the respiratory tract and the digestive tract; systemic symptoms may also occur.

- **Skin:** rash, hives, eczema, itching, tingling lips, swelling around lips and face
- **Respiratory:** runny nose, nasal congestion, difficulty breathing, wheezing
- **Digestive:** vomiting, diarrhea, stomach cramps
- **Systemic:** anaphylaxis (see box, at left), lethargy or fatigue, failure to gain appropriate weight

Diagnosing food allergies

If you suspect that your child has a food allergy, or if you have a strong family history of allergies (at least one parent or sibling has a confirmed food allergy), it is important that you have your child tested. There are several ways to test for allergy.

Elimination diet. With this method, allergenic foods are eliminated from the diet for a 2-week period and are then slowly reintroduced to try and identify which foods are causing symptoms. This diet should be followed under medical supervision. The testing period should not exceed 2 weeks, since nutritional deficiencies may result.

Extreme reaction

Anaphylaxis is an intense, immediate allergic response. Symptoms can include hives, swelling around the mouth and face, itching, difficulty breathing, nausea and diarrhea. Severe cases can lead to anaphylactic shock or even death. Anaphylactic symptoms usually occur within minutes of food ingestion, but can occur up to 1 or 2 hours later. Parents of children with anaphylactic reactions to foods must carry an injection containing epinephrine (for example, Epipen®) at all times. A prescription can be obtained through your physician, pediatrician or immunologist.

tip
Breastfeeding can help to protect against certain allergies. Genetic factors may also play a role in determining which children are at greater risk for developing allergies.

Skin test. Also known as "prick tests," these are widely used to diagnose food allergy. A small amount of an allergen is introduced to the skin by pricking the skin with a small needle. The skin is then monitored for a reaction. Skin tests are not 100% accurate, and false positives (a reaction in the absence of true allergy) may occur. These tests are unreliable for infants and are not used in such cases.

RAST/ImmuneCap. This blood test can be done when a skin test cannot be completed because the child has severe eczema or is on medications that may interfere with a skin test. This test should not replace the skin test, as studies have shown that properly performed skin testing is more reliable than RAST testing. The newer CapRAST is more comparable to skin testing, but it is also more invasive.

Oral food challenge. The gold standard for confirming a food allergy, this test must be performed under controlled circumstances in a doctor's office so that treatment can be given immediately if a reaction occurs. It has significant risks, so other tests are recommended.

Types of food allergies

While any number of foods can cause allergic reactions, the five most common food allergies in North America are to milk, soy, eggs, peanuts and wheat.

Milk allergy and cow's milk colitis

Milk allergy is a reaction to one or more of the proteins found in milk. Cow's milk allergy occurs in about 2 or 3 of every 100 infants, although most grow out of it by the time they are 3 years old. Most children with "traditional" cow's milk allergy (IgE-mediated allergy) are able to tolerate soymilk or formula as an alternative. A breastfeeding mother may need to eliminate cow's milk from her diet, as milk protein can appear in breast milk. Talk to your doctor about more specific recommendations.

Prevention of allergy

There is no evidence at this time to suggest that the avoidance of specific foods either during pregnancy or while breastfeeding will prevent the development of food allergy. Exclusive breastfeeding for a minimum of 4 to 6 months may help to protect against the development of cow's milk allergy and eczema in high-risk infants (where at least one parent or sibling has atopy).

---

tip

You should not immediately eliminate a food from your child's diet because you suspect she is allergic to it. This can result in an unbalanced diet, leading to poor weight gain, as well as possible vitamin or mineral deficiencies. Suspected food allergies should be confirmed before the food is eliminated.

Cow's milk colitis is an intolerance to cow's milk that is sometimes seen in young infants. It is similar to allergy in that an affected infant cannot tolerate cow's milk, but the symptoms tend to be more isolated to the GI tract. Cow's milk colitis is caused by an inflammation in the digestive tract due to an inability to tolerate the proteins in cow's milk. Colitis can also occur in breastfed infants whose mothers consume cow's milk. The symptoms may include vomiting, diarrhea, poor weight gain or blood in the stools. Blood in the diaper of a young infant can be extremely distressing for parents, and blood loss secondary to cow's milk colitis may cause iron-deficiency anemia.

Unlike with cow's milk allergy, infants with cow's milk colitis may not be able to consume soymilk or formula as an alternative, as up to 50% of these infants are also intolerant to soy protein. Infants with cow's milk colitis are typically put on a diet that is free of both cow's milk and soy proteins. For breastfed babies, this means mom has to follow a strict milk-free and soy-free diet. For

Lactose intolerance

Lactose intolerance, an inability to digest the sugar (lactose) found in milk and milk products, results in watery, loose stools. Lactose intolerance is different from and less severe than a milk allergy, which is an immune response to the protein in milk. It is rare for infants to be born with lactose intolerance, as breast milk (nature's perfect food) contains lactose. However, an infant can sometimes have temporary lactose intolerance after a diarrheal illness. This should resolve within 2 weeks or so, and doctors do not generally recommend avoiding lactose in this situation.

Where's the milk?

Milk ingredients are not always clearly indicated as such on food labels. If you see any of the following words on a food label, it means the food contains milk protein.

ammonium caseinate	calcium caseinate	magnesium caseinate
potassium caseinate	sodium caseinate	casein/caseinate
rennet casein	curds	lactate
delactosed/demineralized whey	lactose	lactoferrin
lactoglobulin	milk derivative/protein/fat	modified milk ingredients
hydrolyzed casein	hydrolyzed milk protein	lactalbumin
lactalbumin phosphate	whey protein concentrate	whey

Source: Health Canada. Used with permission.

formula-fed infants, it means that a specialty infant formula in which the proteins are broken down, such as Nutramigen or Alimentum, must be used.

Ultimately, children with either cow's milk colitis or cow's milk allergy must completely avoid foods containing milk protein. As solids are introduced, it is important that you read the food labels on packaged foods to ensure that they do not contain any milk protein. If a physician has diagnosed your child with cow's milk allergy or intolerance, ask to meet with a registered dietitian so you can confirm that your child is consuming the proper nutrients, especially calcium and vitamin D, which are normally supplied by cow's milk and are needed for the development of strong bones and teeth.

Alternative sources of calcium

See page 99 for some non-dairy sources of calcium.

Soy allergy

Soy protein is another common source of food allergy in children. Soy products are a derivative of the soybean, a vegetable that is made into many foods, such as tofu and soymilk, and provides protein, folate, iron, calcium, vitamin D, zinc and B vitamins. Soy allergy can be tricky to manage, as soy is found in many commercial products. Care must be taken to avoid all hidden sources of soy.

What about soy lecithin?

Soy lecithin is a soy fat, not a soy protein. It is often tolerated by children with an allergy to soy protein. However, in rare circumstances, very sensitive children can react to it; these children should avoid soy lecithin in their diet.

Be label-conscious

If your child has been diagnosed with soy allergy, be sure to read the labels of all packaged foods for possible sources of soy. Any of the following words indicate the presence of soy in the product.

edamame	soy protein (isolate/concentrate)	miso
TVP (textured vegetable protein)*	mono-diglyceride	tempeh
natto	TSF (textured soy flour)	tofu (soybean curds)
okara	TSP (textured soy protein)	vegetable protein
soya, soja, soybean, soyabean	yuba	

* Textured vegetable protein may come from different vegetable sources, including soy. If the source is not identified, it may contain soy protein.

Source: Health Canada. Used with permission.

Egg indicators

If you see any of the following words on a food label, it contains egg protein.

albumin/albumen	conalbumin	globulin
egg substitutes (e.g. Egg Beaters®)	livetin	lysozyme
meringue	ovalbumin	ovoglobulin
ovolactohydrolyze proteins	ovomacroglobulin	ovotransferrin
ovomucin, ovomucoid	ovovitellin	silico-albuminate
simplesse®	vitellin	

Source: Health Canada. Used with permission.

Egg allergy

Egg whites contain more than 20 different types of protein, all of which can be a source of egg allergy. Most children will grow out of an egg allergy by their 5th birthday.

For infants who have a confirmed allergy to eggs, avoiding whole eggs is fairly easy. But because eggs are so widely used as an ingredient, it is often much harder to avoid foods that may contain eggs. For example, some common foods that contain eggs include custards, egg nog, Caesar salad, cakes, cookies, pies, pancakes, waffles and battered foods. Eggs may also be used in consommé soup and soft drinks (such as root beer), where it is used as a clarifier. Egg Beaters®, while sold as an egg substitute, is not egg-free and should not be consumed by infants or toddlers with an egg allergy.

Some vaccinations also contain egg protein. Your physician will be able to give you more information if you are concerned about egg allergy and vaccines.

Peanut allergy

Unlike milk and egg allergies, a peanut allergy generally persists beyond childhood. This type of allergy is common — about 1% of children in North America have a peanut allergy — and is one of the most severe, often the cause of anaphylactic shock. While a peanut allergy does not necessarily extend to all nuts, a child

Good to know

Some people who have a peanut allergy may also be allergic to other foods in the legume family, such as soy.

A peanut by any other name ...

If your child has been diagnosed with peanut allergy, you should be aware that peanuts go by many names. Check food labels for the following words.

arachide	arachis oil	beer nuts
cacahouète/cacahouette/cacahuète	goober nuts, goober peas	ground nuts
kernels	mandelonas	Nu-Nuts®
nutmeats	valencias	

Source: Health Canada. Used with permission.

who has had a previous anaphylactic reaction to peanuts should avoid all nuts to be safe. Pure peanut oil should also be avoided, since, although theoretically free of peanut proteins, it may nevertheless contain trace amounts. Peanut oil is widely used in many restaurants (particularly Thai and Chinese), so you may wish to avoid these restaurants altogether. Also, be sure to read labels carefully for foods that "may contain" peanuts. These foods should not be consumed by an infant or toddler with a peanut allergy.

Tree nut allergy

Tree nuts (nuts that grow on trees) include almonds, walnuts, Brazil nuts, cashews, hazelnuts, pecans, pistachios and macadamia nuts. They are not related to peanuts (which are actually part of the legume family), and children with an allergy to peanuts may not be allergic to tree nuts, or vice versa. If a child is allergic to one type of tree nut, her physician will often recommend that she avoid all tree nuts because of the risk of cross-contamination.

Wheat allergy

The most common source of grain allergy in North America is wheat. This allergy is an adverse reaction to the protein component of wheat. It is different from celiac disease, in which affected patients cannot tolerate gluten (a protein found in many grains, including wheat, rye and

Delay the introduction of nuts until 1 year

Consider waiting to introduce nuts to your baby until she is at least 1 year old. Nut allergy is one of the most common food allergies and is more likely to cause anaphylaxis than other allergenic foods. After 1 year of age, children are better able to communicate if something feels funny in their throat. Talk to your doctor if you have any questions about the introduction of nuts.

Other names for wheat

If you see any of the following words on a food label, it means the food contains wheat.

atta	bulgur	couscous
durum	einkorn	emmer
enriched white/whole wheat flour	farina	gluten
graham flour	high gluten/protein flour	Kamut
seitan	semolina	spelt (dinkel, farro)
triticale (a cross between wheat and rye)	triticum aestivum	wheat bran/flour/germ/starch

Source: Health Canada. Used with permission.

tip
If your child has a wheat allergy, try serving quinoa, a gluten-free grain.

barley). Celiac disease requires significant lifelong dietary changes, beyond eliminating wheat from the diet.

Wheat is found in many foods, including breads, cereals, pastas, cakes, luncheon meats and sausage — virtually anything that contains wheat flour. Because wheat flour is fortified with the vitamins riboflavin, thiamin and niacin, as well as iron, the elimination of wheat from an allergic child's diet can result in a nutrient deficiency unless replaced by other foods, including alternative flours such as rye, corn or rice. It is important that the parent of any child with a confirmed allergy to wheat speak to a registered dietitian about the specific dietary changes that are involved.

Food additives

While their effects are uncertain, food additives are often blamed for causing changes in children's behavior. For example, many parents claim they cause conditions such as attention deficit disorder. Food additives include artificial food colorings and flavors, preservatives (such as sulfur dioxide, butylated hydroxytoluene [BHT] and butylated hydroxyanisole [BHA]), nitrates and nitrites, as well as artificial sweeteners.

Many scientific studies have been conducted over the years to assess the effects of additives on children. While some have found that certain additives have an affect on behavior, not all reached the same conclusion. One recent study investigating the effects on children of sodium benzoate and a mixture of food colorings found that only one group of additives increased hyperactivity in 3-year-olds, while both groups increased hyperactivity in 9-year-olds. An easy way to avoid these additives? Choose fresh foods more often; bake your own desserts, using carefully chosen ingredients; and limit your purchases of processed packaged foods, which, in addition to additives, may contain high amounts of sugar, fat and salt, and very little in the way of nutrients.

For parents who believe that eliminating additives will improve a child's behavior, this should be done through objective evaluation, under the supervision of a family doctor. This will require taking certain measurements of their child's behavior before the new diet is started, and several days after it is started. Objective measures may include recording the exact amount of time (in minutes or hours) that certain behaviors are observed over a defined period of days.

Overstimulated?

Sugar and chocolate may be considered additives, and many parents claim these also cause an increase in hyperactivity in their children. Caffeine, a known stimulant found in varying amounts in chocolate, has a metabolic reason for its effects on increasing activity. There is no scientific evidence that sugar causes hyperactivity or disruptive behavior in children.

Dealing with diarrhea

The primary cause of diarrhea is infection. The condition is defined as when infants or children have excessive stool — that is, greater than 4 to 10 tsp (20 to 50 mL) per kilogram of body weight per day or 1 to 2 cups (250 to 500 mL) per day for a 1-year-old — and where the output is changed from its normal consistency. (Keep in mind that infants' stools can vary in frequency and consistency from day to day, and from infant to infant.) Typically, this means the stool has more water than usual and is more frequent.

Infants younger than 6 to 8 months are especially vulnerable to the consequences of diarrhea. This is because of the risk of dehydration, due to the potentially large fluid losses. A family doctor should always be consulted when diarrhea lasts longer than 24 hours in young infants.

What are the most common childhood gastrointestinal complaints?

Infants in the first 6 months of life most commonly experience regurgitation, colic, constipation, vomiting and diarrhea. In the second year of life, up to 10% of children may experience constipation, one of the most common causes of complaints of abdominal pain in children. In most cases, dietary changes, such as increased fiber intake, can help resolve constipation.

The consistency of diarrhea can be watery, mucusy or oily. Each provides an indication as to the cause of the diarrhea.

Watery diarrhea usually occurs as a result of intolerance to carbohydrate (sugar), often lactose or sorbitol. Intolerance to lactose (found in cow's milk) can occur temporarily following a viral infection that affects the gut lining, decreasing the amount of the enzyme lactase. (Lactase is needed to break down lactose.) Sorbitol is found in some juices (non-citrus varieties, such as apple, pear and prune juices), which, if ingested in large amounts, can also cause watery diarrhea.

Mucusy stools can be caused by a viral or bacterial infection. It may indicate inflammation of the colon. Sometimes a change in formula (to a more predigested formula, for example) can also result in more mucusy stool, although volume is not usually increased. With a viral infection, stools increase in volume.

Oily stools are a sign that fats are not being digested properly. Causes of this can include disorders of the pancreas or intolerance of gluten (protein found in bread and other cereals). Stools may be formed or loose, and are usually excessive and foul-smelling.

Other causes of diarrhea include cow's milk protein sensitivity, which is the most common milk-related illness among infants. Diarrhea (and vomiting) can occur as soon as milk protein is ingested, with a typical onset being anywhere between 2 days and 4 months of age. For more information on milk allergies, see pages 83–85.

Treatment

The first step in treating diarrhea is to replace the fluid and electrolytes (salts) that have been lost. If the diarrhea lasts for longer than a day (depending on the age of the infant), rehydration solutions (such as Pedialyte®) may be used for a period of 24 hours. After this, a normal diet can be

---

Soothing sore bums

Diaper rash is a common aftereffect of diarrhea. If the rash is severe, try Ihle's Paste, which contains cornstarch and zinc, or another cream with zinc (preferably with a zinc content of more than 10%), and use it liberally with each diaper change. When wiping buttocks, use only tissue and water. Cotton balls or make-up-remover pads are also good. Keep a plastic container of water in a drawer or near the change table area for convenience. The astringent in commercial diaper wipes (even those that are scent-free) can irritate sensitive infant skin, so avoid using these when your child has a rash.

resumed. (Note: if vomiting was associated with the diarrhea, then refeeding should begin as soon as vomiting has stopped.) Your doctor will guide you on the type, volume and duration of rehydration solution to give your child. Remember to ask how long the solution is to be used for, and when a full diet can be reintroduced.

Child constipation

Constipation is defined as a reduced water content in the stool and is caused by insufficient water in the colon. It is one of the most common disorders in Western society, affecting children and adults alike. Despite numerous studies, the dietary factors leading to constipation remain unclear. One study concluded that insufficient calorie and nutrient intake, as well as a decrease in body weight, were associated with constipation. Cow's milk allergy may cause constipation and reflux, but this cause is rare.

tip
Keep in mind that stooling patterns in young children can vary from day to day. Less frequent stooling may not necessarily mean they are constipated.

Symptoms

How do you know if your child is constipated? Stools may appear like small pellets, or they may be in the form of one very large round ball. They are usually difficult for your child to pass. Mucus may also appear in the stool, and it may be slightly blood-streaked. This is not normally a cause for concern. The mucus is from the lining of the intestine and the blood may represent a small tear in the lining. If the bleeding persists or appears heavier than a slight streak, contact your doctor.

Eat more fiber

A lack of fiber in the diet is a leading cause of both childhood and adult constipation. According to some studies, we generally consume only about half the recommended amount of fiber.

There are medical causes for chronic constipation (other than dietary), and these will be investigated if your doctor has reason for concern. In most cases, however, diet is the source of the problem.

Treatment

Providing an adequate supply of fluids may help in the treatment of constipation. If your house is kept very warm in the winter, or is hot in the summer months, then extra fluid must be provided. Daily fluid intake (including all sources of fluid) should be approximately 4 to 6 cups (1 to 1.5 L).

If your child is on solids, offer a varied diet, with plenty of fresh fruits and vegetables. Offer cereals daily, and try a few teaspoons of bran cereal mixed in with oatmeal or infant cereal for children older than 12 to 18 months.

If your child shows signs of difficulty with a bowel movement — straining or grunting, for example, or becoming red in the face and crying — you can provide some relief by laying the infant on the change area and pulling her legs up, then massaging the stomach gently.

If constipation cannot be relieved through dietary measures, or if it is very severe, then lactulose (an undigestable sugar) may be prescribed by your family doctor or pediatrician. Only a small amount of the lactulose is required to promote fecal movement and softer stools. Glycerin suppositories may also be prescribed.

CHAPTER 7

Nutrition Facts

It goes without saying (particularly in a book like this one) that good nutrition is essential to the health of a child. And while today's parents are generally more diet-conscious than any generation before them, the task of sorting out all the information now available about nutrition can be a little overwhelming. Our advice to worried parents? Relax. A balance of good, nutritious foods and regular exercise is generally all your child needs. It is only in a small number of circumstances — for example, in cases of iron deficiency or where a strict vegetarian diet is being followed — that special dietary measures may be required. In this chapter, we'll look at some of these issues, as well as the basic components of a healthy, balanced diet.

> ## Viva Variety!
>
> "With smiling faces, my boys have enthusiastically stuffed the following into their mouths over the last little while: tofu (plain, with soy/sesame oil and red curry), eggplant miso, steak, lamb, chicken and beef burgers, papaya, chopped liver, beets, goat cheese, salmon, avocado, mango, gnocchi, and ravioli filled with squash and gorgonzola sauce."
>
> —Proud mom of 13-month-old twins

Food Fundamentals

Food provides the essential elements that the body requires for growth and metabolism. These include carbohydrates, proteins, fats, minerals and vitamins.

Carbohydrate

Carbohydrates are sugars of various types that provide the body with energy. They also help to keep bowel movements soft and regular, by way of fiber. Common sources include breads and cereals, as well as fruits and vegetables. Carbohydrates supply about 4 calories for every gram of weight.

Simple carbohydrates, or simple sugars, are short chains of sugars known as monosaccharides and disaccharides. The monosaccharides are glucose, fructose and galactose. The disaccharides are sucrose (made up of glucose and fructose), lactose (made up of glucose and galactose) and maltose (made up of two molecules of glucose). Sucrose is found in fruits and vegetables and in table sugar; lactose is found in breast milk, cow's milk and milk products; and maltose is found in cereals such as wheat and barley.

The more complex, or longer-chain, carbohydrates are called polysaccharides. These include starches and modified starches, such as those found in vegetables, rice, beans and potatoes. Modified starch is used as a thickening agent in foods.

Fiber is a very important polysaccharide that we, young and old, generally do not get enough of in our daily North American diet. Fiber helps to keep bowel movements soft and easy to pass and blood cholesterol levels low. It also helps people with diabetes regulate blood sugars. In adults, a high-fiber diet has been associated with a reduced risk of colon cancer, heart disease, diabetes and constipation. Children who eat a high-fiber diet will experience even more of the protective benefits of fiber as they reach adulthood. (See page 96 for more on fiber.)

Protein

Proteins are complex structures of amino acids that the body uses to build tissue and to carry out specific functions, such as fighting infections. Certain essential amino acids cannot be produced by the body, so must be taken in through the diet. Like carbohydrate, protein provides 4 calories for each gram of weight. Examples of protein foods include eggs, meat and fish. Proteins are also found in many plant sources, but a combination of plant foods is required to supply all of the amino acids the body needs. Including foods that contain protein in a meal or snack can help kids (and adults!) feel full longer. The typical North American diet provides more than enough protein.

Fat

Fats are an important component of a healthy diet. They serve as a good source of energy, transport fat-soluble vitamins, produce hormones and form part of the structure of cell membranes. Fats provide 9 calories per gram.

Fat is made up of smaller components called fatty acids. Depending on their chemical structure and how many double bonds they have, fats are classified as monounsaturated, polyunsaturated or saturated. Saturated fats, which have no double bonds, are found in animal foods, such as milk, butter and meat. Monounsaturated and polyunsaturated fats, which have double bonds, are considered healthy fats and are found in a variety of sources, such as vegetable oils, nuts and seeds, avocados and fish.

Trans fats are found naturally in small amounts in meat and some dairy foods, but are not a significant part of the diet. Manufactured trans fats, which can make up a larger part of the diet, are considered to have a negative affect on health. These hydrogenated fats are added to many snack foods, such as crackers, chips and pastries, to create a crispy texture. Food manufacturers are now limiting or removing trans fats from their products.

The omega 3 and omega 6 fatty acids (which are polyunsaturated fats) are considered essential because the body cannot make them on its own; they must be taken in through the foods we eat. Together, they are involved in regulating the inflammation process, among other functions. Consumption of omega 3 fatty acids is limited

Joanne Saab on nutrition for kids

Armed with a little knowledge, parents can provide their children with healthy alternatives to the sugar-laden convenience foods available in grocery stores. Given our busy lives, it is often difficult to prepare home-cooked meals and eat as a family. But a great time to lay down the groundwork for family meals is while your children are young. Eating out infrequently and having family meals around the dinner table can reduce the risk of obesity, and studies have shown that children communicate more with their parents in families that eat together. As a working mom, I understand how challenging it can be to balance work life and family life, but I always make family meals a priority.

I am also a firm believer in "everything in moderation." My children do have sweets occasionally, but dessert is almost always fruit and they drink very little fruit juice. As an alternative to candies on holidays such as Valentine's Day, try giving them a small outdoor toy such as a soccer ball or sidewalk chalk. Children learn by watching you, so set an example by making good nutrition a part of your everyday life.

in the North American diet, and it is recommended that individuals increase their intake. Breast milk naturally contains DHA, an omega 3 fatty acid known to help with brain development. DHA is also found in fatty fish, such as sardines, trout, salmon and herring.

Minerals and vitamins

Minerals and vitamins are essential to the proper functioning of the body's metabolism, especially when the body is growing quickly, as it does in infancy and childhood. These nutrients help establish a foundation for a healthy adult life.

Dietary fiber

Dietary fiber is a component of plant-based foods, including fruits, vegetables, legumes and whole grains such as oats, rye, barley, whole wheat and wheat bran. Our bodies do not have the enzyme needed to break fiber down into small enough parts to be absorbed, so fiber passes through the digestive tract without being digested. This allows it to do a few things:

1. It reduces the speed at which food passes through the small intestine, which increases the amount of nutrients absorbed from food.
2. It lowers blood cholesterol, mainly the "bad" low-density lipoprotein (LDL) cholesterol. (Although babies do not typically have high blood cholesterol levels, eating a high-fiber diet now will help them prevent high cholesterol later in life.)
3. It helps to increase stool bulk.

Certain types of dietary fiber also increase the speed at which food moves through the colon, or large intestine. This prevents excess water from being removed from stools and keeps stools soft and moving through your body. Basically, fiber helps to prevent constipation and keep you regular.

How much is enough fiber for babies and young children?

Fiber is not required in the first 6 months of life, when only breast milk or formula is consumed. As solid food is introduced after 6 months, fiber intake gradually increases. In general, children get only about half the fiber they need. By 1 to 3 years of age, children should be eating at least 19 grams of fiber daily. Here is an example of a day's worth of foods that would supply this amount of fiber:

2 slices whole-grain bread + ½ pear + ½ peach + ½ cup (125 mL) blueberries + ¼ cup (50 mL) peas + ½ cup (125 mL) whole-grain pasta + ¼ cup (50 mL) chickpeas + ¼ cup (50 mL) quinoa

---

tip

Constipation is the leading cause of abdominal pain in children. A healthy intake of fiber can help prevent this distressing pain. Look for breads or cereals that have at least 2 to 4 grams of fiber per serving.

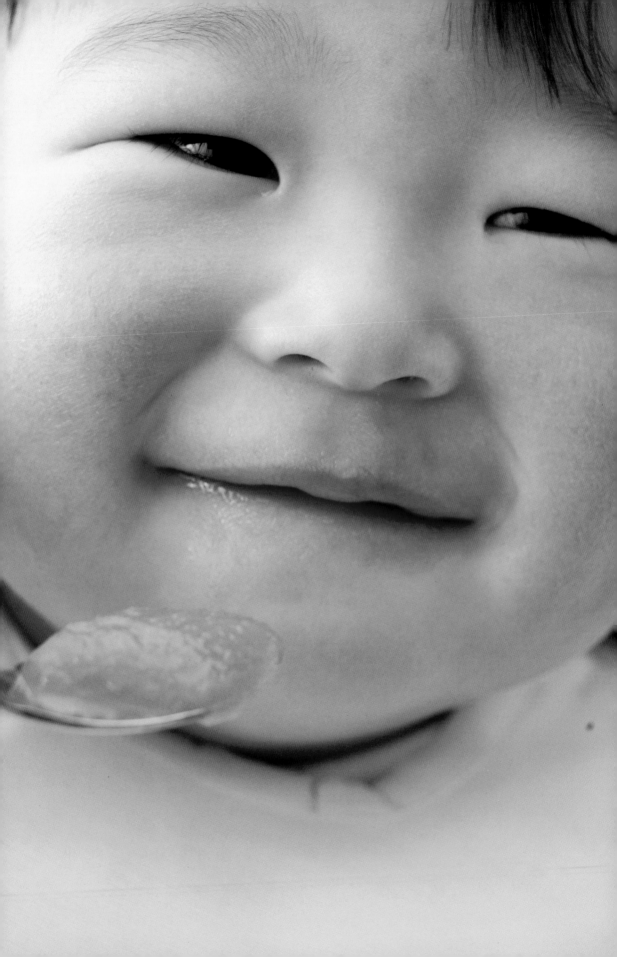

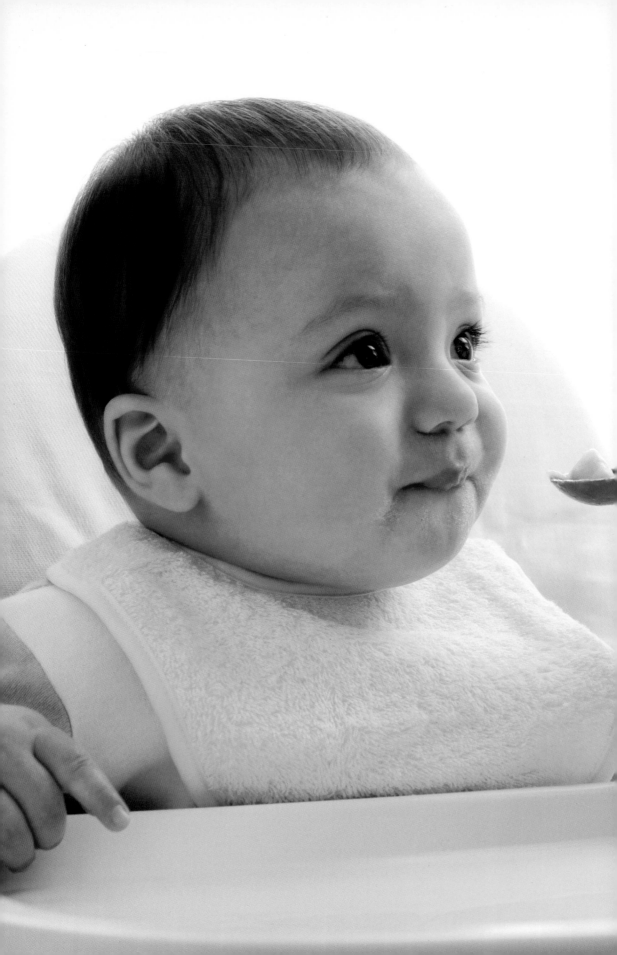

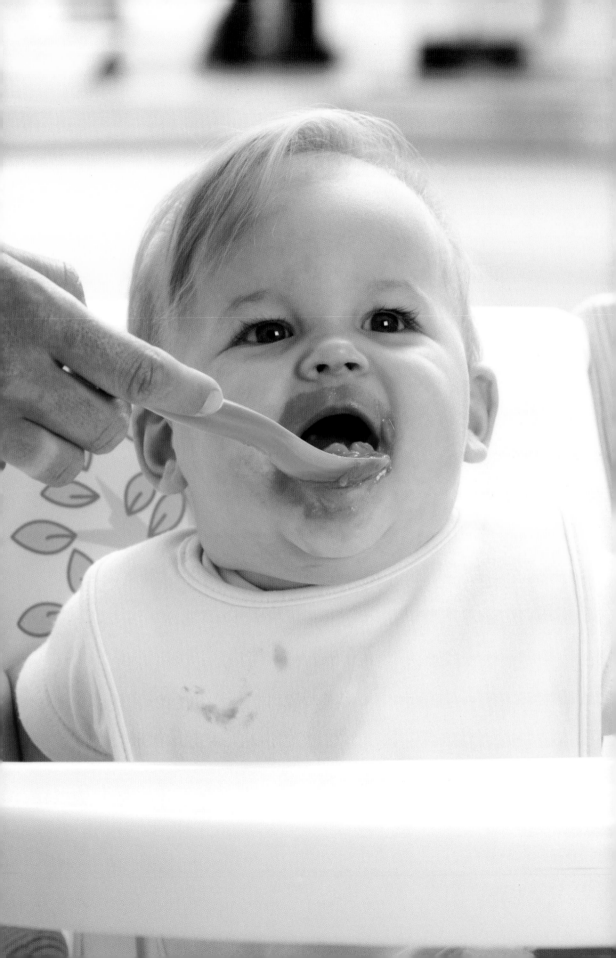

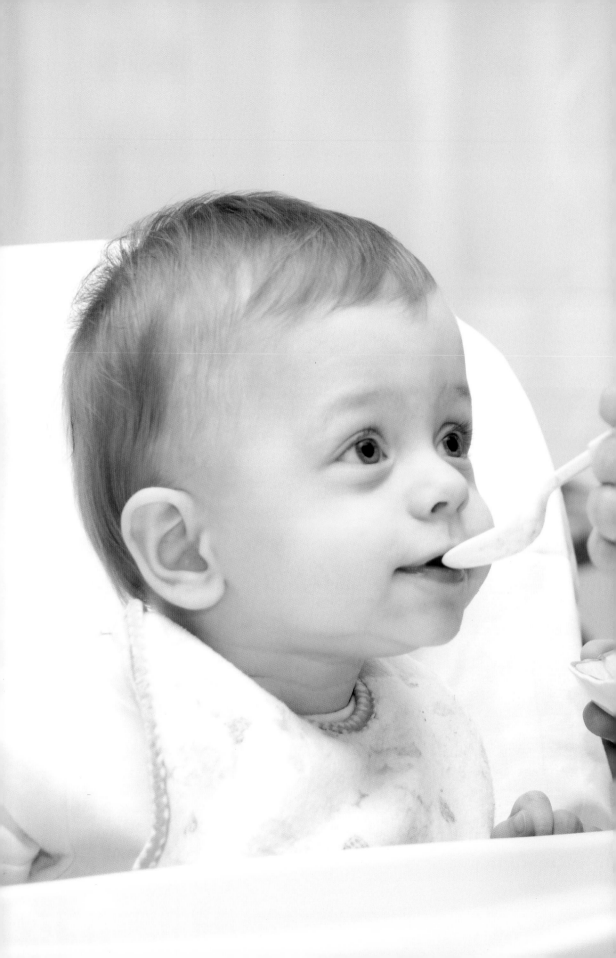

Food sources of fiber

FOOD	SERVING SIZE	TOTAL FIBER (G)
Almonds, whole	½ cup (125 mL)	8.7
Lentils	½ cup (125 mL) cooked	7.8
Baked beans, canned	½ cup (125 mL)	7.0
Avocado	½ medium	6.8
Chickpeas	½ cup (125 mL) mashed	5.3
Apricots, dried	½ cup (125 mL) halves	4.8
Whole wheat pasta	½ cup (125 mL)	3.2
Pear	½ medium	2.8
Raisins	½ cup (125 mL)	2.7
Peas	¼ cup (50 mL)	2.2
Oatmeal	½ cup (125 mL) cooked	1.9
Whole wheat bread	1 slice	1.9
Rye bread	1 slice	1.9
Blueberries	½ cup (125 mL)	1.8
Apple, unpeeled	½ medium	1.7
Orange	½ medium	1.6
Strawberries	½ cup (125 mL)	1.5
Corn	¼ cup (50 mL) kernels	1.2
Green beans	¼ cup (50 mL)	1.0
Carrot	½ medium	0.9
Broccoli	¼ cup (50 mL)	0.6

Dietary recommended intake of fiber

Most North American children aren't eating enough fiber. Current recommendations suggest that children between 1 and 3 years should aim for an intake of 19 grams of fiber a day. It has been estimated that the average toddler consumes about 8 grams of fiber a day — less than half the suggested amount. (There are no recommendations set for infants because of their largely fluid-based diet.)

When increasing the amount of fiber in your child's diet, be sure to offer him plenty of fluids (such as water or milk). Fiber intake should be increased gradually; if done too quickly, it can cause flatulence (gas).

Although it is rare for anyone to eat too much fiber, this can also be problematic, as it can reduce the absorption of certain minerals, such as calcium, iron, magnesium and zinc.

Vitamins and minerals to watch

While all vitamins and many minerals are important for the growing needs of a healthy child, there are some that deserve special attention, since they may be deficient in a poorly balanced North American diet. For a list of other vitamins and minerals and their role in metabolism, see pages 103–104.

see pages 103–104.

Dairy-free dilemma

Children who can't drink milk because of a milk protein allergy or lactose intolerance may require a supplement of calcium and vitamin D. Soy beverages, which may be given to replace cow's milk, may not be adequate to prevent the development of rickets unless they are fortified with supplemental vitamin D and calcium. Be sure to check any milk-free substitutes to ensure that they contain sufficient amounts of these essential nutrients. If you are unsure, check with your doctor or dietitian. Keep in mind, too, that dairy-free beverages may also contain less fat (and energy) than cow's milk. For a list of non-dairy sources of calcium, check out "Food sources of calcium" (page 99).

Calcium and vitamin D

Calcium and vitamin D are essential for growth and maintenance of healthy bones and teeth. If a child does not receive adequate amounts of these nutrients daily, then the deficiency can lead to rickets — a condition in which the bones soften, making them more susceptible to breakage or to a bowing of the legs when the child learns to walk. Rickets can occur in exclusively breastfed infants who are not provided with a vitamin D supplement (see page 22).

Good dietary sources of calcium and vitamin D include milk and cheese. Sunshine is also a good source of vitamin D (which is produced when skin absorbs the sun rays).

Iron

Iron is a very important nutrient for growing children. It is part of a blood component called hemoglobin, which is necessary for the transport, storage and use of oxygen throughout the body. All babies are born with a supply of iron, which takes them through the first 6 months of life. After that, iron must be obtained through the diet.

For infants and young children, iron-fortified infant cereals are often the primary source of iron from solid foods. Meats are also an excellent source of iron (see tip, page 102). Iron is also supplied by tofu, spinach, peas

Food sources of calcium

FOOD	SERVING SIZE	CALCIUM (mg)
Dairy		
Cheese, ricotta	½ cup (125 mL)	337
Cheese, Cheddar	1½ oz (45 g)	307
Yogurt, plain	½ cup (125 mL)	148
Custard (made with whole milk)	½ cup (125 mL)	139
Milk, whole	½ cup (125 mL)	138
Cheese, Parmesan, grated	2 tbsp (25 mL)	111
Ice cream, vanilla	½ cup (125 mL)	84
Cottage cheese	½ cup (125 mL)	78
Cream cheese	2 tbsp (25 mL)	23
Non-dairy		
Tofu, raw, firm, pressed with calcium sulfate	½ cup (125 mL)	861
Sardines canned in tomato sauce, with bones	4 sardines (152 g)	365 mg
Almonds	½ cup (125 mL) whole	189
Almond butter	2 tbsp (25 mL)	86
Soymilk, fortified	1 cup (250 mL)	310
Broccoli	1 cup (250 mL)	43
Kale	½ cup (125 mL) cooked	47
Salmon, canned with bones	3 oz (90 g)	188
White beans	½ cup (125 mL) cooked	81

How much calcium?
Recommended daily calcium intakes

AGE	DRI (US/CAN)
0 to 6 months	210 mg
6 months to 1 year	270 mg
1 to 2 years	500 mg
2 to 3 years	500 mg

Food sources of vitamin D

FOOD	SERVING SIZE	VITAMIN D (IU)
Fish liver oil (cod liver oil)	1 tbsp (15 mL)	1,360
Salmon, canned, pink	3 oz (90 g)	530
Salmon, cooked	3½ oz (105 g)	360
Mackerel, cooked	3½ oz (105 g)	345
Sardines, canned	3½ oz (105 g)	270
Herring, pickled	2 oz (30 g)	204
Tuna, canned, light	3 oz (90 g)	200
Eel, cooked	3½ oz (105 g)	200
Milk (all types including chocolate)	1 cup (250 mL)	100
Soy or rice beverage, fortified	1 cup (250 mL)	100
Margarine, fortified	2 tsp (10 mL)	53
Egg, whole	1 medium	25
Beef liver, cooked	3½ oz (105 g)	15

How much vitamin D?
Recommended daily vitamin D intakes

AGE	DRI (US/CAN)
0 to 6 months	5 µg (200 IU)
6 to 12 months	5 µg (200 IU)
1 to 3 years	5 µg (200 IU)

Note: The DRIs for vitamin D for infants, children and adults may be revised (to higher levels) in the near future as studies are completed.

and dark green vegetables — although the type of iron found in these plant foods is not as readily absorbed as that found in meats.

Iron from meats is called heme iron; the type found in vegetables and grains is called non-heme iron. This distinction is generally not provided on food labels, but it is an important one to remember, since heme iron is absorbed two to three times better than the non-heme form.

Children who do not obtain an adequate supply of iron in their diet run the risk of developing iron-deficiency anemia, a condition that arises when hemoglobin falls below normal levels. A child with this condition is typically pale, tires easily and has a lower tolerance for exercise. Other symptoms include irritability and decreased appetite.

Iron-deficiency anemia is most common worldwide among infants and children from 6 months to 3 years of age — a period during which the child's natural stores of iron have been exhausted (and must be obtained through diet), and during which the child requires substantial amounts of iron to fuel his rapid growth.

Typically, the danger period is most acute between the ages of 12 to 18 months, when children make the transition from iron-fortified foods (such as formula

tip

To enhance iron absorption from non-heme sources such as vegetables and grains, serve these foods with other foods that are high in vitamin C, such as oranges or strawberries.

Food sources of iron

FOOD	SERVING SIZE	IRON (mg)
Liver	1½ oz (45 g)	9.0
Infant cereal	8 tbsp (120 mL)	6.7
Infant formula, fortified	8 oz (250 mL)	5.0
Cream of wheat	¼ cup (50 mL)	3.0
Spinach, cooked	¼ cup (50 mL)	1.6
Prune juice	½ cup (125 mL)	1.5
Beef, lean broiled	2 oz (60 g)	1.3
Beans, navy, canned	¼ cup (50 mL)	1.2
Raisins, seedless	⅓ cup (75 mL)	1.0
Avocado	½ medium	1.0
Potato, baked, skin on	3¼ oz (95 g)	0.9
Broccoli, cooked	½ cup (125 mL)	0.9
Whole wheat bread	1 slice	0.9
Strained infant meat	4 tbsp (60 mL)	0.8
Chicken, light/dark, no skin	2 oz (60 g)	0.7
White bread	1 slice	0.7
Halibut	2 oz (60 g)	0.6
Rice, white, enriched	¼ cup (50 mL)	0.4
Apricots, raw	1 medium	0.2

tip

While meats are a good source of iron, they may not always appeal to younger children, who may also find these foods hard to chew. Good choices include moist pieces of chicken and beef that have been prepared with a variety of herbs and flavors. Meatballs are always a favorite. (See pages 226, 227 and 268 for recipes.) Or try tofu, which is soft and takes on the flavors of whatever foods it is prepared with.

tip

It is essential to ensure adequate amounts of iron in the diet. Recent studies show that iron deficiency in infants and young children, even if treated, can cause developmental changes that continue until past 10 years of age.

How much iron?

Recommended daily iron intakes

AGE	DRI (US/CAN)
0 to 6 months	0.27 mg
7 to 12 months	11 mg
1 to 3 years	7 mg

Notes: The recommended daily intake for pregnant women is 27 mg; for breastfeeding women, it is 9 mg. For those following a vegetarian diet, iron needs may be higher because iron from plant sources is less bioavailable.

and infant rice cereal) to solids that, while otherwise nutritious, may contain less iron. It is also at this age that children switch to cow's milk, which can displace iron-rich foods and has the effect of reducing iron absorption from other foods. (This effect can be minimized by restricting milk intake to between meals.)

Treatment of iron-deficiency anemia usually requires an oral supplement of iron. If the response to this treatment is poor (that is, if hemoglobin levels do not return to normal), other causes of iron deficiency must be ruled out. Once hemoglobin levels return to normal, then iron supplementation can be discontinued, provided the diet supplies an adequate amount. (See table, page 101.)

Vitamin C

Vitamin C is essential for healing. It is also helpful in enhancing iron absorption and, many believe, in fighting colds (although there is no definitive clinical evidence to support this). A diet that includes fresh fruits containing large amounts of vitamin C — such as mangos, oranges and strawberries — will help to ensure that your child is getting enough. Fruit juices, such as orange and apple juice, also contain vitamin C, but are less nutritious than fresh fruit. Excess amounts of vitamin C, as with most vitamins, can be dangerous, and can actually lead to a deficiency when discontinued. This is called rebound scurvy, which can cause bleeding gums and lips.

How much vitamin C?
Recommended daily vitamin C intakes

AGE	DRI (US/CAN)
0 to 6 months	40 mg
6 months to 1 year	50 mg
1 to 3 years	15 mg

Zinc

Zinc, a mineral found in many foods, is important for the immune system, normal growth and development, reproduction and the neurological system. Many enzyme systems depend on zinc, and proteins and cell membranes need zinc for their structure. While breast milk provides all the zinc an infant needs in the first few months of life, by 6 months, the zinc supply in breast milk is lower, and foods such as meat, poultry and eggs become important complements, supplying zinc and iron, as well as protein.

The ABCs of vitamins and minerals
Essential nutrients at a glance

VITAMIN/MINERAL	TYPE	ASSISTS IN	SOURCES
Vitamin A (from beta-carotene)	Fat-soluble	Vision, growth, bone development, healthy skin	Liver, eggs, whole milk, dark green leafy vegetables, yellow and orange vegetables and fruit
Vitamin B_1 (thiamin)	Water-soluble	Enzyme activity, metabolism of nutrients	Oatmeal, enriched breads and grains, rice, dairy products, fish, pork, liver, nuts, legumes
Vitamin B_2 (riboflavin)	Water-soluble	Growth, metabolism of nutrients	Dairy products, eggs, organ meats, enriched breads and grains, green leafy vegetables
Vitamin B_3 (niacin)	Water-soluble	Tissue repair, metabolism of nutrients	Organ meats, peanuts, brewer's yeast, enriched breads and grains, meats, poultry, fish and nuts

VITAMIN/MINERAL	TYPE	ASSISTS IN	SOURCES
Vitamin B_6 (pyridoxine)	Water-soluble	Metabolism of nutrients (primary role)	Brewer's yeast, wheat, germ, pork, liver, whole-grain cereals, potatoes, milk, fruits and vegetables
Folate (part of B vitamin group)	Water-soluble	Growth, enzyme activity, prevents neural tube defects	Liver, lima and kidney beans, dark green leafy vegetables, beef, potatoes, whole wheat bread
Vitamin B_{12}	Water-soluble	Metabolism of nutrients, prevents anemia	Liver, kidneys, meat, fish, dairy products, eggs
Biotin (part of B vitamin group)	Water-soluble	Enzyme activity; deficiency can lead to a type of dermatitis	Liver, milk, meat, egg yolk, vegetables, fruit, peanuts, brewer's yeast
Vitamin C	Water-soluble	Many cellular functions, promotes healthy teeth, skin and tissue repair	Citrus fruits such as oranges and grapefruit, leafy vegetables, tomatoes, strawberries
Vitamin D	Fat-soluble	Essential for normal growth, development, bones and teeth; helps protect against immune diseases	Liver, butter, fortified milk, fatty fish (fish liver oils), exposure to sunlight
Vitamin E	Fat-soluble	Antioxidant function protects cells; assists neurological function, prevents anemia	Vegetable and fish oils, nuts, seeds, egg yolk, whole grains
Vitamin K	Fat-soluble	Blood clotting	Green leafy vegetables, liver, wheat bran, tomatoes, cheese, egg yolk
Iron	Mineral	Formation of hundreds of proteins and enzymes; it is part of the protein hemoglobin, which carries oxygen from the lungs to the rest of the body's tissues, by way of blood circulation	Liver, meat, chicken, fish, tofu, infant cereal, spinach, lentils, beans, raisins, apricots, nuts
Calcium	Mineral	Signaling within nerves, muscle tissue and blood vessels; it is the main structural component of bones and teeth	Milk, cheese, yogurt, tofu, broccoli, spinach, chickpeas, beans, nuts, seaweed, sunflower seeds, sesame seeds
Zinc	Mineral	Growth and development, immune, reproductive and neurological system function; almost 100 enzymes require zinc to function; it is an important part of proteins and cell membranes	Meat, poultry, eggs, dairy products

Limit salt, sugar and caffeine

Salt and sugar are often added to processed and packaged foods to enhance flavor, so it is easy to see why people who rely on processed foods get too much salt and sugar in their diet. Caffeine is a natural component of some plants, and is also added to some beverages to provide the energized feeling that many people need in the morning. Salt, sugar and caffeine should be minimized in your young child's diet.

Salt (sodium)

Salt is made up of sodium and chloride, two very important minerals that are required for health. One teaspoon (5 mL) of table salt contains 2,300 mg of sodium. The amount of sodium that adults need in a day is only 1,500 mg, so you can see how easy it is to get too much salt just by using that salt shaker at the table.

Both children and adults typically take in *more than double* the amount of sodium they require every day. The health consequences of high sodium intake include high blood pressure and heart disease.

Salt is used to flavor food, and much of our packaged food is loaded with it. To reduce your salt intake, prepare fresh foods, choose processed and packaged foods less often and remove the salt shaker from the table.

It is easy to avoid giving your baby too much salt, especially in the first year of life, when breast milk or formula are the main sources of nutrition, followed by solid foods. Typically, commercial baby foods do not contain salt, and salt should not be added to homemade baby foods. Once regular table foods are introduced, children will be exposed to a higher intake of salt.

Infants between 7 and 12 months of age need only 370 mg of sodium a day, while 1- to 3-year-olds need 1,000 mg a day (with a maximum of 1,500 mg a day). The table on page 106 indicates the amount of sodium in some common foods.

> ### Tips to keep sodium intake low
>
> - Choose fresh fruits, vegetables, meats, chicken and fish more often.
> - Choose processed foods less often.
> - Use the salt shaker sparingly.
> - When making a recipe that calls for chicken or beef stock, use a homemade low-sodium vegetable broth or chicken stock instead (see pages 154 and 155 for recipes).
> - Rinse canned vegetables and legumes before cooking, or purchase low-sodium varieties.
> - Limit your use of ketchup.
> - Choose low-sodium soy sauce.
> - Avoid rice mixes and noodle mixes.

Sodium content of food

FOOD	SERVING SIZE	SODIUM (MG)
Bacon	4 slices (3 oz/90 g)	1,442
Lean ham	3 oz (90 g)	1,194
Wiener, pork or beef	1 medium	638
Chicken breast, skinless	3 oz (90 g)	67
Fish, fresh	3 oz (90 g)	50–95
Tuna or salmon, canned in water	3 oz (90 g)	340–470
Tofu, firm, raw	3 oz (90 g)	13
Egg, whole	1 medium	63
Milk or yogurt	1 cup (250 mL)	125
Soymilk	1 cup (250 mL)	29
Mozzarella cheese	1 oz (30 g)	130
Feta cheese	1 oz (30 g)	335
Sliced processed cheese	1 slice	406
Butter	1 tbsp (15 mL)	124
Legumes, boiled without added salt	1 cup (250 mL)	<12
Fresh vegetables	1 cup (250 mL)	0–100
Fresh fruits	1 cup (250 mL)	0–20
Oatmeal, cooked	1 cup (250 mL)	2
Table salt	1 tsp (5 mL)	2,325
Ketchup	1 tbsp (15 mL)	120–190
Salad dressing, regular	1 tbsp (15 mL)	100–220
Mayonnaise	1 tbsp (15 mL)	75–110
Soy sauce, regular	1 tbsp (15 mL)	1,029
Soy sauce, 40% reduced sodium	1 tbsp (15 mL)	600
Peanut butter, salted	½ cup (125 mL)	594
Potato chips, salted	20 chips	230–350
Popcorn, air-popped	1 cup (250 mL)	0
Pizza, plain cheese, regular crust	1 slice (103 g)	551
Cheeseburger	1 regular patty, no condiments	589
Soup, canned	1 cup (250 mL)	1,000–1,200
Pickle, dill	2 small (74 g total)	648
Club soda	1 cup (250 mL)	50

Sugar

Surveys reveal that foods with added sugars, such as candy and sweetened drinks, make up a significant part of children's diets. For some kids, sugary drinks account for about 25% of the calories they consume in a day. That's a lot of calories! And it isn't the best way to provide the body with energy, that's for sure. When reading labels, keep your eye out for "-ose" ingredients, such as sucrose, fructose, glucose and high-fructose corn syrup, which are all simple sugars.

To keep your young child's sugar intake to a minimum, choose appropriate snacks, such as fresh fruits and vegetables and homemade cookies or muffins, where you control the amount of sugar added. The table below indicates the amount of sugar in some common foods and drinks.

Sugar content of food and drinks

FOOD	SERVING SIZE	SUGAR
Soda pop	12 oz (341 mL)	10 tsp (50 mL)
Grape juice, sweetened	8 oz (227 mL)	10 tsp (50 mL)
Apple juice, sweetened	8 oz (227 mL)	6 tsp (30 mL)
Chocolate milk	1 cup (250 mL)	6 tsp (30 mL)
Fruit beverage (e.g., Kool-Aid, Sunny Delight)	6¾ oz (200 mL)	5 tsp (25 mL)
Ice cream bar	1	17 tsp (85 mL)
Cupcake, iced	1	16 tsp (80 mL)
Doughnut, with glaze	1	6 tsp (30 mL)

Caffeine

Many adults enjoy the kick-start of a good cup of coffee or tea in the morning, but infants and young children do not need caffeine to start their day. While there is no maximum recommended amount of caffeine for infants or young children, it would certainly be much less than the maximum amount recommended for children 4 to 6 years of age, which is 45 mg a day. This is about the amount found in 5 cups (1.25 L) of chocolate milk, 1 can (12 oz/341 mL) of cola, 1 cup (250 mL) of tea or ⅓ cup (75 mL) of coffee (milk chocolate has only about 7 mg per 2 oz/30 g, depending on the chocolate bar).

tip
Moms who are pregnant or breastfeeding should consume no more than 300 mg of caffeine a day (about 2 cups/ 500 mL of coffee).

tip

While excessive doses of vitamins have become popular with some adults, they should never be given to children. Check with your pediatrician, family doctor, dietitian or pharmacist to learn what amounts are safe for your child and if any vitamins are necessary.

The fab four food groups

While many foods are important sources of nutrients, there is no single food that provides everything you need for a healthy diet. That's why it's important to enjoy a balanced diet that includes all four food groups.

Grain products are an essential source of carbohydrates, vitamins and minerals, and provide fiber as well.

Fruits and vegetables provide another variety of carbohydrates, vitamins (particularly vitamin C) and minerals, as well as fiber.

Meat and alternatives are an important source of proteins, fats, vitamins and minerals (particularly iron).

Milk and dairy products provide a balance of proteins, carbohydrates and fats, and are an important source of calcium and vitamin D.

In both the U.S. and Canada, health authorities have devised charts that recommend a range of servings from each of the four food groups. Whether it's MyPyramid (in the U.S.) or Eating Well with Canada's Food Guide, the message is very much the same: enjoy a variety of healthy foods every day.

Being vegetarian

A vegetarian lifestyle has become increasingly popular among North Americans in recent years. When parents follow a vegetarian diet, their children often do too. Vegetarian diets have many health benefits. They are typically lower in saturated fat and dietary cholesterol and higher in dietary fiber. Vegetarians may have lower rates of certain types of cancer and are less likely to suffer from obesity and type 2 diabetes. Infants and young children can grow and thrive on a vegetarian diet; however, careful planning is needed to ensure that all of your little one's nutrient needs are being met.

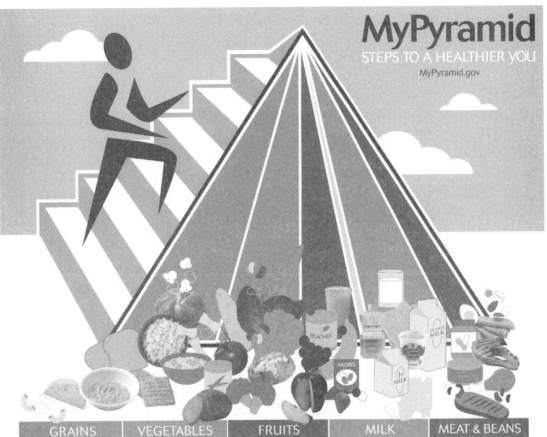

MyPyramid
STEPS TO A HEALTHIER YOU
MyPyramid.gov

GRAINS	VEGETABLES	FRUITS	MILK	MEAT & BEANS
GRAINS Make half your grains whole	**VEGETABLES** Vary your veggies	**FRUITS** Focus on fruits	**MILK** Get your calcium-rich foods	**MEAT & BEANS** Go lean with protein
Eat at least 3 oz. of whole-grain cereals, breads, crackers, rice, or pasta every day 1 oz. is about 1 slice of bread, about 1 cup of breakfast cereal, or ½ cup of cooked rice, cereal, or pasta	Eat more dark-green veggies like broccoli, spinach, and other dark leafy greens Eat more orange vegetables like carrots and sweetpotatoes Eat more dry beans and peas like pinto beans, kidney beans, and lentils	Eat a variety of fruit Choose fresh, frozen, canned, or dried fruit Go easy on fruit juices	Go low-fat or fat-free when you choose milk, yogurt, and other milk products If you don't or can't consume milk, choose lactose-free products or other calcium sources such as fortified foods and beverages	Choose low-fat or lean meats and poultry Bake it, broil it, or grill it Vary your protein routine — choose more fish, beans, peas, nuts, and seeds

For a 2,000-calorie diet, you need the amounts below from each food group. To find the amounts that are right for you, go to MyPyramid.gov.

Eat 6 oz. every day	Eat 2½ cups every day	Eat 2 cups every day	Get 3 cups every day; for kids aged 2 to 8, it's 2	Eat 5½ oz. every day

Find your balance between food and physical activity
- Be sure to stay within your daily calorie needs.
- Be physically active for at least 30 minutes most days of the week.
- About 60 minutes a day of physical activity may be needed to prevent weight gain.
- For sustaining weight loss, at least 60 to 90 minutes a day of physical activity may be required.
- Children and teenagers should be physically active for 60 minutes every day, or most days.

Know the limits on fats, sugars, and salt (sodium)
- Make most of your fat sources from fish, nuts, and vegetable oils.
- Limit solid fats like butter, stick margarine, shortening, and lard, as well as foods that contain these.
- Check the Nutrition Facts label to keep saturated fats, trans fats, and sodium low.
- Choose food and beverages low in added sugars. Added sugars contribute calories with few, if any, nutrients.

MyPyramid.gov
STEPS TO A HEALTHIER YOU

U.S. Department of Agriculture
Center for Nutrition Policy and Promotion
April 2005
CNPP-15

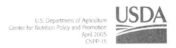

Eating Well with Canada's Food Guide

Recommended Number of *Food Guide Servings* per Day

What is One Food Guide Serving?
Look at the examples below.

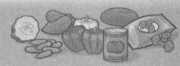

	Children			Teens		Adults			
Age in Years	2-3	4-8	9-13	14-18		19-50		51+	
Sex	Girls and Boys			Females	Males	Females	Males	Females	Males
Vegetables and Fruit	4	5	6	7	8	7-8	8-10	7	7
Grain Products	3	4	6	6	7	6-7	8	6	7
Milk and Alternatives	2	2	3-4	3-4	3-4	2	2	3	3
Meat and Alternatives	1	1	1-2	2	3	2	3	2	3

Fresh, frozen or canned vegetables
125 mL (½ cup)

Bread
1 slice (35 g)

Bagel
½ bagel (45 g)

Milk or powdered milk (reconstituted)
250 mL (1 cup)

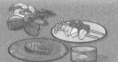

Cooked fish, shellfish, poultry, lean meat
75 g (2 ½ oz.)/125 mL (½ cup)

The chart above shows how many Food Guide Servings you need from each of the four food groups every day.

Having the amount and type of food recommended and following the tips in *Canada's Food Guide* will help:

- Meet your needs for vitamins, minerals and other nutrients.
- Reduce your risk of obesity, type 2 diabetes, heart disease, certain types of cancer and osteoporosis.
- Contribute to your overall health and vitality.

For the full guide, please contact Health Canada or visit their website.

Source: Health Canada. Used with permission.

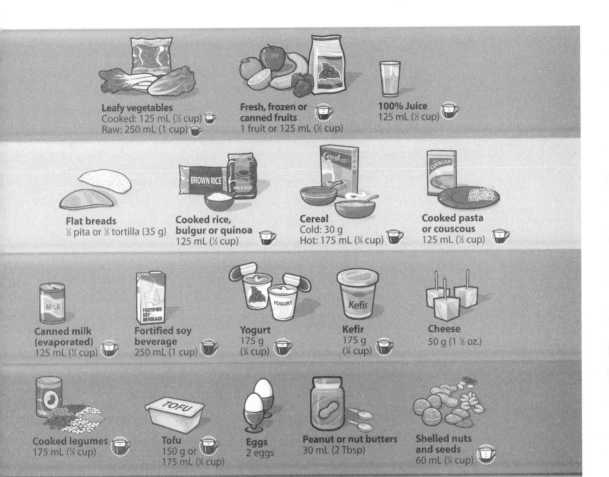

Leafy vegetables
Cooked: 125 mL (½ cup)
Raw: 250 mL (1 cup)

Fresh, frozen or canned fruits
1 fruit or 125 mL (½ cup)

100% Juice
125 mL (½ cup)

Flat breads
½ pita or ½ tortilla (35 g)

Cooked rice, bulgur or quinoa
125 mL (½ cup)

Cereal
Cold: 30 g
Hot: 175 mL (¾ cup)

Cooked pasta or couscous
125 mL (½ cup)

Canned milk (evaporated)
125 mL (½ cup)

Fortified soy beverage
250 mL (1 cup)

Yogurt
175 g (¾ cup)

Kefir
175 g (¾ cup)

Cheese
50 g (1 ½ oz.)

Cooked legumes
175 mL (¾ cup)

Tofu
150 g or 175 mL (¾ cup)

Eggs
2 eggs

Peanut or nut butters
30 mL (2 Tbsp)

Shelled nuts and seeds
60 mL (¼ cup)

Oils and Fats

- Include a small amount – 30 to 45 mL (2 to 3 Tbsp) – of unsaturated fat each day. This includes oil used for cooking, salad dressings, margarine and mayonnaise.
- Use vegetable oils such as canola, olive and soybean.
- Choose soft margarines that are low in saturated and trans fats.
- Limit butter, hard margarine, lard and shortening.

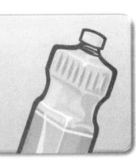

What is a vegetarian?

There are many variations of the vegetarian diet, ranging from the simple elimination of red meat to the complete avoidance of any item of animal origin. The type of vegetarian lifestyle practiced will affect the nutrients of concern for young vegetarians.

Semi-, or partial, vegetarians generally avoid red meat but may continue to eat some poultry and fish while primarily eating plant-based foods.

Pesco-vegetarians avoid red meat and poultry but continue to consume fish and seafood.

Lacto-ovo-vegetarians avoid all animal flesh, including meat, poultry and fish. However, they still include dairy (lacto) and egg (ovo) products in their diet.

Vegans avoid all foods of animal origin, including meat, poultry, fish, eggs, dairy, gelatin and honey. Many vegans also avoid animal-based non-food items, such as leather, wool and tallow candles.

Macrobiotic vegetarians often follow very restrictive diets that may include the elimination of entire food groups. These types of diets are not recommended for children.

Within these subgroups of vegetarianism there can be many variations in diet, and individual circumstances should be considered when meal planning. On the whole, children will grow and develop well on lacto-ovo-, pesco- and semi-vegetarian diets, which are varied enough to meet their nutrient requirements for protein, calcium and vitamin D. Vegan diets, however, must be carefully planned to ensure adequate intake of all essential nutrients. An infant following a vegan diet who is no longer breastfeeding should continue to consume an iron-fortified soy formula until he is at least 2 years old in order to get the additional vitamins and minerals he needs.

Vegetarian diets for children

Given all the touted benefits of a vegetarian lifestyle, why do we not recommend that all children follow a meat-free diet?

Vegetarian diets are not for everyone. While they can be healthy, they need to be planned for young children to ensure they provide all the nutrients required for normal growth and development. When their diets are well planned, vegetarian (including vegan) children can be well nourished. Let's review some of the specific nutrient considerations.

Energy

Because many plant foods are not concentrated sources of calories, vegetarian diets have the potential to be low in energy. This is less of a challenge for lacto-ovo-vegetarians, who continue to choose energy-dense foods containing milk and eggs. Examples of higher-calorie options include whole milk and yogurt, many varieties of cheese and whole eggs. Vegan children must boost their energy intake by eating high-calorie plant foods, such as avocados, nuts and nut butters, every day.

Protein

The diets of semi-, pesco- and lacto-ovo-vegetarians generally contain enough protein from animal sources. Plant proteins are incomplete proteins (quinoa is an exception), which means they are deficient in one or more of the essential amino acids (the building blocks of protein). So vegan children must eat a wide variety of plant proteins to ensure that their diet includes all of the essential amino acids the body needs to make other proteins.

Vitamin B_{12}

Vitamin B_{12}, found only in foods derived from animal sources, is important for the process of cell division. Vitamin B_{12} deficiency can lead to megaloblastic anemia, which can result in permanent neurological damage. In general, lacto-ovo-vegetarians have no difficulty consuming enough vitamin B_{12}. Children under the age of 2 years can get an adequate amount by consuming the equivalent of 3 cups (750 mL) of cow's milk per day or 2 cups (500 mL) of cow's milk plus 1 egg per day. The breast milk of a vegan mother should contain sufficient vitamin B_{12} as long as she is eating fortified foods or taking a supplement. Once a vegan infant has been weaned from the breast, fortified foods (such as soy formula) or a supplement should be provided. Speak with your family doctor or pediatrician for more information.

Calcium

This important mineral works with vitamin D to promote the growth of strong, healthy bones and teeth, and helps to prevent osteoporosis later in life. As such, it is important to ensure that children receive adequate dietary calcium in their growing years. Lacto-ovo-vegetarian children should consume the equivalent of 2 cups (500 mL) of milk daily. Vegan children should consume calcium-fortified foods, such as fortified soy formula or soymilk.

Vitamin D

Like calcium, vitamin D is important for the development of healthy bones and teeth. More recently, an adequate supply of vitamin D has been associated with protection against immune diseases. All breastfed infants, regardless of their mothers' dietary choices, should receive a vitamin D supplement to prevent deficiency. Infant formula and cow's milk also contain vitamin D. Vegetarian sources of vitamin D include fortified soy formula or soymilk. For those vegetarians who eat fish, cod liver oil is another good source. While the body can use sunlight to produce vitamin D, most breastfed infants in the northern U.S. and Canada are not exposed to enough sunlight during the day to produce adequate amounts.

Our favorite veggie-friendly recipes

We have included many vegetarian-friendly recipes in *Better Baby Food*. Here are a few of our favorites:

Breakfast
* Baby's Fruit Smoothie (page 128)
* Big-Batch Oatmeal Pancakes (page 132)
* Oat Bran Applesauce Muffins (page 139)

Lunch
* Crazy for Quinoa (page 157)
* Fantastic Black Bean Soup (page 164)
* Carrot 'n' Cheese Crustless Quiche (page 179)
* Vegetable Burritos (page 189)

Dinner
* Ratatouille (page 204)
* Vegetarian Stir-Fry (page 218)
* Vegetarian Chili (page 251)

Iron

This mineral is essential for the formation of red blood cells, and a lack of it can lead to iron-deficiency anemia, the most common nutritional deficiency in children around the globe (see pages 101–102 for more information). Iron is a concern in vegetarian diets, though not because plant foods lack iron. In fact, whole grains, legumes and dark green and orange vegetables (such as spinach and squash) are good sources of iron. The difficulty lies in the chemistry of plant-based iron, which the body does not absorb as well as the iron from animal-based foods. While ensuring adequate iron intake is of particular concern for vegans, it is important for all vegetarians. Iron-rich vegetarian foods include iron-fortified infant cereals and infant formulas.

Childhood obesity

Obesity — and specifically childhood obesity — has been on the rise since 1965. In 1980, about 25% of the adult population in the U.S. was obese; by 2006, that figure had increased to about 34%. It is estimated that the number of overweight children between the ages of 2 and 5 increased to nearly 14% in 2003–04 from 5% in 1976–80. The trend was even more significant for children between the ages of 6 and 19. As of 2004, the number of overweight children in this age range was estimated at between 17% and 19%.

These statistics may be depressingly familiar to adults, particularly those who are engaged in the difficult business of trying to lose weight. But surely, you might ask, shouldn't young children be spared dietary restrictions?

Absolutely. While most nutritionists agree that an adult diet should consist of no more than 30% of calories from fat (and less than 10% of calories from saturated fats), these restrictions need not apply to children from birth to 2 years of age. Indeed, during infancy, a high-fat diet (about 50% of calories from fat) is actually beneficial, providing all the caloric and fatty acid intakes needed for growth and development.

tip
Foods rich in vitamin C increase the absorption of plant-based iron, so eating mangos or oranges with cereals or legumes is a good idea!

tip
When it comes to obesity, prevention is key!

The freedom from restriction can extend into the preschool years when children have high activity levels and fluctuating appetites. Small frequent feedings play an important role in meeting the energy needs of young children. Preschoolers are dependent on their caregivers to make food choices for them, and parents should promote healthy eating patterns and choices, as well as frequent physical exercise.

The transition from the high-fat diet of infancy to the lower-fat diet of adulthood should occur gradually from the age of 2 until adolescence, when a child has reached his height potential. This is also a critical period for the development of healthy eating habits and a positive attitude toward food. During this transition, it is important for parents to make healthy food choices for their children while providing them with sufficient calories to promote normal growth and development. Children should consume a variety of foods from the four food groups, including complex carbohydrates and lower-fat foods. (However, keep in mind that healthy fats, such as those found in nuts, seeds, vegetable oils, avocados and olives, should be included in a healthy diet.)

Remember, a slightly chubby infant or toddler will not necessarily become an obese adult. Children experience rapid growth spurts. Your family doctor or pediatrician should be plotting your child's growth on a growth chart to ensure that he is growing at an appropriate rate.

Complications of obesity

Some of the complications of obesity that used to be seen only in adults are now being observed in overweight and obese children. These include higher rates of

- type 2 diabetes;
- high blood pressure;
- dyslipidemias, including problems with blood cholesterol and triglycerides;
- respiratory problems, including asthma and obstructive sleep apnea;
- fatty liver;
- orthopedic problems, including problems with the hips and knees;
- social stigma, leading to low self-esteem and depression.

What causes obesity in children?

Many factors contribute to the development of obesity in children, including

- genetic factors;
- increased dietary intakes;
- decreased physical activity;
- increased sedentary activities (including TV and computer time);
- environmental factors (including home, daycare, school and community).

We cannot control our genetics. Children born to obese parents are more likely to become obese adults themselves. But this is influenced by many factors, including lifestyle and dietary choices. What is important is to reduce your child's controllable risk factors to decrease the influence that genetics plays on his growth potential.

Preventing obesity

Prevention is the cornerstone of pediatric practice. Now is the time to forge healthy behaviors for your child and the entire family that can last a lifetime. Although there are factors you cannot control, such as genetics, there is much you can do to encourage a healthy lifestyle for your family.

Diet: Prepare home-cooked meals; serve less prepackaged food; offer foods high in fiber, including lots of fruits and veggies; choose foods low in sodium; make sure all of your child's caretakers, at home and at daycare, are aware of your dietary guidelines.

Activity: Babies should get some activity every day, and TV use should be kept to a minimum.

How much TV should my toddler be watching?

The American Academy of Pediatrics recommends no TV time for children under the age of 2. Try to avoid using the television as an electronic babysitter. By keeping the TV turned off, you will encourage other fun activities that you and your child can do together, such as reading books, doing crafts or solving simple board puzzles. As children get a little older, TV time (including time spent on the computer or playing video games) should be limited to no more than 2 hours per day. (We cover this in more detail in *Better Food for Kids*.)

Encourage healthy eating habits

As your infant is introduced to new foods, make sure to offer plenty of fruits and vegetables. Choose whole-grain breads, cereals and pastas in place of their white alternatives. As your child ages, slowly transition from high-fat dairy products, such as whole milk and yogurts, to lower-fat options, including 2% or skim milk products; this transition should be completed by the time your child is 5 years old. Do not offer juice to your toddler. Once he is over 9 months old, he can drink water from a cup or sippy cup for thirst. Avoid sugar-sweetened beverages, including sweetened juices or fruit punches. Choose leaner cuts of meats and try to include other protein choices, such as white fish and vegetarian legume dishes. As much as possible, avoid prepackaged foods.

Toddlers have variable appetites and may not always be hungry at mealtimes. Do not force your child to eat or to clear his plate. Your child is in charge of how much he puts into his tummy. If he is telling you he is full by turning his head or refusing to open his mouth, then it is important to listen to his cues. But don't offer cookies or other foods 5 minutes later! He does not need anything in place of the meal until the next scheduled meal or snack time, which should be no more than about 2 to 3 hours later.

Toddlers eat frequent small meals, and what may seem like very little food to you is likely more than enough for your toddler to grow on. Toddlers are very good at regulating their own intake, and they know when they have had enough to eat; no amount of cajoling or force from mom or dad (or grandma) is going to change their mind. Only as we get older, and begin to ignore the little voice in our head that tells us when we are full, do we find ourselves unable to recognize our own satiety cues.

Encourage physical activity

Babies and toddlers are naturally active. They seem to have a boundless amount of energy, and it is up to us as

tip

Research has shown that families that cook meals and eat together eat healthier.

Diet and daycare

If you're a working mom, a large proportion of your child's daily calories may be consumed at daycare. When choosing a daycare for your infant or toddler, be sure that the menu is part of your selection criteria. Here are some questions you may want to ask:

① How much juice is offered?
② Is milk offered with meals and snacks?
③ Are fruits and vegetables offered as snack options?

A daycare that is committed to offering good nutrition to your child will provide milk with meals and/or snacks. Minimal juice (a maximum of $\frac{1}{2}$ cup/125 mL a day) should be included, and water should be offered for thirst to infants over 9 months. Good meal options will include at least three of the four food groups. Snacks should include fruits or vegetables at least once every day.

You may also want to ask how much TV the children watch during the day. This is particularly important for home daycares. Remember that children under the age of 2 should not watch any TV.

their parents and caregivers to foster this endless energy and give them opportunities to play, run, laugh and explore. While your child is a baby, take him out for a daily walk. Even if it is cold, bundle him up and head outdoors. A few minutes of fresh air can be invigorating for both of you. As your baby heads into toddlerhood, do things together that he will enjoy. Continue to take him out for a walk in the stroller, go to the park and help him practice climbing the small stairs up to the baby slide, where he can sit and slide down. In the summer, head out to the local splash pad or simply turn on the outside hose and watch your child have fun soaking himself, as well as you. Small children can play for what seems like forever with the simplest toy — a ball. Toss a large beach ball back and forth with your youngster and let him run after it. Activity doesn't need to be complicated or cost a lot of money to be fun.

tip
Toddlers need at least 90 minutes of physical activity each day and should not sit still for longer than 60 minutes at a time.

Activity ideas for babies and toddlers

6 to 12 months

- Practice lots of "tummy time" on a blanket.
- Encourage him to spend lots of time on the floor, practicing rolling, crawling, pulling up to a standing position, cruising the furniture and eventually walking.
- Roll a ball back and forth between you and baby.
- Crawl around on the floor with your baby, encouraging him to follow you.
- Place an object just out of reach and encourage your baby to get it.

12 to 18 months

- Give him pull toys to encourage walking.
- Go to the park.
- Play catch with soft balls.
- Have him move objects (inside or outside) from one place to another.
- Teach him to pound wooden pegs with a hammer.

18 to 24 months

- Kick and throw balls of different sizes back and forth.
- Encourage him to walk up and down stairs, both inside and outside.
- Dance and move to music together.
- Walk, hop, run and jump with your toddler.
- Begin to ride a tricycle.

Breakfast

Makes 1¼ cups (300 mL)

Kitchen Tip

For infants just starting fruits, you can use a sweeter eating apple (such as Golden Delicious) and eliminate the sugar. When adding sugar, do it 1 tbsp (15 mL) at a time, tasting after each addition so applesauce does not become too sweet. For older infants, try mashing to a thicker texture.

Applesauce

| 3 | medium cooking apples, washed, peeled, cored and cut into quarters | 3 |
| ⅔ cup | water | 150 mL |

1. In a saucepan, combine apples and water. Bring to a boil and cook for about 10 minutes or until apples are tender. Drain.
2. Mash with fork to desired texture or, for a smoother texture, purée in a food processor and strain through a sieve.

NUTRITIONAL ANALYSIS (PER ¼ CUP/50 ML)

Energy	Protein	Carbohydrate	Fat	Fiber	Calcium	Iron	Sodium
46 kcal	0.3 g	12 g	0.1 g	1 g	5 mg	0.1 mg	–

Makes ¾ cup (175 mL)

Oats and Banana Cereal

¼ cup	quick-cooking rolled oats	50 mL
½ cup	2% milk (approx.)	125 mL
½	banana, mashed	½

1. In a small saucepan, combine oats and milk. Bring to a boil over medium-high heat. Reduce heat and simmer, stirring occasionally, for 5 minutes or until thick.
2. Stir in mashed banana and let cool. Serve topped with additional milk, if desired.

NUTRITIONAL ANALYSIS (PER ¼ CUP/50 ML)

Energy	Protein	Carbohydrate	Fat	Fiber	Calcium	Iron	Sodium
81 kcal	3 g	14 g	2 g	2 g	57 mg	1 mg	18 mg

Makes 2 cups (500 mL)

Steel-cut oats are a delicious whole grain that can be found in most grocery stores, often in the organic section, along with other whole grains. Oats in the morning provide long-lasting satiety.

Kitchen Tip

Any leftover oatmeal can be refrigerated (without the yogurt and berries) and enjoyed the next morning, warmed in the microwave.

Variation

Moms, dads and older siblings can top with 1 tbsp (15 mL) sunflower or pumpkin seeds for added flavor, protein and fiber!

Berrilicious Oatmeal Starter

1½ cups	water	375 mL
½ cup	steel-cut oats	125 mL
2 tbsp	vanilla-flavored or plain yogurt	25 mL
2 tbsp	fresh or frozen raspberries or blueberries (thawed if frozen)	25 mL

1. In a saucepan, bring water to a boil. Add oats; reduce heat and simmer, stirring frequently, for about 15 minutes or until cooked to desired tenderness.

2. Divide oatmeal among four bowls and mix in yogurt and berries. Serve while still warm. Any leftovers can be refrigerated and enjoyed the next morning, warmed in the microwave.

NUTRITIONAL ANALYSIS (PER ½ CUP/125 ML)

Energy	Protein	Carbohydrate	Fat	Fiber	Calcium	Iron	Sodium
86 kcal	4 g	15 g	2 g	2 g	25 mg	1 mg	7 mg

It's nice to introduce your infant to different hot cooked cereals. It can lead to a lifetime of enjoying the pleasure and comfort of a hot cereal start to the day. These single-serve amounts can be easily increased according to the child's appetite. Serve with extra milk and sugar as desired.

Hot Breakfast Ideas

Cooked Rolled Oats or Cream of Wheat

Microwave

1. In a small microwave-safe bowl, combine 1 tbsp (15 mL) quick-cooking rolled oats with 2 tbsp (25 mL) water, milk or formula. Microwave, uncovered, on High, for about 1 minute; stir. Let stand until appropriate serving temperature is reached and mixture has thickened. Stir and serve.

Stovetop

1. In a small saucepan, use same measurements as above. Cook, stirring frequently, over medium-low heat for 2 to 4 minutes.

NUTRITIONAL ANALYSIS

Energy	Protein	Carbohydrate	Fat	Fiber	Calcium	Iron	Sodium
38 kcal	2 g	5 g	1 g	1 g	32 mg	0.3 mg	10 mg

Cooked Oat Bran

Microwave

1. In a small microwave-safe bowl, combine 1 tbsp (15 mL) oat bran with 3 tbsp (45 mL) water, milk or formula. Microwave, uncovered, on High for about minute; stir. Let stand until appropriate serving temperature is reached and mixture has thickened. Stir and serve.

Stovetop

1. In a small saucepan, use same measurements as above. Cook, stirring frequently, over medium-low heat for 2 to 4 minutes.

NUTRITIONAL ANALYSIS

Energy	Protein	Carbohydrate	Fat	Fiber	Calcium	Iron	Sodium
43 kcal	2 g	6 g	2 g	1 g	56 mg	0.3 mg	19 mg

Whole-Grain Cereal Mix

1. Combine ½ cup (125 mL) each quick-cooking rolled oats, oat bran and whole wheat cereal. Store in a tightly sealed container. Makes 1½ cups (375 mL).

Microwave

2. In a small microwave-safe bowl, combine 1 tbsp (15 mL) cereal mix with 3 tbsp (45 mL) water, milk or formula. Microwave, uncovered, on High for about 1 minute; stir. Microwave, uncovered, on Low for 1 minute. Let stand until appropriate serving temperature is reached and mixture has thickened. Stir and serve.

Stovetop

2. In a small saucepan, use same measurements as above. Cook over medium-low heat for 2 to 4 minutes; stir frequently. Cover and remove from heat; let stand a few minutes.

NUTRITIONAL ANALYSIS

Energy	Protein	Carbohydrate	Fat	Fiber	Calcium	Iron	Sodium
55 kcal	3 g	7 g	2 g	1 g	56 mg	0.4 mg	19 mg

Variations

For a treat, add a sprinkle of ground nutmeg or cinnamon. For children older than 12 months, try adding raisins and chopped dried fruit. Prunes, apricots or apples are appropriate, a few to each serving during cooking.

**Makes 12 large or
24 small muffins**

Kitchen Tip

These freeze well for up to
3 months, and can be enjoyed
as a quick snack or as a part
of breakfast.

Cornmeal Berry Muffins

Preheat oven to 400°F (200°C)
12-cup muffin tin or 24-cup mini muffin tin, greased or
paper-lined

1 cup	all purpose flour	250 mL
½ cup	whole wheat flour	125 mL
½ cup	granulated sugar	125 mL
⅓ cup	cornmeal	75 mL
2½ tsp	baking powder	12 mL
¼ tsp	salt	1 mL
1	egg	1
¾ cup	2% milk	175 mL
¼ cup	butter, melted	50 mL
1 tsp	grated lemon zest	5 mL
1 cup	fresh or frozen blueberries	250 mL

1. In a large bowl, combine all-purpose flour, whole
wheat flour, sugar, cornmeal, baking powder and salt.

2. In another bowl, beat egg and stir in milk, butter
and lemon zest. Add to dry ingredients; stir until
just moistened. Stir in blueberries.

3. Spoon into prepared muffin cups. Bake in preheated
oven for 25 to 30 minutes for large (or 20 to 25 minutes
for small), until muffins are lightly browned. Cool in
pan on a wire rack for 10 minutes before removing to
rack to cool completely.

NUTRITIONAL ANALYSIS (PER SMALL MUFFIN)

Energy	Protein	Carbohydrate	Fat	Fiber	Calcium	Iron	Sodium
85 kcal	2 g	15 g	2 g	1 g	26 mg	1 mg	49 mg

Makes 1 serving

This combination makes a great breakfast or meatless lunch dish. Its very soft texture makes it ideal for children who are just starting textures.

Fruity Cottage Cheese

¼ cup	cottage cheese	50 mL
2 tbsp	unsweetened canned fruit	25 mL

1. In a small bowl, combine cottage cheese and fruit. Serve.

NUTRITIONAL ANALYSIS

Energy	Protein	Carbohydrate	Fat	Fiber	Calcium	Iron	Sodium
54 kcal	7 g	5 g	1 g	0.3 g	34 mg	0.1 mg	195 mg

Makes 1 serving

This recipe works well with many kinds of fruit. Choose the ones most popular with your infant. Serve with toast squares for a healthy breakfast.

Kitchen Tip

If you wish, substitute plain or fruit-flavored yogurt for the sour cream.

Cottage Cheese 'n' Fruit

¼ cup	cottage cheese	50 mL
2 tbsp	sour cream (see tip)	25 mL
¼ cup	chopped fresh fruit (such as orange, pineapple, banana, apple, strawberry, kiwifruit, peach, pear)	50 mL
Pinch	ground cinnamon	Pinch

1. In a small bowl, stir together cottage cheese, sour cream and fruit of your choice. Sprinkle lightly with cinnamon.

NUTRITIONAL ANALYSIS

Energy	Protein	Carbohydrate	Fat	Fiber	Calcium	Iron	Sodium
101 kcal	8 g	6 g	5 g	1 g	83 mg	0.4 mg	255 mg

Makes 2 cups (500 mL)

Just like a milkshake — but even better. Start with cold milk, fruit and yogurt, then blend until smooth.

Kitchen Tips

Busy parents can have this smoothie ready in the refrigerator the night before to serve at breakfast. You may even find you'll enjoy it as well.

If your baby is over 12 months and you wish to sweeten this recipe, you can add 1 tbsp (15 mL) liquid honey with the yogurt.

Baby's Fruit Smoothie

1	large banana	1
1 cup	raspberries or strawberries	250 mL
¾ cup	2% milk	175 mL
⅓ cup	plain yogurt	75 mL

1. In a blender, combine banana and berries; purée until smooth. Add milk and yogurt; blend for 1 minute or until smooth and frothy. Chill before serving or enjoy immediately.

NUTRITIONAL ANALYSIS (PER ¼ CUP/50 ML)

Energy	Protein	Carbohydrate	Fat	Fiber	Calcium	Iron	Sodium
36 kcal	2 g	6 g	1 g	1 g	47 mg	0.1 mg	16 mg

Makes 3¼ cups (800 mL)

This makes a healthy meal or snack that can be enjoyed by everyone! Experiment with different berries and fruits. Add more or less milk to make the consistency thinner or thicker. Older kids can make their own, with the newly designed smaller blenders.

Kitchen Tips

This is a great way to use up ripe fruits.

Freeze ripe bananas if you are not ready to use them and place in the blender right from the freezer when needed.

Another Fruity Smoothie

1 cup	vanilla-flavored or plain 1% to 2% yogurt	250 mL
1 cup	2% milk	250 mL
1 cup	fresh or frozen blueberries	250 mL
1	ripe banana or pear, chopped	1

1. In a blender, combine yogurt, milk, blueberries and banana; purée until smooth. Serve immediately.

NUTRITIONAL ANALYSIS (PER ½ CUP/125 ML)

Energy	Protein	Carbohydrate	Fat	Fiber	Calcium	Iron	Sodium
68 kcal	3 g	11 g	1 g	1 g	111 mg	0.1 mg	40 mg

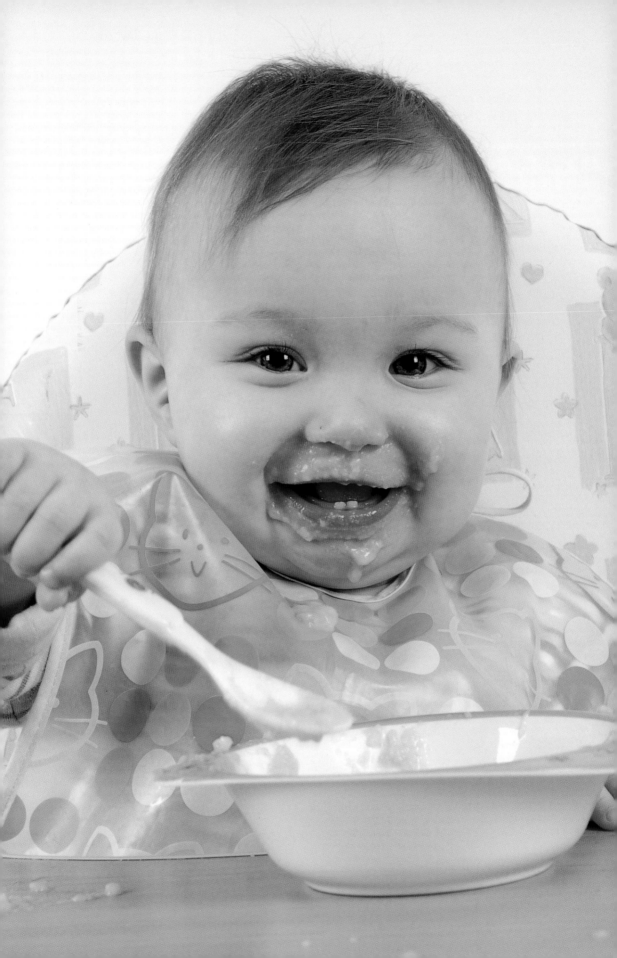

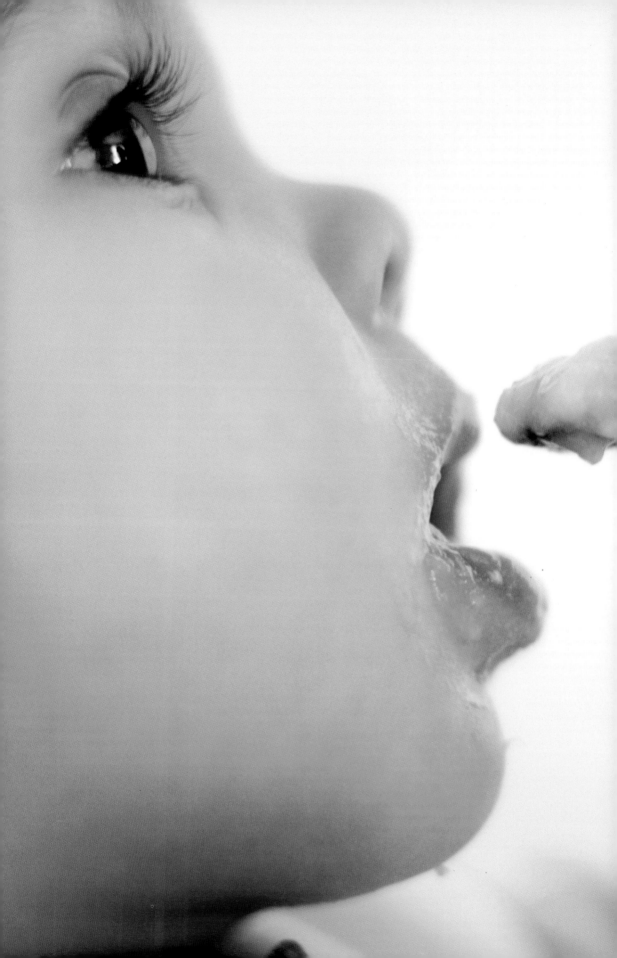

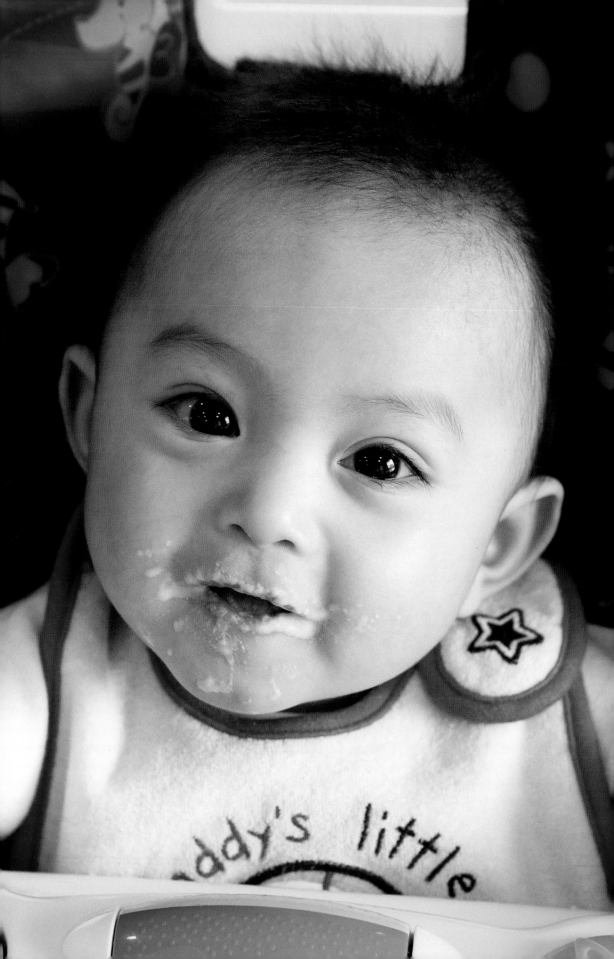

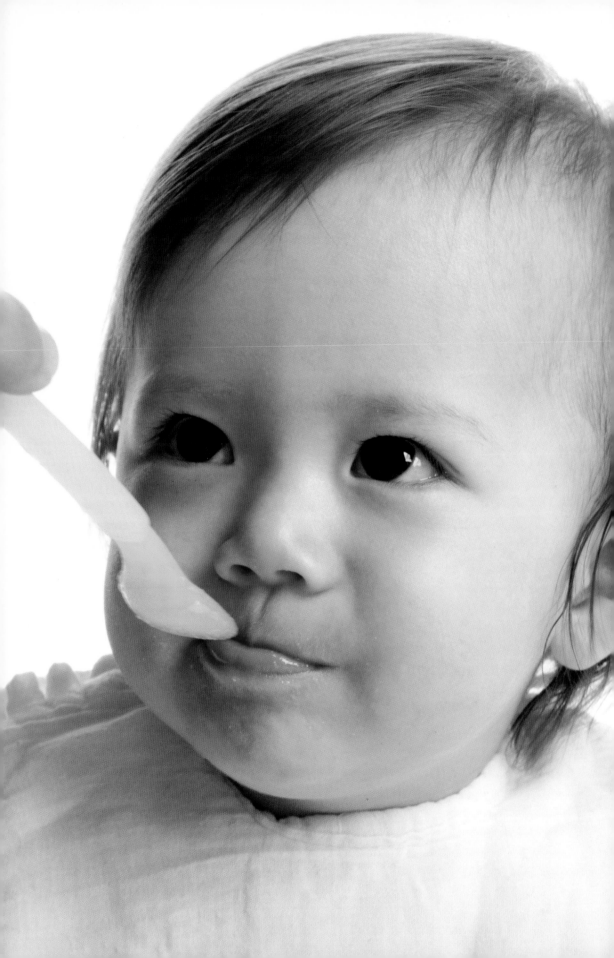

Makes 1 cup (250 mL)

Kitchen Tips

Any favorite fruit-flavored yogurt may be used

Choose any fruit jam that will be compatible with the yogurt.

Food Safety Tip

When it comes to food safety, cold temperatures can keep most harmful bacteria from growing or multiplying on food.

Yogurt Orange Fruit Dip

1/2	package (8 oz/250 g) softened cream cheese	1/2
1/2 cup	peach yogurt (see tip)	125 mL
1/4 cup	orange marmalade (see tip)	50 mL
1/4 tsp	vanilla or maple extract	1 mL
Pinch	ground ginger	Pinch
	Assorted fresh fruit	

1. In a small bowl, beat cream cheese, yogurt, marmalade, vanilla and ginger until blended. Spoon into a covered container and store in the refrigerator for up to 2 days.
2. Let soften slightly before serving with fruit.

NUTRITIONAL ANALYSIS (PER 1 TBSP/15 ML)

Energy	Protein	Carbohydrate	Fat	Fiber	Calcium	Iron	Sodium
47 kcal	1 g	4 g	3 g	–	16 mg	0.1 mg	28 mg

Makes 2 servings

This oatmeal is not only a great source of iron, but its thick, "stay in the spoon" consistency makes it easy for children to feed themselves.

Iron-Boosted Oatmeal

2/3 cup	water	150 mL
1/3 cup	quick-cooking rolled oats	75 mL
1/8 tsp	salt	0.5 mL
3 tbsp	infant rice cereal (iron-fortified)	45 mL
2 tbsp	whole milk	25 mL

1. In a large saucepan, bring water to a boil. Add oatmeal and salt; return to a boil, reduce heat and simmer for 3 to 5 minutes. Stir in rice cereal and milk (adjust quantities, if you wish, to achieve desired consistency). Let cool before serving.

NUTRITIONAL ANALYSIS (PER SERVING)

Energy	Protein	Carbohydrate	Fat	Fiber	Calcium	Iron	Sodium
89 kcal	3 g	16 g	1.5 g	2 g	24 mg	2.3 mg	153 mg

This healthy breakfast will keep up the energy level of active children and their parents for several hours. Serve with extra milk, if desired.

Creamy Egg 'n' Oatmeal Porridge

½ cup	water	125 mL
2	eggs	2
½ cup	2% milk	125 mL
¼ tsp	vanilla extract	1 mL
Pinch	ground nutmeg	Pinch
⅔ cup	quick-cooking rolled oats	150 mL

1. In a saucepan, bring water to a boil over high heat.

2. In a bowl, whisk together eggs, milk, vanilla and nutmeg; gradually stir into boiling water and return to a boil. Reduce heat to low. Stir in rolled oats. Cook, stirring constantly to prevent sticking, for 5 minutes or until mixture thickens. Let cool to a temperature suitable for your child to enjoy.

NUTRITIONAL ANALYSIS (PER ½ CUP/125 ML)

Energy	Protein	Carbohydrate	Fat	Fiber	Calcium	Iron	Sodium
146 kcal	8 g	16 g	6 g	2 g	78 mg	1 mg	60 mg

Here's a fast-start recipe for those "what am I going to feed my child for breakfast" mornings. It can easily be multiplied to serve the entire family.

Kitchen Tip

For a change of taste — or for children who cannot tolerate peanut butter — substitute cream cheese, a fruit spread or processed Cheddar cheese.

Fruit and Raisin Toast

1	slice raisin bread	1
1 tbsp	smooth peanut butter (see tip)	15 mL
¼ cup	diced apple	50 mL
Pinch	ground cinnamon	Pinch

1. Toast bread; spread with peanut butter. Top with apple and sprinkle with cinnamon. Fold in half so apple is secure inside. Cut into fingers and serve.

NUTRITIONAL ANALYSIS

Energy	Protein	Carbohydrate	Fat	Fiber	Calcium	Iron	Sodium
179 kcal	6 g	21 g	9 g	3 g	38 mg	1 mg	211 mg

Makes 12 bars

These moist, fruit-filled bars make a nice change from muffins.

Kitchen Tip

If you can't find date snacking cake, use another variety. Make sure the package size is the same and that it does not contain nuts.

Apple Breakfast Bars

Preheat oven to 350°F (180°C)
9-inch (2.5 L) square cake pan, greased

3 cups	finely chopped peeled apples, divided (about 2 large apples)	750 mL
1	package (14 oz/400 g) date snacking cake mix (see tip)	1
¼ cup	wheat germ	50 mL
¼ cup	natural wheat bran	50 mL
1 tsp	ground cinnamon	5 mL
1 cup	2% milk	250 mL
2 tbsp	packed brown sugar	25 mL

1. In a medium bowl, stir together 2 cups (500 mL) apples, cake mix, wheat germ, bran and cinnamon; stir in milk just until blended. Spread into prepared cake pan.

2. Top with remaining apples; sprinkle with sugar.

3. Bake in preheated oven for 45 minutes or until a tester inserted in the center comes out clean. Move to wire rack to cool. Cut into bars.

NUTRITIONAL ANALYSIS (PER BAR)							
Energy	Protein	Carbohydrate	Fat	Fiber	Calcium	Iron	Sodium
182 kcal	3 g	34 g	4 g	1 g	77 mg	1 mg	229 mg

Makes 32 pancakes

The young and the not-so-young will enjoy these whole-grain pancakes. Try them plain or with a topping of fresh fruit (such as sliced bananas and blueberries), along with plain or vanilla yogurt. This large-scale pancake mix can be kept on hand for a day when you're short on time.

Kitchen Tips

For great pancakes, do not overmix, as they will become tough. Let the batter stand for a few minutes before cooking.

Cook all of the pancake batter, then freeze pancakes by separating each between sheets of waxed paper and wrapping tightly in plastic wrap or placing in a resealable freezer bag. These will make a fast-start meal another day. Pop in the toaster to heat them up.

To add the flavor of maple syrup, mix about 1 tbsp (15 mL) maple syrup with 1 cup (250 mL) plain yogurt and use as topping for the pancakes. You'll get more nutrients and less sugar than you would with plain syrup.

Big-Batch Oatmeal Pancakes

Pancake Mix

2½ cups	whole wheat flour	625 mL
1½ cups	quick-cooking rolled oats	375 mL
½ cup	wheat germ	125 mL
½ cup	instant skim milk powder	125 mL
¼ cup	packed brown sugar	50 mL
2 tsp	baking powder	10 mL
¼ tsp	salt	1 mL

1. In a bowl, combine flour, rolled oats, wheat germ, milk powder, sugar, baking powder and salt. Store in a cool place in a tightly sealed container until ready to use, for up to 2 weeks. Makes about 5 cups (1.25 mL)

To make 8 pancakes:

1. In a bowl, place 1¼ cups (300 mL) pancake mix.

2. In another bowl, beat together 1 egg, 1 cup (250 mL) buttermilk and 3 tbsp (45 mL) vegetable oil. Pour into dry ingredients; stir just until moistened.

3. In a nonstick skillet, heat 1 tbsp (15 mL) oil over medium heat. Using ¼ cup (50 mL) batter for each pancake, pour into hot skillet; cook for 3 minutes or until bubbles break on surface and underside is golden brown. Turn pancakes with a spatula and cook just until bottom is lightly browned. Repeat with remaining batter.

NUTRITIONAL ANALYSIS (PER PANCAKE)

Energy	Protein	Carbohydrate	Fat	Fiber	Calcium	Iron	Sodium
169 kcal	6 g	17 g	9 g	2 g	83 mg	1 mg	88 mg

Serves 4
Makes 8 slices

Children love toast — so they'll really enjoy this "toast with an egg twist." (Parents will enjoy this classic breakfast dish too!) French toast is normally quite time-consuming, and is hard to fit into busy morning schedules. So try this overnight version. Accompany it with a fruit sauce or maple syrup mixed with plain yogurt, or just serve it plain and enjoy its marvelous flavor and crisp texture alone.

Overnight French Toast

2	eggs	2
½ cup	whole milk	125 mL
½ tsp	grated orange zest	2 mL
¼ tsp	ground cinnamon	1 mL
8	slices French bread stick	8
1 tbsp	butter or margarine	15 mL

1. In a small bowl, whisk together eggs, milk, orange zest and cinnamon until blended.

2. Place bread slices in a shallow baking dish large enough to hold the 8 slices in a single layer. Pour egg mixture evenly over bread; turn each slice to coat. Cover and refrigerate overnight.

3. Heat butter in a large nonstick skillet over medium-high heat. Add bread; cook for 2 minutes per side or until each side is golden brown.

NUTRITIONAL ANALYSIS (PER SLICE)

Energy	Protein	Carbohydrate	Fat	Fiber	Calcium	Iron	Sodium
130 kcal	5 g	20 g	3 g	2 g	71 mg	2 mg	453 mg

Makes 1 serving

Serve this fast and easy dish with toast, a bagel or an English muffin.

Variation
Add ¼ cup (50 mL) cooked chopped broccoli.

Quick Cheese Omelet

1	egg	1
1 tbsp	whole milk	15 mL
1 oz	Cheddar cheese, cut into 1-inch (2.5 cm) pieces	30 g

1. In a small microwave-safe dish, whisk together egg and milk. Add cheese.

2. Microwave, uncovered, on High for 1½ to 2 minutes, stirring at the halfway point to ensure that all of egg is cooked. (Actual cooking time will vary according to the power of your microwave.) Let stand for 5 minutes before serving.

NUTRITIONAL ANALYSIS

Energy	Protein	Carbohydrate	Fat	Fiber	Calcium	Iron	Sodium
182 kcal	13 g	1 g	14 g	–	223 mg	1 mg	222 mg

The following quick egg ideas make ideal breakfasts or lunches for your child. Add a light sprinkle of chopped parsley for visual appeal. Enjoy the same meal with your child by doubling any of the recipes for an adult helping.

Variations

Replace cottage cheese with 1 tbsp (15 mL) grated Cheddar, mozzarella, Swiss, Monterey Jack, ricotta or other available cheese or diced tofu.

Vegetable Variations

Replace asparagus with other cooked vegetables, such as small amounts of chopped carrot, green beans, broccoli, corn kernels, red or green bell pepper, chopped tomato or mashed sweet potatoes.

Egg Starters

Egg and Cottage Cheese

1 tsp	butter or margarine	5 mL
1	egg	1
1 tbsp	cottage cheese	15 mL
	Salt and freshly ground black pepper to taste	

1. In a small skillet, melt butter over medium-low heat.

2. In a small bowl, stir together egg and cottage cheese. Pour into skillet; cook, stirring frequently, until egg is cooked to desired consistency. Lightly season to taste with salt and pepper.

NUTRITIONAL ANALYSIS

Energy	Protein	Carbohydrate	Fat	Fiber	Calcium	Iron	Sodium
121 kcal	8 g	1 g	9 g	–	36 mg	1 mg	148 mg

Scrambled Egg with Asparagus

1 tsp	butter or margarine	5 mL
1 tsp	finely chopped onion	5 mL
1	egg, lightly beaten	1
1 tbsp	whole milk	15 mL
1	stalk cooked asparagus, cut into small pieces	1
	Salt and freshly ground black pepper	

1. In a small skillet, melt butter over medium-low heat. Add onion and sauté for 1 minute or until softened.

2. Whisk egg with milk; add to skillet. Cook, stirring frequently, until egg is cooked to desired consistency. Top with asparagus pieces, cover and remove from heat. Let stand a few minutes until asparagus is warm. Lightly season to taste with salt and pepper.

NUTRITIONAL ANALYSIS

Energy	Protein	Carbohydrate	Fat	Fiber	Calcium	Iron	Sodium
122 kcal	7 g	2 g	9 g	0.3 g	48 mg	1 mg	98 mg

Makes 4 servings

Enjoy this flavorful egg recipe on mornings when you have a little more time to cook. It is easy to serve just the right amount for infant appetites.

Food Safety Tip

Bacteria are found on all raw agricultural products. Wash all produce under cool running water prior to eating or cooking.

Mushroom Scrambled Eggs

4	eggs, beaten	4
3 tbsp	whole milk	45 mL
¼ tsp	salt	1 mL
Pinch	freshly ground black pepper	Pinch
1 tbsp	butter or margarine	15 mL
1	green onion, thinly sliced	1
1 cup	sliced mushrooms	250 mL

1. In a small bowl, whisk together eggs, milk, salt and pepper; set aside.

2. In a large nonstick skillet, melt butter over medium-high heat. Add onions and mushrooms; cook, stirring frequently, for 2 minutes or until just tender.

3. Reduce heat to medium-low. Pour egg mixture into skillet. Cook for 3 minutes, stirring frequently, or until eggs begin to set. Continue to cook until eggs reach desired consistency.

NUTRITIONAL ANALYSIS (PER SERVING)							
Energy	Protein	Carbohydrate	Fat	Fiber	Calcium	Iron	Sodium
111 kcal	8 g	2 g	8 g	0.3 g	41 mg	1 mg	207 mg

Makes 4 servings

This recipe may be too much to prepare during the week, but a lazy weekend would be the perfect time to enjoy it. And it's a great way to start the wee ones appreciating fine dining.

Kitchen Tip

If there are only three people in the family, you may want to reserve some of the spinach mixture for another meal.

Microwave Breakfast Eggs Florentine

1	package (10 oz/300 g) frozen chopped spinach, thawed	1
2 tbsp	finely chopped onion	25 mL
4	eggs	4
1 tbsp	grated Parmesan cheese	15 mL
¼ tsp	salt	1 mL
¼ tsp	dried basil	1 mL
4	whole wheat English muffins, halved	4

1. Squeeze excess moisture from spinach.

2. In a small microwave-safe bowl, combine spinach and onion. Cover and microwave on High for 3 minutes. Spoon mixture into 4 medium-size custard cups, using more spinach for adult servings (see tip).

3. Break 1 egg into each dish; pierce with a fork. Sprinkle with cheese, salt and basil. Cover and microwave on Medium-High for 6 minutes or until eggs are cooked to desired consistency.

4. Meanwhile, toast muffin halves. Using a rubber spatula, slide cooked egg and spinach onto muffin halves. Serve with second muffin half.

NUTRITIONAL ANALYSIS (PER SERVING)

Energy	Protein	Carbohydrate	Fat	Fiber	Calcium	Iron	Sodium
223 kcal	15 g	29 g	7 g	7 g	353 mg	6 mg	662 mg

Makes 12 baby servings, or 4 adult servings

Make this terrific recipe the night before, then pop into the oven about 30 minutes before serving. Useful when weekend guests are expected. Let small cubes of the strata cool before serving to little fingers and mouths.

Kitchen Tip

Add your choice of assorted chopped vegetables — such as sliced mushrooms, broccoli florets, or red or green bell peppers. Arrange over bread cubes in Step 1 and proceed with recipe.

Food Safety Tip

Refrigerate leftovers within 2 hours. This is one simple way that you can give bacteria the cold shoulder!

Overnight Cheese Strata

Preheat oven to 350°F (180°C)
13- by 9-inch (3 L) baking pan, greased

6	slices whole wheat bread, crusts removed	6
2 cups	shredded medium Cheddar cheese, divided	500 mL
6	eggs, beaten	6
2 cups	2% milk	500 mL
2	green onions, sliced	2
½ tsp	dried oregano	2 mL
½ tsp	salt	2 mL
¼ tsp	freshly ground black pepper	1 mL
1	large tomato, cut into wedges	1
	Chopped fresh parsley	

1. Cut bread into cubes. Arrange cubes in prepared baking dish. Sprinkle with one-half the cheese.
2. In a medium bowl, combine eggs, milk, onions, oregano, salt and pepper. Pour over bread. Sprinkle with remaining cheese. Cover with plastic wrap and refrigerate for several hours or overnight.
3. Arrange tomato wedges on top of strata. Bake in preheated oven for 35 minutes or until light golden brown and center is set. Let stand for 5 minutes before cutting into squares.

NUTRITIONAL ANALYSIS (PER BABY SERVING)							
Energy	Protein	Carbohydrate	Fat	Fiber	Calcium	Iron	Sodium
179 kcal	11 g	11 g	8 g	1 g	214 mg	1 mg	337 mg

Makes 1 serving

Here we have egg and toast in one convenient package that tastes great. It's an old favorite that never goes out of style.

Kitchen Tip

Some children may prefer this dish without cheese. Try it both ways.

Egg in a Hole

1	slice whole wheat bread	1
1 tsp	butter or margarine	5 mL
1	medium egg	1
1 tbsp	shredded Cheddar cheese (see tip)	15 mL

1. Using a cookie cutter or the rim of a glass, cut a circle from middle of bread.

2. In nonstick skillet, melt butter over medium-low heat. Place bread and bread round separately in skillet. Break egg into hole, cover skillet and cook for 5 minutes or until egg is almost set. Sprinkle with cheese. Continue to cook until cheese starts to melt. Top with bread round and serve.

NUTRITIONAL ANALYSIS

Energy	Protein	Carbohydrate	Fat	Fiber	Calcium	Iron	Sodium
223 kcal	11 g	16 g	13 g	2 g	102 mg	2 mg	318 mg

Makes 2 servings

Kitchen Tip

To prevent the muffin tin from warping, place a little water in each unused cup before placing in oven.

Ham and Egg Muffin

Preheat oven to 350°F (180°C)
Muffin tin

1	slice whole wheat bread	1
1 tsp	butter or margarine	5 mL
1	slice ham, chopped	1
1	egg	1
1 tbsp	grated Cheddar cheese	15 mL

1. Remove crusts from bread and butter one side. Press bread into muffin tin, buttered side down. Insert ham pieces and egg. Top with cheese. Bake for 15 minutes, until egg is cooked.

NUTRITIONAL ANALYSIS (PER ½ MUFFIN)

Energy	Protein	Carbohydrate	Fat	Fiber	Calcium	Iron	Sodium
124 kcal	7 g	9 g	7 g	1 g	54 mg	1 mg	93 mg

Makes 12 muffins

Nourishing oat bran in combination with applesauce makes a healthy breakfast wake-up for all ages. If you or your little one are feeling a bit peckish between meals, these muffins are also an ideal snack with milk or juice.

Oat Bran Applesauce Muffins

Preheat oven to 350°F (180°C)
12-cup muffin tin, greased or paper-lined

1⅓ cups	whole wheat flour	325 mL
½ cup	oat bran	125 mL
½ cup	loosely packed brown sugar	125 mL
2 tsp	baking powder	10 mL
½ tsp	baking soda	2 mL
½ tsp	ground cinnamon	2 mL
½ tsp	ground nutmeg	2 mL
¼ cup	vegetable oil	50 mL
1 cup	applesauce	250 mL
1	egg, beaten	1
¼ cup	finely chopped raisins (optional)	50 mL

1. In a large bowl, combine flour, oat bran, brown sugar, baking powder, baking soda and spices.

2. In another bowl, stir together oil, applesauce and egg. Stir in raisins. Add applesauce mixture to dry ingredients; stir just until moistened.

3. Spoon batter into prepared muffin cups. Bake in preheated oven for 15 minutes or until muffins are firm to the touch. Let cool for 10 minutes before removing from pan to wire rack to cool completely.

NUTRITIONAL ANALYSIS (PER MUFFIN)

Energy	Protein	Carbohydrate	Fat	Fiber	Calcium	Iron	Sodium
152 kcal	3 g	27 g	5 g	2 g	43 mg	1 mg	105 mg

Makes 12 muffins

Most people enjoy muffins for breakfast or as a snack — and kids are no exception. Rolled oats add extra fiber to these tasty-healthy muffins.

Kitchen Tips

Because it contains honey, this recipe is only appropriate for children over 12 months. For younger children, replace honey with an equal quantity of granulated sugar.

Honey does not stick to the measuring cup if oil is measured first.

Don't have buttermilk? Sour milk makes a good substitute and it's easy to make: For the quantity needed in this recipe, add 1½ tsp (7 mL) lemon juice or vinegar to a measuring cup, then add enough milk to make up ¾ cup (175 mL); let mixture stand for 5 minutes.

Banana Oat Muffins

Preheat oven to 400°F (200°C)
12-cup muffin tin, greased or paper-lined

1 cup	all-purpose flour	250 mL
½ cup	whole wheat flour	125 mL
½ cup	quick-cooking rolled oats	125 mL
1 tsp	baking powder	5 mL
½ tsp	baking soda	2 mL
½ tsp	ground cinnamon	2 mL
¾ cup	buttermilk or sour milk (see tip)	175 mL
¼ cup	vegetable oil	50 mL
1	egg	1
⅓ cup	liquid honey (see tip)	75 mL
1	medium banana, mashed	1

1. In a large bowl, combine all-purpose and whole wheat flour, rolled oats, baking powder, baking soda and cinnamon.

2. In another bowl, combine buttermilk, oil, egg, honey and banana. Add to dry ingredients; stir just until moistened.

3. Spoon batter into prepared muffin cups. Bake in preheated oven for 18 minutes or until muffins are firm to the touch.

NUTRITIONAL ANALYSIS (PER MUFFIN)

Energy	Protein	Carbohydrate	Fat	Fiber	Calcium	Iron	Sodium
167 kcal	4 g	27 g	5 g	2 g	40 mg	1 mg	91 mg

Makes 18 muffins

Whole wheat flour adds extra nutrition to these tasty, moist muffins. They're great for breakfast or as a snack.

Spiced Pumpkin Muffins

Preheat oven to 400°F (200°C)
Two 12-cup muffin tins, 18 cups paper-lined or greased

1 cup	all purpose flour	250 mL
¾ cup	whole wheat flour	175 mL
½ cup	granulated sugar	125 mL
1 tsp	baking powder	5 mL
1 tsp	baking soda	5 mL
1 tsp	ground cinnamon	5 mL
½ tsp	ground nutmeg	2 mL
½ tsp	ground ginger	2 mL
2	eggs	2
1 cup	canned pumpkin purée (not pie filling)	250 mL
½ cup	canola oil	125 mL
⅓ cup	buttermilk	75 mL
1 tsp	vanilla extract	5 mL

1. In a large bowl, combine all purpose flour, whole wheat flour, sugar, baking powder, baking soda, cinnamon, nutmeg and ginger.

2. In another bowl, whisk together eggs, pumpkin, oil, buttermilk and vanilla. Add to dry ingredients; stir just until moistened.

3. Spoon batter into prepared muffin cups. Bake in preheated oven for 18 minutes or until muffins are firm to the touch. Cool in pan on a wire rack for 10 minutes before removing to rack to cool completely.

NUTRITIONAL ANALYSIS (PER MUFFIN)							
Energy	Protein	Carbohydrate	Fat	Fiber	Calcium	Iron	Sodium
138 kcal	2 g	16 g	7 g	1 g	24 mg	1 mg	101 mg

Makes one 12-slice loaf

Kitchen Tips

Because it contains honey, this recipe is only appropriate for children over 12 months. For younger children, use maple syrup instead of the honey.

Try half whole wheat flour and half all-purpose flour.

Honey Loaf

Preheat oven to 350°F (180°C)
9- by 5-inch (2 L) loaf pan, lightly greased

½ cup	butter or margarine	125 mL
½ cup	granulated sugar	125 mL
1	egg	1
⅓ cup	liquid honey	75 mL
1 tsp	salt	5 mL
2½ cups	all-purpose flour	625 mL
1 tbsp	baking powder	15 mL
⅔ cup	2% milk	150 mL

1. In a large bowl, cream together butter and sugar. Add egg, honey and salt; mix well.
2. In another smaller bowl, combine flour and baking powder; add to butter mixture. Add milk, stirring, until just moistened.
3. Pour into prepared loaf pan and bake in preheated oven for 1¼ hours.

NUTRITIONAL ANALYSIS (PER SLICE)							
Energy	Protein	Carbohydrate	Fat	Fiber	Calcium	Iron	Sodium
250 kcal	4 g	38 g	9 g	1 g	59 mg	1 mg	346 mg

Makes 4 servings

Orange Smoothie Shake

¾ cup	frozen orange juice concentrate, thawed	175 mL
1 cup	2% milk	250 mL
1 cup	water	250 mL
2 tbsp	granulated sugar	25 mL
½ tsp	vanilla extract	2 mL
5	ice cubes	5

1. In a blender, combine orange juice concentrate, milk, water, sugar and vanilla. With motor running, add ice cubes one at a time. Blend until smooth.

NUTRITIONAL ANALYSIS (PER SERVING)

Energy	Protein	Carbohydrate	Fat	Fiber	Calcium	Iron	Sodium
66 kcal	2 g	11 g	1 g	0.1 g	81 mg	0.1 mg	28 mg

Makes 2⅓ cups (575 mL)

Both children and adults will love these fruit sauces. They make handy toppings for pancakes, milk or rice pudding, cottage cheese or ice cream or other fresh fruits. Use your favorite fruits when they are at their freshest best. Make lots of sauce and freeze what you can't use now.

Kitchen Tip

Prepared fruits are stemmed, pitted, peeled (if necessary) and sliced.

Food Safety Tip

All produce should be washed under cool running water prior to eating or cooking.

Basic Fast Fruit Sauce

2 cups	prepared fruit, such as strawberries, blueberries, raspberries, Saskatoon berries, peaches and plums (see tip)	500 mL
1 cup	water, divided	250 mL
2 tbsp	cornstarch	25 mL
1 tbsp	lemon juice	15 mL

1. In a saucepan, bring ¾ cup (175 mL) of the water to a boil. Add fruit. Return to a boil, reduce heat to low and cook, uncovered, for 5 minutes.

2. Blend together cornstarch and remaining ¼ cup (50 mL) water. Add slowly to fruit and boil until thick and clear, stirring constantly.

3. Stir lemon juice into fruit. Sauce may be served warm or cooled and stored in the refrigerator.

NUTRITIONAL ANALYSIS (PER 1 TBSP/15 ML)

Energy	Protein	Carbohydrate	Fat	Fiber	Calcium	Iron	Sodium
6 kcal	–	2 g	–	0.2 g	1 mg	–	–

Makes 1½ cups (375 mL)

This topping is excellent for pancakes, frozen waffles or French toast. It combines two all-time child favorites — bananas and cream cheese.

Serving Suggestion

Cut pancakes, waffles or French toast into baby-bite-size pieces. Top with sauce.

Variations

Pineapple Sauce: Replace banana with ½ cup (125 mL) drained canned crushed pineapple.

Strawberry Sauce: Replace banana with 1½ cups (375 mL) sliced strawberries.

Spiced Banana Sauce

2 tbsp	frozen orange juice concentrate, thawed	25 mL
2 tbsp	water	25 mL
¼ cup	cream cheese (at room temperature)	50 mL
½ to 1 tsp	granulated sugar	2 to 5 mL
⅛ tsp	ground cinnamon	0.5 mL
⅛ tsp	ground nutmeg	0.5 mL
2	bananas, cut into slices	2
	Frozen waffles	

1. In a small nonstick skillet, combine orange juice, water, cream cheese, sugar, cinnamon and nutmeg. Cook over medium heat for about 5 minutes or until heated and smooth; stir frequently. Add bananas and cook for 1 minute, until slices are coated with sauce.

2. Toast waffles. Spoon some warm sauce over each.

NUTRITIONAL ANALYSIS (PER ¼ CUP/50 ML)							
Energy	Protein	Carbohydrate	Fat	Fiber	Calcium	Iron	Sodium
73 kcal	1 g	12 g	3 g	1 g	11 mg	0.2 mg	25 mg

Enjoy this sauce as a breakfast fruit dip or serve over cut-up fresh fruit at another meal.

Ricotta Cream Sauce

1 cup	smooth 2% ricotta cheese	250 mL
1 tbsp	confectioner's (icing) sugar	15 mL
1 tsp	grated orange zest	5 mL
½ tsp	vanilla extract	2 mL
	Fresh fruit pieces (banana chunks, seedless grapes, melon pieces, whole strawberries, kiwi slices, or any other fresh fruit suitable for dipping)	

1. In a small bowl, beat together cheese and sugar until smooth. Stir in orange zest and vanilla. Spoon into a tightly sealed container and store in the refrigerator for up to 1 week.

2. Serve in a small container suitable for dipping fruit.

NUTRITIONAL ANALYSIS (PER 1 TBSP/15 ML)

Energy	Protein	Carbohydrate	Fat	Fiber	Calcium	Iron	Sodium
25 kcal	2 g	1 g	1 g	–	44 mg	0.1 mg	20 mg

This quick, easy recipe can easily be multiplied to serve the entire family.

Pineapple Toast

Preheat broiler

2	slices whole-grain bread	2
2 tbsp	cream cheese	25 mL
2	slices unsweetened canned pineapple, drained	2
Pinch	ground cinnamon	Pinch

1. Spread each slice of bread with 1 tbsp (15 mL) cheese. Top each with 1 pineapple slice; sprinkle lightly with cinnamon.

2. Place on a baking pan; broil under preheated broiler for 1 minute or until cheese starts to melt. Let cool slightly before cutting into child-size portions.

NUTRITIONAL ANALYSIS (PER SERVING)

Energy	Protein	Carbohydrate	Fat	Fiber	Calcium	Iron	Sodium
80 kcal	2.4 g	11 g	3 g	2 g	28 mg	1 mg	107 mg

Makes 30 muffins

This reliable and healthy recipe brings back childhood memories of muffins served after school.

Kitchen Tip

If buttermilk is not available, simply add 1 tsp (5 mL) vinegar or lemon juice to each ½ cup (125 mL) low-fat milk to sour it.

Bran Muffins

Preheat oven to 375°F (190°C)
Two or three 12-cup muffin tins, greased or paper-lined

1½ cups	whole wheat flour	375 mL
1½ cups	natural wheat bran	375 mL
1¼ cups	all-purpose flour	300 mL
2 tsp	baking powder	10 mL
2 tsp	baking soda	10 mL
½ tsp	salt	2 mL
¾ cup	soft margarine	175 mL
⅔ cup	lightly packed brown sugar	150 mL
2 cups	buttermilk or sour milk (see tip)	500 mL
½ cup	raisins	125 mL
¼ cup	light (fancy) molasses	50 mL
2	eggs, well beaten	2

1. In a large bowl, combine whole wheat flour, bran, all-purpose flour, baking powder, baking soda and salt.

2. In another bowl, cream together margarine and brown sugar. Stir in milk, raisins and molasses. Stir in beaten eggs. Add mixture to dry ingredients; stir just until moistened.

3. Spoon batter into prepared muffins cups. Bake in preheated oven, in batches as necessary, for 20 minutes or until muffins are firm to the touch. Cool in pan on a wire rack for 10 minutes before removing to rack to cool completely.

NUTRITIONAL ANALYSIS (PER 1 TBSP/15 ML)

Energy	Protein	Carbohydrate	Fat	Fiber	Calcium	Iron	Sodium
137 kcal	3 g	21 g	6 g	2 g	49 mg	1.2 mg	231 mg

Lunch

Makes 1 to 2 servings

Kitchen Tips

Vegetable and fruit purées will keep in the freezer for 4 to 6 months. Be sure to label with date before freezing.

For older infants, fork-mash cooked fruit for a thicker texture.

Puréed Baby Fruit

| 1⁄3 to 1⁄2 cup | cooked fruit, chopped into small pieces | 75 to 125 mL |
| 2 tsp | water or fruit juice | 10 mL |

1. In a small bowl, microwave fruit on High for about 1 minute. Stir in water. Transfer to a food processor or blender; process for 30 to 60 seconds, until purée is smooth.
2. Serve immediately or freeze in an ice-cube tray for later use (see page 51).

NUTRITIONAL ANALYSIS

Varies with fruit used

Makes 2 cups (500 mL)

Kitchen Tip

Try different varieties of apples for different flavors!

Puréed Apples

| 6 | apples, peeled and sliced | 6 |

1. In a saucepan of boiling water, boil apples for 5 to 10 minutes or until tender. Drain, reserving 2 tbsp (25 mL) of the cooking liquid.
2. Transfer apples to a food processor or blender and purée, adding reserved cooking liquid about 1 tsp (5 mL) at a time until apples are smooth. Serve immediately or freeze in ice-cube trays for later use (see page 51).

NUTRITIONAL ANALYSIS (PER 1⁄4 CUP/50 ML)

Energy	Protein	Carbohydrate	Fat	Fiber	Calcium	Iron	Sodium
47 kcal	0.3 g	12 g	–	1 g	5 mg	–	–

Makes ⅓ cup (75 mL)

Kitchen Tips

This recipe makes enough for about half an ice-cube tray. Try different varieties of pears for different flavors.

Cooked pears do not generally require added water for processing.

Puréed Pears

| 1 | medium pear, peeled, cored and cut into small pieces (about 1 cup/250 mL) | 1 |

1. In a saucepan of boiling water, cook pear for about 15 minutes or until tender. Drain. Transfer to a food processor or blender; process for 30 to 60 seconds, until purée is smooth.

2. Serve immediately or freeze in an ice-cube tray for later use (see page 51).

NUTRITIONAL ANALYSIS (PER ¼ CUP/50 ML)

Energy	Protein	Carbohydrate	Fat	Fiber	Calcium	Iron	Sodium
49 kcal	1 g	13 g	0.1 g	2 g	8 mg	0.2 mg	1 mg

Makes ½ cup (125 mL)

Puréed Peaches

| 2 | small peaches, peeled, pitted and cut into small pieces (about 1 cup/250 mL) | 2 |
| 1 to 2 tsp | water or cooking liquid | 5 to 10 mL |

1. In a saucepan of boiling water, cook peaches for about 10 minutes or until tender. Drain. Transfer to a food processor or blender; process for 30 to 60 seconds, adding water as needed until purée is smooth.

2. Serve immediately or freeze in an ice-cube tray for later use (see page 51).

NUTRITIONAL ANALYSIS (PER ¼ CUP/50 ML)

Energy	Protein	Carbohydrate	Fat	Fiber	Calcium	Iron	Sodium
34 kcal	1 g	8 g	0.2 g	2 g	6 mg	0.2 mg	–

Makes 1½ cups (375 mL)

Kitchen Tip

No additional water is required to process ripe mangos. If ripe mangos aren't available, unripe mangos can be cooked in a pot of boiling water for 5 to 10 minutes, until tender. Drain and purée.

Mango Purée

| 2 | ripe mangos, cubed | 2 |

1. In a food processor or blender, purée mango until smooth. Serve immediately or freeze in an ice-cube tray for later use (see page 51).

NUTRITIONAL ANALYSIS (PER ¼ CUP/50 ML)

Energy	Protein	Carbohydrate	Fat	Fiber	Calcium	Iron	Sodium
55 kcal	0.4 g	14 g	0.2 g	2 g	8 mg	0.1 mg	2 mg

Makes 1¼ cups (300 mL)

This is a quick and easy starter recipe. For babies who are still on a much smoother texture, this recipe can be also be puréed.

Kitchen Tip

For teething infants, try putting some diced melon pieces in the freezer for about 15 minutes. Makes a cool and soothing treat for sore gums.

Melon Mash

½ cup	cubed cantaloupe	125 mL
1	banana, sliced	1
½ cup	plain yogurt	125 mL
Pinch	ground ginger	Pinch

1. In a bowl, combine cantaloupe and banana; mash until desired consistency. Stir in yogurt and ginger. Serve immediately or freeze in an ice-cube tray for later use (see page 51).

NUTRITIONAL ANALYSIS (PER ¼ CUP/50 ML)

Energy	Protein	Carbohydrate	Fat	Fiber	Calcium	Iron	Sodium
42 kcal	2 g	8 g	0.5 g	0.5 g	48 mg	0.1 mg	20 mg

Makes 1 cup (250 mL)

Bananas and avocados are both great first foods. Their soft texture makes them easy to mash or cube, with no cooking required.

Kitchen Tip

To keep unused avocado from turning brown, try storing the unused portion face down on a plate in the fridge, or store in a covered container *with* the pit.

Although this recipe freezes well, the exposed areas will turn brown.

Variations

You can try other fruits in combination with the avocado, including soft ripe peeled peaches or a peeled and cooked apple.

Mashed Banana and Avocado

1	banana, sliced	1
1	avocado, cubed	1

1. In a small bowl, using a potato masher or fork, mash banana and avocado to desired consistency. Serve immediately or freeze in an ice-cube tray for later use (see page 51).

NUTRITIONAL ANALYSIS (PER ¼ CUP/50 ML)

Energy	Protein	Carbohydrate	Fat	Fiber	Calcium	Iron	Sodium
106 kcal	1 g	11 g	8 g	4 g	8 mg	0.4 mg	4 mg

Makes 3 to 4 servings

Puréed Baby Vegetables

¾ cup	cooked vegetables, chopped into small pieces	175 mL
3 tbsp	water or cooking liquid	45 mL

1. In a small bowl, microwave vegetables on High for about 1 minute or until tender. Stir in water. Transfer to a food processor or blender; process for 1 to 2 minutes, until purée is smooth.

2. Serve immediately or freeze in an ice-cube tray for later use (see page 51).

NUTRITIONAL ANALYSIS

Varies with vegetables used

Puréed Green Beans

Kitchen Tip

This recipe makes enough for about half an ice-cube tray. Frozen or fresh varieties of beans work equally well.

| 1 cup | chopped green beans (washed and trimmed) | 250 mL |
| 2 tbsp | water or cooking liquid | 25 mL |

1. In a saucepan of boiling water, cook beans for about 15 minutes or until tender. Drain. Transfer to a food processor or blender; process for 30 to 60 seconds, adding water as needed until purée is smooth.

2. Serve immediately or freeze in an ice-cube tray for later use (see page 51).

NUTRITIONAL ANALYSIS (PER ¼ CUP/50 ML)

Energy	Protein	Carbohydrate	Fat	Fiber	Calcium	Iron	Sodium
23 kcal	1 g	5 g	0.2 g	2 g	28 mg	0.5 mg	1 mg

Puréed Carrots

| 2 | medium carrots, peeled and thinly sliced (about 1 cup/250 mL) | 2 |
| 2 tbsp | water or cooking liquid | 25 mL |

1. In a saucepan of boiling water, cook carrots for 12 to 15 minutes or until tender. Drain. Transfer to a food processor or blender; process for 30 to 60 seconds, adding water as needed until purée is smooth.

2. Serve immediately or freeze in an ice-cube tray for later use (see page 51).

NUTRITIONAL ANALYSIS (PER ¼ CUP/50 ML)

Energy	Protein	Carbohydrate	Fat	Fiber	Calcium	Iron	Sodium
29 kcal	1 g	7 g	0.2 g	2 g	25 mg	0.5 mg	48 mg

Puréed Broccoli

Kitchen Tips

This recipe makes enough for about half an ice-cube tray.

Try steaming broccoli instead of boiling it — more vitamins will be retained as a result.

| 1 cup | chopped broccoli florets (washed and trimmed) | 250 mL |
| 2 tbsp | water or cooking liquid | 25 mL |

1. In a saucepan of boiling water, cook broccoli for 5 to 10 minutes or until tender. Drain. Transfer to a food processor or blender; process for 30 to 60 seconds, adding water as needed until purée is smooth.

2. Serve immediately or freeze in an ice-cube tray for later use (see page 51).

NUTRITIONAL ANALYSIS (PER ¼ CUP/50 ML)

Energy	Protein	Carbohydrate	Fat	Fiber	Calcium	Iron	Sodium
38 kcal	2 g	7 g	1 g	2 g	40 mg	0.5 mg	41 mg

Puréed Sweet Potatoes

Kitchen Tip

Using the reserved cooking liquid in lieu of water saves some of the nutrients that are lost during the cooking process.

| 2 | large sweet potatoes, peeled and cubed (about 5 cups/1.25 L) | 2 |

1. In a saucepan of boiling water, boil sweet potatoes for about 20 minutes or until tender. Drain, reserving ⅔ cup (150 mL) of the cooking liquid.

2. Transfer potatoes to a food processor or blender and purée for 30 to 60 seconds, adding reserved cooking liquid as needed until smooth. Serve immediately or freeze in ice-cube trays for later use (see page 51).

NUTRITIONAL ANALYSIS (PER ¼ CUP/50 ML)

Energy	Protein	Carbohydrate	Fat	Fiber	Calcium	Iron	Sodium
74 kcal	1 g	18 g	0.1 g	2 g	11 mg	0.3 mg	6 mg

Makes 2 cups (500 mL) broth and 2½ cups (625 mL) vegetable purée

This broth is worth making — you won't believe how tasty it is — and the bonus is, you get puréed veggies too. The broth is a much better choice for soups and other dishes than regular chicken or beef broths, which are usually high in sodium.

Kitchen Tips

Freeze broth in 1-cup (250 mL) portions for use in recipes.

You can use the puréed vegetables to make a cream soup too! Add about ½ cup (125 mL) whole milk to ½ cup (125 mL) of the vegetables. Simply delicious!

Vegetable Broth and Puréed Veggies

1 cup	sliced celery	250 mL
1 cup	sliced broccoli	250 mL
1 cup	sliced parsnips (or 1 medium)	250 mL
1 cup	sliced onions (or 1 small)	250 mL
1 cup	sliced leeks	250 mL
1 cup	sliced carrots (or 4 medium)	250 mL
4 cups	water	1 L

1. In a large pot, combine celery, broccoli, parsnips, onions, leeks, carrots and water. Bring to a boil over high heat. Reduce heat and boil gently for about 30 minutes or until vegetables are soft.

2. Strain, reserving vegetables and broth separately. Use broth immediately or transfer to containers for storage.

3. In a food processor or blender, or in a bowl, purée or mash vegetables to desired consistency. Serve immediately or transfer to containers for storage.

NUTRITIONAL ANALYSIS (PER ½ CUP/125 ML SOUP, INCLUDING PURÉED VEGETABLES)							
Energy	Protein	Carbohydrate	Fat	Fiber	Calcium	Iron	Sodium
39 kcal	1 g	9 g	0.2 g	2 g	33 mg	0.5 mg	32 mg

Makes 8 cups (2 L)

It is always nice to have homemade chicken or beef stocks on hand for soups or other recipes. It freezes well and will defrost overnight.

Kitchen Tip

You can purchase stewing chickens specifically for the purpose of making stock or you can also use a leftover carcass from a chicken or turkey dinner.

Chicken Stock

12-cup (3 L) stockpot

2 lbs	chicken pieces and/or bones	1 kg
1	onion, thinly sliced	1
1	stalk celery, sliced	1
8 cups	cold water	2 L
	Salt and freshly ground black pepper to taste	
1	sprig parsley	1

1. Add all ingredients to stockpot and bring to a boil. Reduce heat, cover and simmer for $2\frac{1}{2}$ to 3 hours. Drain through a sieve to remove solids.

NUTRITIONAL ANALYSIS (PER 1 CUP/250 ML)

Energy	Protein	Carbohydrate	Fat	Fiber	Calcium	Iron	Sodium
160 kcal	23 g	1 g	6 g	0.2 g	20 mg	1 mg	98 mg

Italian Harvest Soup

This vegetarian soup will appeal to all members of the family — cheese for the kids, lots of vegetables for all members. For babies, this flavorful soup can be puréed.

2 tbsp	olive oil	25 mL
6	mushrooms, chopped	6
1	carrot, shredded	1
1	clove garlic, minced	1
2 cups	diced zucchini	500 mL
1 cup	shredded cabbage	250 mL
½ cup	chopped onion	125 mL
2 cups	reduced-sodium or homemade vegetable broth	500 mL
1 to 2 tsp	dried basil	5 to 10 mL
¼ tsp	freshly ground black pepper	1 mL
¼ cup	grated Parmesan cheese, optional	50 mL

1. In a large saucepan, heat oil over medium-high heat. Add mushrooms, carrot, garlic zucchini, cabbage and onion; sauté for 5 minutes or until tender.
2. Add broth, basil and pepper. Cover and bring to a boil; reduce heat to medium-low and cook for 15 minutes or until vegetables are tender.
3. Stir in cheese (if using) and cook until cheese is melted.

NUTRITIONAL ANALYSIS (PER ½ CUP/125 ML)							
Energy	Protein	Carbohydrate	Fat	Fiber	Calcium	Iron	Sodium
57 kcal	2.5 g	4 g	4 g	1 g	43 mg	0.5 mg	207 mg

Easy Cheesy Spinach

Kitchen Tip

This recipe is a great source of calcium.

½ cup	water	125 mL
1	package (10 oz/284 g) fresh spinach	1
1 cup	2% cottage cheese	250 mL

1. In a large pot, bring water to a boil over medium heat. Add spinach, cover and cook for about 4 minutes or until tender. Drain spinach well.

2. In a bowl, combine spinach and cottage cheese. Stir well.

NUTRITIONAL ANALYSIS (PER ¼ CUP/50 ML)

Energy	Protein	Carbohydrate	Fat	Fiber	Calcium	Iron	Sodium
27 kcal	4 g	2 g	1 g	1 g	44 mg	1 mg	114 mg

Crazy for Quinoa

Kitchen Tips

Some people prefer washing the quinoa first to remove the sometimes bitter flavor, while others prefer to heat it in oil. Experiment to see what works best for your taste buds.

Store leftovers in an airtight container in the refrigerator for up to 3 days.

Great source of fiber, iron, and protein.

1 tbsp	olive oil	15 mL
½ cup	quinoa	125 mL
1	clove garlic, minced	1
3 cups	reduced-sodium vegetable broth (store-bought or see recipe, page 154)	750 mL
½ cup	green peas, cooked or thawed if frozen	125 mL
½ cup	shelled edamame	125 mL
½	tomato, diced	½

1. In a saucepan, heat oil over medium heat. Add quinoa and toast, stirring constantly, for about 2 minutes or until lightly browned. Add garlic and sauté for 1 minute. Remove from heat.

2. Gradually pour in vegetable stock. Return pan to low heat, cover and cook for about 10 minutes or until water is absorbed and quinoa appears fluffy. Gently stir in peas, edamame and tomato.

NUTRITIONAL ANALYSIS (PER ¼ CUP/50 ML)

Energy	Protein	Carbohydrate	Fat	Fiber	Calcium	Iron	Sodium
50 kcal	3 g	6 g	2 g	1 g	9 mg	1 mg	159 mg

Makes 3½ cups (875 mL)

As it cooks, the soup mix thickens the liquid, making this hearty soup more like a stew. Prepare during morning naptime to have ready for lunch. For infants, purée until smooth. Toddlers and their elders will love it straight from the pot.

Kitchen Tips

Purchase premixed bags of assorted dried legumes or mix your own.

Look for reduced-sodium bouillon cubes.

Food Safety Tip

Bacteria thrive in foods left out at room temperature. To reduce the chance of food-borne illnesses, refrigerate any leftover soup within 2 hours.

Barley Vegetable Soup

3 cups	water	750 mL
⅓ cup	mixed dried lentils, split peas, barley (see tip)	75 mL
1	bouillon cube, beef or vegetable	1
1	medium carrot, diced	1
1	medium potato, diced	1
1	stalk celery, chopped	1
½ cup	tomato sauce	125 mL
½ tsp	dried basil	2 mL

1. In a large saucepan, combine water, soup mix, bouillon cube, carrot, potato and celery. Bring to a boil, reduce heat and simmer, covered, for about 1 hour or until legumes are tender. Add more water if soup is too thick.

2. Add tomato sauce and basil. Heat until warmed through.

NUTRITIONAL ANALYSIS (PER ½ CUP/125 ML)							
Energy	Protein	Carbohydrate	Fat	Fiber	Calcium	Iron	Sodium
66 kcal	3 g	13 g	0.5 g	2 g	19 mg	1.1 mg	485 mg

Broccoli Soup

Kitchen Tips

This recipe can be prepared in advance, up to the point of adding milk in Step 3. Purée can be frozen in portion sizes until ready to eat. Just defrost and add milk; season to taste with salt and pepper. Warm until heated through.

Use homemade or reduced-sodium stock to lower the sodium content of this recipe.

1 tbsp	butter or margarine	15 mL
½	onion, chopped	½
1 lb	broccoli, chopped	500 g
2 cups	chicken stock, divided	500 mL
2 tbsp	all-purpose flour	25 mL
1 cup	water	250 mL
1	bay leaf	1
2 tbsp	chopped parsley	25 mL
1 cup	whole milk	250 mL
¼ tsp	salt	1 mL
¼ tsp	freshly ground black pepper	1 mL

1. In a large saucepan, melt butter over medium heat. Add onion and cook for about 5 minutes or until soft. Add broccoli and a few tablespoons of the chicken stock; cook, covered, for another 10 minutes. Sprinkle flour over mixture and blend well.

2. In a medium bowl, combine remaining chicken stock with water. Stir mixture into saucepan with bay leaf and parsley; cook, covered, for about 20 minutes longer. Remove and discard bay leaf.

3. Transfer soup to a food processor or blender; purée until smooth. Return mixture to saucepan and stir in milk, salt and pepper. Cook over medium-low heat for about 5 minutes or until heated through.

NUTRITIONAL ANALYSIS (PER ½ CUP/125 ML)

Energy	Protein	Carbohydrate	Fat	Fiber	Calcium	Iron	Sodium
76 kcal	4 g	9 g	3 g	2 g	67 mg	1 mg	171 mg

Makes 8 cups (2 L)

Kitchen Tips

For additional protein, add tofu or cheese to soup. Serve with hot bread or buns.

This recipe can be prepared in advance, up to the point of adding milk in Step 2. Purée can be frozen in portion sizes until ready to eat. Just defrost and add milk. Warm until heated through.

For a richer texture, use cream instead of milk.

Use homemade or reduced-sodium stock to lower the sodium content of this recipe.

Colorful Carrot Soup

2 tbsp	butter or margarine	25 mL
1 cup	finely chopped onions	250 mL
3 cups	thickly sliced carrots	750 mL
4 cups	chicken stock	1 L
2 tbsp	tomato paste	25 mL
2 tbsp	long-grain rice	25 mL
½ cup	whole milk	125 mL
¼ tsp	salt	1 mL
¼ tsp	freshly ground black pepper	1 mL
2 cups	water	500 mL

1. In a large skillet, melt butter over medium heat. Add onions and cook until soft. Add carrots, stock, tomato paste and rice; reduce heat and simmer for 30 minutes.
2. In a food processor or blender, purée soup in batches until smooth, transferring each batch to a saucepan. Stir in milk, salt and pepper. Add water. Heat until warmed through before serving.

NUTRITIONAL ANALYSIS (PER ½ CUP/125 ML)

Energy	Protein	Carbohydrate	Fat	Fiber	Calcium	Iron	Sodium
53 kcal	2 g	6 g	2 g	1 g	22 mg	0.2 mg	144 mg

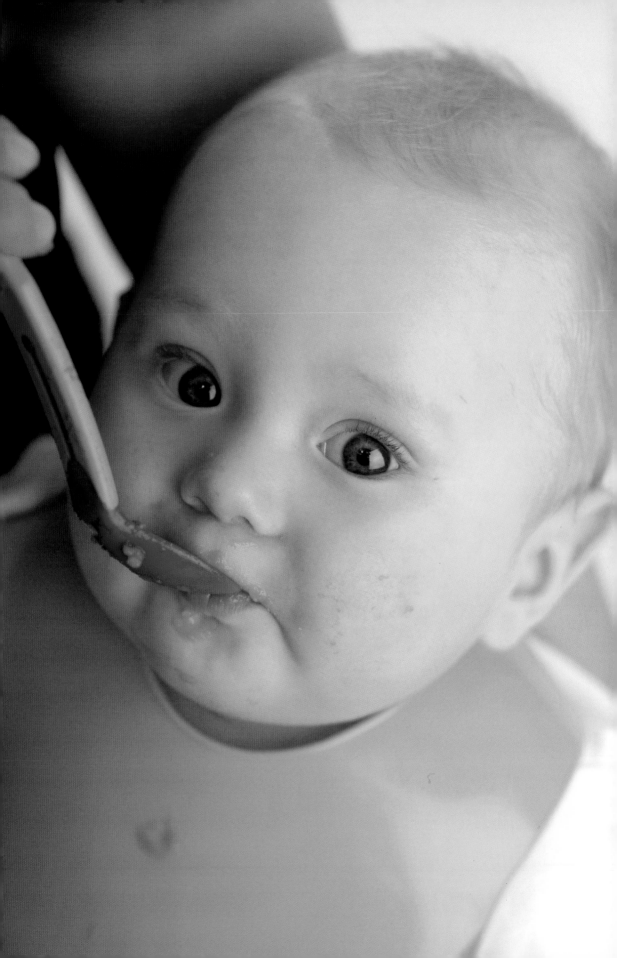

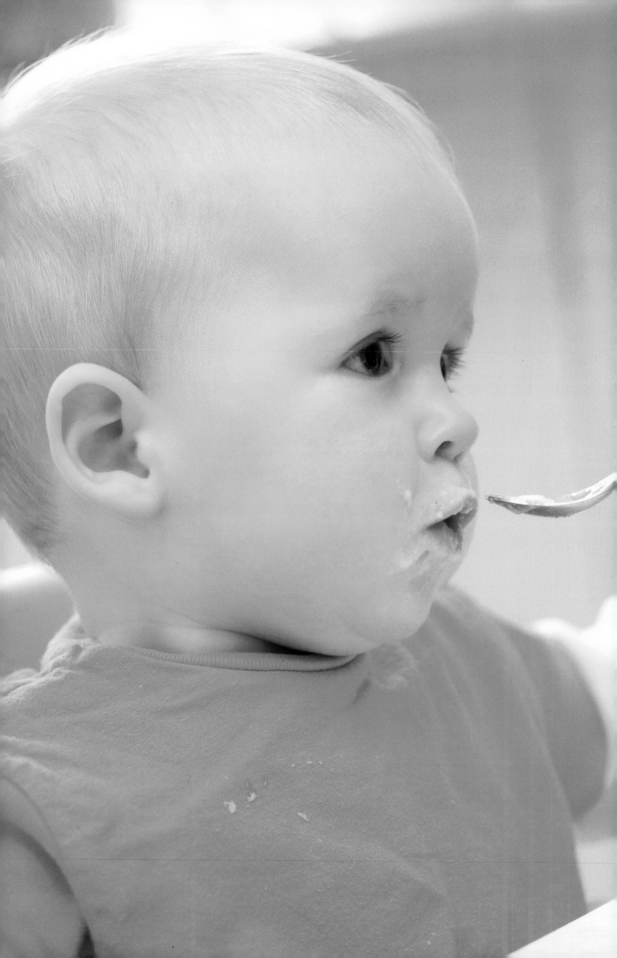

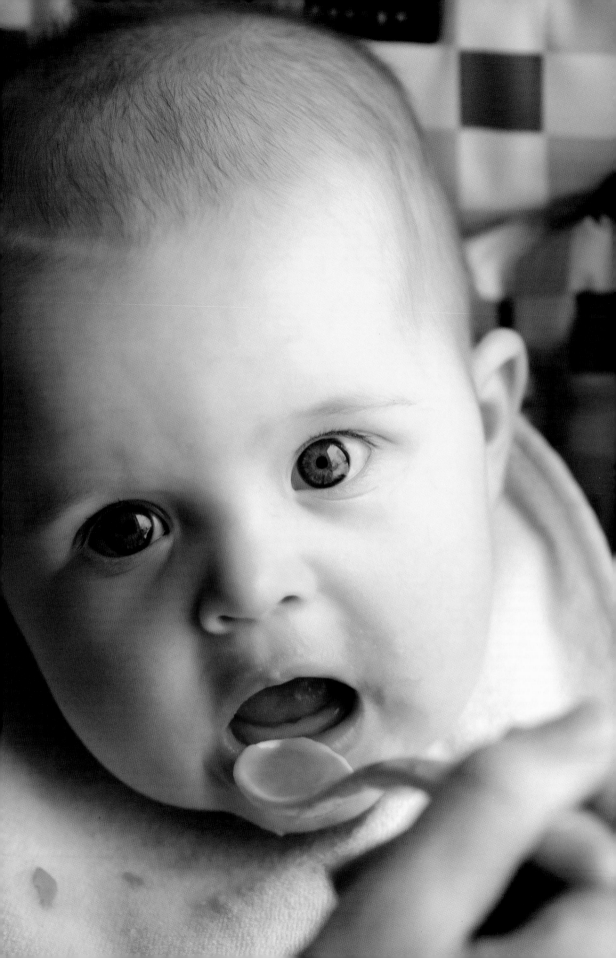

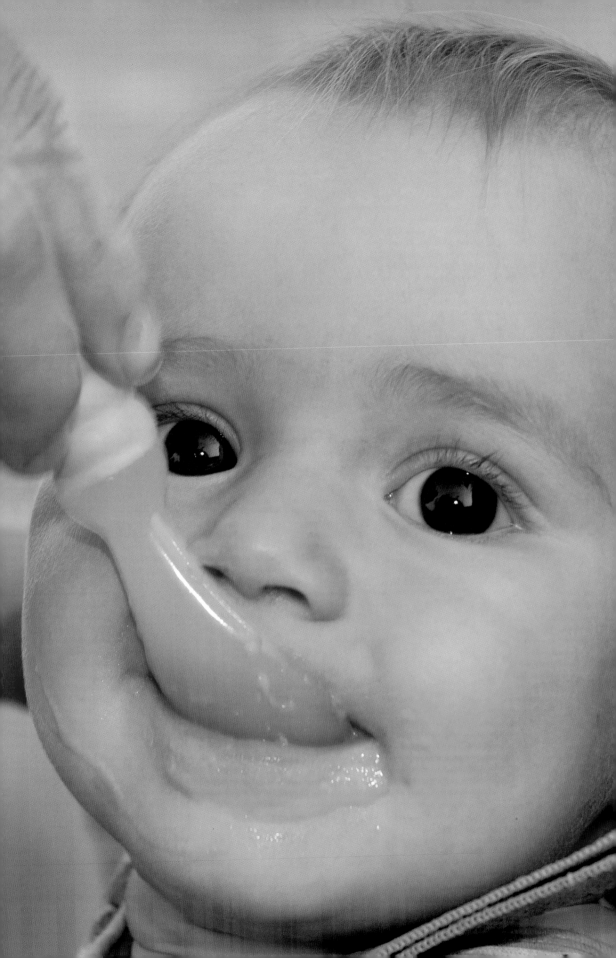

Corn Chowder

Great corn chowder was never easier than this!

1	can (10 oz/284 mL) cream of potato soup	1
½ cup	2% milk	125 mL
½ cup	canned cream-style corn	125 mL
1	small seeded and diced tomato	1
¼ tsp	dried thyme	1 mL
⅛ tsp	freshly ground black pepper	0.5 mL
¼ cup	shredded Cheddar or Monterey Jack cheese	50 mL

1. In a medium saucepan, combine soup, milk, corn, tomato, thyme and pepper. Bring to a boil, stirring constantly. Spoon into serving bowls. Sprinkle each with cheese. Let infant servings cool to a safe temperature.

NUTRITIONAL ANALYSIS (PER ½ CUP/125 ML)

Energy	Protein	Carbohydrate	Fat	Fiber	Calcium	Iron	Sodium
78 kcal	3 g	10 g	3 g	1 g	70 mg	0.4 mg	480 mg

Spinach Soup

Kitchen Tips

This recipe can be prepared in advance, up to the point of adding milk in Step 2. Purée can be frozen in portion sizes until ready to eat. Just defrost and add milk; season to taste with salt and pepper. Warm until heated through.

Use homemade or reduced-sodium stock to lower the sodium content of this recipe.

1 tbsp	butter or margarine	15 mL
½	medium onion, chopped	½
1	package (10 oz/284 mL) fresh spinach, washed, coarse stems removed	1
2 tbsp	all-purpose flour	25 mL
2 cups	chicken stock	500 mL
1	bay leaf	1
2 tbsp	chopped parsley	25 mL
1 cup	whole milk	250 mL
	Salt and freshly ground black pepper to taste	

1. In a large saucepan, melt butter over medium heat. Add onion and cook for about 5 minutes or until soft. Add spinach and cook, covered, for about 10 minutes longer. Sprinkle flour over mixture. Blend well. Add chicken stock, bay leaf and parsley; cook, uncovered, for about 15 minutes longer. Remove and discard bay leaf.
2. In a food processor or blender, purée soup in batches until smooth, transferring each batch to a saucepan. Stir in milk, salt and pepper. Heat until warmed through before serving.

NUTRITIONAL ANALYSIS (PER ½ CUP/125 ML)

Energy	Protein	Carbohydrate	Fat	Fiber	Calcium	Iron	Sodium
66 kcal	4 g	6 g	3 g	1 g	64 mg	0.1 mg	339 mg

Makes 4 cups (1 L)

Kitchen Tips

Chicken stock can be replaced by an equal quantity of canned reduced-sodium chicken broth, or water mixed with reduced-sodium chicken bouillon cubes or sachets. In the latter case, extra salt may not be needed.

For faster cooking time, use red lentils rather than brown or green ones.

Serving Suggestions

For extra calcium (and flavor), add a spoonful of plain yogurt or sour cream to each bowl.

Younger children may prefer this soup puréed in a blender or food processor for a smoother consistency.

Vegetable Lentil Soup

1 cup	shredded carrots	250 mL
½	small onion, finely chopped	½
1 cup	diced rutabaga or turnip	250 mL
1	small potato, cubed	1
1	clove garlic, minced	1
½ cup	red lentils (see tip)	125 mL
3 cups	chicken stock (see tip)	750 mL
1	bay leaf	1
	Salt and freshly ground black pepper	

1. In a large saucepan, combine carrots, onion, rutabaga, potato, garlic, lentils, stock and bay leaf. Bring to a boil. Reduce heat to low and simmer, covered, for 20 minutes or until vegetables and lentils are tender. Season to taste with salt and pepper. Remove and discard bay leaf before serving.

NUTRITIONAL ANALYSIS (PER ½ CUP/125 ML)

Energy	Protein	Carbohydrate	Fat	Fiber	Calcium	Iron	Sodium
107 kcal	6 g	18 g	1 g	2 g	25 mg	2 mg	157 mg

Makes 5½ cups (1.375 L)

Fantastic Black Bean Soup

2 tsp	vegetable oil	10 mL
2 tsp	minced garlic	10 mL
1 cup	chopped onions	250 mL
1 cup	chopped carrots	250 mL
1	can (19 oz/540 mL) black beans, rinsed and drained	1
3 cups	chicken stock	750 mL
¾ tsp	ground cumin	4 mL
¼ cup	chopped parsley	50 mL

1. In a large skillet, heat oil over medium-high heat. Add garlic, onions and carrots; cook for 4 to 5 minutes or until onions are softened. Stir in beans, chicken stock and cumin; bring to a boil. Reduce heat to medium-low and simmer, covered, for about 20 to 25 minutes or until the carrots are soft.

2. In a food processor or blender, purée soup in batches until smooth. Sprinkle with parsley before serving.

NUTRITIONAL ANALYSIS (PER ½ CUP/125 ML)

Energy	Protein	Carbohydrate	Fat	Fiber	Calcium	Iron	Sodium
94 kcal	5 g	14 g	2 g	3 g	28 mg	1 mg	107 mg

Tomato Minestrone

Most versions of minestrone — Italy's national soup — contain tomatoes, macaroni and, frequently, beans. This version features plenty of vegetables and macaroni, but no beans.

Kitchen Tips

Beef stock can be replaced by an equal quantity of canned reduced-sodium beef broth, or water mixed with reduced-sodium beef bouillon cubes or sachets.

For younger children, this soup can be puréed (or pressed through a sieve) to give it a smoother, thicker consistency.

1 tsp	olive oil	5 mL
½ cup	finely chopped onions	125 mL
1	small carrot, chopped	1
1	small zucchini, chopped	1
1	stalk celery, sliced	1
1 cup	diced tomatoes	250 mL
1	clove garlic, minced	1
3 cups	beef stock (see tip)	750 mL
¼ tsp	dried basil	1 mL
¼ tsp	dried oregano	1 mL
¼ tsp	salt	1 mL
¼ cup	dry macaroni	50 mL
	Grated Parmesan cheese (optional)	

1. In a large saucepan, heat oil over medium heat. Add onions and cook for 5 minutes or until softened. Add carrot, zucchini, celery, tomatoes, garlic, stock, basil, oregano and salt. Cover and bring to a boil. Reduce heat and simmer for about 15 minutes.

2. Add macaroni and cook for 10 minutes or until macaroni is tender. Serve sprinkled with Parmesan, if using.

NUTRITIONAL ANALYSIS (PER ½ CUP/125 ML)							
Energy	Protein	Carbohydrate	Fat	Fiber	Calcium	Iron	Sodium
51 kcal	2.5 g	8 g	1 g	1 g	15 mg	0.3 mg	87 mg

Makes 6½ cups (1.625 L)

Kitchen Tips

Serve with hot bread or buns.

Use homemade or reduced-sodium stock to lower the sodium content of this recipe.

Apple and Butternut Squash Soup

4 cups	chicken stock	1 L
1	medium butternut squash, peeled, seeded and cut into 2-inch (5 cm) cubes	1
2	medium tart apples, peeled, cored and sliced	2
1¼ cups	chopped onions	300 mL
1 tsp	salt	5 mL
½ tsp	freshly ground black pepper	2 mL
½ tsp	dried rosemary	2 mL
½ tsp	dried thyme	2 mL
¼ cup	milk	50 mL

1. In a large pot, combine stock, squash, apples, onions, salt, pepper, rosemary and thyme. Bring to a boil. Reduce heat and simmer for 15 minutes or until vegetables are tender. Remove from heat and stir in milk. Let soup cool slightly

2. In a food processor or blender, purée soup in batches until smooth, transferring each batch to a saucepan. Bring to a boil before serving.

NUTRITIONAL ANALYSIS (PER ½ CUP/125 ML)

Energy	Protein	Carbohydrate	Fat	Fiber	Calcium	Iron	Sodium
45 kcal	1 g	10 g	1 g	1 g	32 mg	0.5 mg	486 mg

Makes 4 cups (1 L)

Enjoy this easy-to-prepare soup on cold days. The aroma and flavors are classic.

Kitchen Tip

Depending on the age of your child, you can purée this soup or serve it as is. Because it cooks for so long, the soup has a very smooth, thick consistency, with just a few tender chunks.

Split Pea Soup

1 cup	dried split peas, washed	250 mL
6 cups	water	1.5 L
1 cup	finely chopped ham or 4 slices bacon, diced	250 mL
1	medium onion, chopped	1
1	stalk celery, chopped	1
1	medium carrot, peeled and chopped	1
	Salt and freshly ground black pepper to taste	

1. In a large saucepan, combine peas, water, ham, onion, celery and carrot. Bring to a boil; reduce heat to low and simmer for 2 hours or until vegetables and peas are tender. Remove from heat and let cool slightly.

2. In a food processor or blender, purée soup in batches until smooth (see tip). Season to taste with salt and pepper before serving.

NUTRITIONAL ANALYSIS (PER ½ CUP/125 ML)

Energy	Protein	Carbohydrate	Fat	Fiber	Calcium	Iron	Sodium
126 kcal	10 g	19 g	2 g	2 g	30 mg	1 mg	246 mg

Makes 8 cups (2 L)

This soup is really easy to make and freezes well.

Kitchen Tips

This soup is great for preparing in a slow cooker. Just add all ingredients and cook on High for 8 to 10 hours or Low for 10 to 12 hours.

Beef stock can be replaced with canned reduced-sodium beef stock or reduced-sodium bouillon cubes; in this case, you may not need additional salt.

Beef Barley Soup

¼ cup	pearl barley	50 mL
6 cups	beef stock or bouillon, divided	1.5 L
2 tbsp	butter or margarine	25 mL
1	onion, chopped	1
2	carrots, chopped	2
½	turnip, chopped	½
1	stalk celery, chopped	1
2 cups	diced cooked stewing beef	500 mL
	Salt and freshly ground black pepper to taste	

1. In a large pot, combine barley with 3 cups (750 mL) of the beef stock. Simmer over low heat for 1½ to 2 hours. Add butter.
2. In a saucepan, combine onion, carrots, turnip, celery and remaining beef stock. Cook over medium heat for 20 minutes or until tender. Pour vegetables and stock into pot with barley mixture. Season to taste with the salt and pepper. Add cooked meat just before serving.

NUTRITIONAL ANALYSIS (PER ½ CUP/125 ML)

Energy	Protein	Carbohydrate	Fat	Fiber	Calcium	Iron	Sodium
90 kcal	10 g	4 g	3 g	1 g	16 mg	1 mg	578 mg

Makes 7 cups (1.75 L)

Kitchen Tips

This recipe is easily converted into chicken noodle soup by omitting the rice and adding 1½ cups (375) cooked egg noodles.

Use homemade or reduced-sodium stock to lower the sodium content of this recipe.

Chicken Rice Soup

5 cups	chicken stock	1.25 L
¼ cup	chopped onion	50 mL
½ cup	chopped celery	125 mL
½ cup	chopped carrots	125 mL
¾ tsp	salt	4 mL
⅛ tsp	freshly ground black pepper	0.5 mL
3 tbsp	long-grain rice	50 mL
1 cup	chopped cooked chicken	250 mL

1. In a large pot, combine stock. onion, celery, carrots, salt and pepper. Bring to a boil. Reduce heat and simmer until the vegetables are tender. Add rice and cook for about 15 minutes or until tender. Add cooked chicken and simmer for another 5 minutes.

NUTRITIONAL ANALYSIS (PER ½ CUP/125 ML)

Energy	Protein	Carbohydrate	Fat	Fiber	Calcium	Iron	Sodium
62 kcal	5 g	6 g	1 g	0.3 g	9 mg	0.4 mg	274 mg

Makes 7 cups (1.75 L)

Kitchen Tip
Use homemade or reduced-sodium stock to lower the sodium content of this recipe.

Cauliflower Soup

1 tbsp	butter or margarine	15 mL
8 oz	cauliflower, chopped	250 g
2	onions, chopped	2
4	stalks celery, chopped	4
3 tbsp	all-purpose flour	45 mL
4 cups	chicken stock or vegetable stock	1 L
1	bay leaf	1
	Salt and freshly ground black pepper to taste	
⅔ cup	milk or cream	150 mL
1 tbsp	chopped parsley	15 mL

1. In a large saucepan, melt butter over medium heat. Add cauliflower, onions and celery and cook for 2 minutes. Do *not* brown. Stir in flour and cook for another minute. Remove from heat. Add stock, bay leaf, salt and pepper. Simmer for about 1 hour, until vegetables are tender. Remove and discard bay leaf.

2. If desired, transfer in batches to a food processor and process until smooth. Add milk and parsley. Reheat and serve.

NUTRITIONAL ANALYSIS (PER ½ CUP/125 ML)

Energy	Protein	Carbohydrate	Fat	Fiber	Calcium	Iron	Sodium
52 kcal	3 g	6 g	2 g	0.5 g	25 mg	0.3 mg	121 mg

Makes 4 cups (1 L)

This easy-to-prepare vegetarian soup is made from ingredients usually found in your kitchen cupboard.

Kitchen Tips

If you prefer, the soup can be cooked in the microwave oven on High for about 5 minutes; stir once. Let cool, checking temperature before serving to infants.

Save any leftovers for another meal.

Sandwich 'n' Soup in a Bowl

1	can (14 oz/398 mL) diced tomatoes	1
1	can (14 oz/398 mL) beans in tomato sauce	1
¾ cup	water	175 mL
½ tsp	dried basil	2 mL
½ tsp	dried oregano	2 mL
⅛ tsp	salt	0.5 mL
⅛ tsp	freshly ground black pepper	0.5 mL
4	slices whole wheat bread	4
½ cup	shredded mozzarella cheese	125 mL

1. In a large saucepan, combine tomatoes, beans, water, basil, oregano and salt. Bring to a boil. Reduce heat to low and simmer, covered, for 10 minutes. (Soup can also be cooked in microwave; see tip.)
2. Meanwhile, toast bread. Cut each slice into cubes.
3. Spoon 1 cup (250 mL) soup into each bowl (or about ¼ cup/50 mL for an infant's portion). Garnish with bread cubes and sprinkle with cheese. For larger portions, microwave bowls for a few seconds on High or until cheese melts. Infant portions need not be heated; cheese will melt from the heat of the soup as it cools to a baby-friendly serving temperature.

NUTRITIONAL ANALYSIS (PER ½ CUP/125 ML)

Energy	Protein	Carbohydrate	Fat	Fiber	Calcium	Iron	Sodium
128 kcal	6 g	23 g	2 g	4 g	102 mg	2 mg	448 mg

Cock-a-Leekie Soup

Makes 7 cups (1.75 L)

Kitchen Tips

For a hearty, chunky soup, serve without puréeing.

If you'd prefer a clearer soup, replace milk with additional chicken stock.

Do not add salt if using canned broth.

Use homemade or reduced-sodium stock to lower the sodium content of this recipe.

1 tbsp	butter or margarine	15 mL
3	leeks, washed and sliced	3
1½ tbsp	all-purpose flour	22 mL
3	large potatoes, peeled and chopped	3
2 or 3	stalks celery, chopped	2 or 3
2½ cups	chicken stock	625 mL
1	bay leaf	1
	Salt and freshly ground black pepper to taste	
1¼ cups	milk or cream	300 mL
1 tbsp	chopped parsley	15 mL

1. In a large saucepan, melt butter over medium heat. Add leeks and cook for 1 minute. Add flour and cook for another minute. Stir in potatoes and celery. Add chicken stock, bay leaf, salt and pepper. Simmer for 1 hour or until vegetables are very tender. Remove and discard bay leaf.
2. Transfer soup in batches to a food processor and process until smooth. (Alternatively, you can mash the solids by hand). Add milk and parsley. Reheat and serve.

NUTRITIONAL ANALYSIS (PER ½ CUP/125 ML)

Energy	Protein	Carbohydrate	Fat	Fiber	Calcium	Iron	Sodium
81 kcal	3 g	13 g	2 g	1 g	45 mg	1 mg	87 mg

Mexican Bean Tortilla Soup

2 tbsp	canola oil	25 mL
4	6-inch (15 cm) corn tortillas, cut into thin strips	4
½ cup	finely chopped onion	125 mL
1	clove garlic, minced	1
½ cup	diced celery	125 mL
1	can (14 oz/398 mL) stewed tomatoes	1
2 cups	reduced-sodium or homemade chicken or vegetable broth	500 mL
1 cup	drained and rinsed canned black beans	250 mL
1 to 2 tsp	chili powder	5 to 10 mL
½ cup	diced Cheddar or mozzarella cheese (about 4 oz/125 g)	125 mL

1. In a nonstick skillet, heat oil over medium-high heat. Add tortilla strips and fry for about 2 minutes or until crisp but not brown. Remove to paper towels to drain, leaving remaining oil in the pan.

2. Add onion to skillet and sauté for 5 minutes or until tender. Add garlic, celery, tomatoes, broth, black beans and chili powder and bring to a boil. Cover, reduce heat and simmer for about 10 minutes or until vegetables are tender. Stir in cheese until melted.

3. Divide the tortilla strips among serving bowls and top with soup.

NUTRITIONAL ANALYSIS (PER ½ CUP/125 ML)

Energy	Protein	Carbohydrate	Fat	Fiber	Calcium	Iron	Sodium
158 kcal	5 g	18 g	8 g	1 g	105 mg	2 mg	387 mg

Makes 8 servings

Deviled eggs are a favorite with all ages — particularly infants. The eggs are somewhat "squishy" when held in small hands (which is half the fun), and the messy fingers are great for licking.

Kitchen Tips

If you or your family don't care for cottage cheese, omit it and use extra mayonnaise.

To hard-cook eggs: Place cold eggs in a single layer in a saucepan. Add enough water to cover eggs by at least 1 inch (2.5 cm). Bring to a full boil. Remove pan from heat, cover and let eggs stand in hot water for 20 to 25 minutes. Run cold water over eggs until they are completely cooled. Hard-cooked eggs, peeled or in their shells, can be refrigerated for up to 1 week. If peeled, they are best stored in a plastic bag or other airtight plastic container.

Food Safety Tip

Refrigerating prepared eggs will help reduce the risk of food-borne illnesses. Make sure the refrigerator is set to a temperature of 40°F (4°C).

Deviled Eggs

4	hard-cooked eggs (see tip), peeled	4
½ cup	cottage cheese (see tip)	125 mL
2 tbsp	mayonnaise	25 mL
1 tbsp	finely diced onion	15 mL
¼ tsp	salt	1 mL
⅛ tsp	freshly ground black pepper	0.5 mL
⅛ tsp	paprika	0.5 mL

1. Cut each egg in half lengthwise. Remove yolks and transfer to a small bowl; mash together with cottage cheese, mayonnaise and onion. Stir in salt and pepper.

2. Fill egg whites with yolk mixture; sprinkle lightly with paprika. For best flavor, cover and refrigerate for about 1 hour before serving.

NUTRITIONAL ANALYSIS (PER ½ EGG)

Energy	Protein	Carbohydrate	Fat	Fiber	Calcium	Iron	Sodium
65 kcal	5 g	2 g	4 g	–	24 mg	0.3 mg	173 mg

Makes 32 bites

Serve these small quiche-like squares for baby lunches or snacks — or as appetizers for parents.

Kitchen Tip

Leave salmon bones in — they're an excellent source of calcium — but mash well before serving to a small child.

Food Safety Tip

Prepare foods quickly, cook them thoroughly and serve immediately. Don't let potentially unsafe foods linger at room temperature, where bacteria can grow quickly.

Salmon Bites

Preheat oven to 350°F (180°C)
8-inch (2 L) square baking pan, greased

1 cup	cottage cheese	250 mL
½	package (8 oz/250 g) cream cheese	½
3	eggs	3
1 tbsp	lemon juice	15 mL
¼ tsp	salt	1 mL
¼ tsp	dried thyme	1 mL
1	can (7½ oz/213 g) salmon, drained	1
¼ cup	finely chopped onion	50 mL

1. In a food processor or blender, combine cottage cheese, cream cheese, eggs, lemon juice, salt and thyme; process until smooth. Transfer mixture to a bowl.

2. In another bowl, flake salmon; mash bones. Stir salmon into cheese-egg mixture. Stir in onion.

3. Spoon mixture into prepared pan. Bake in a preheated oven for 40 minutes or until a knife inserted in center comes out clean. Remove from oven and let stand for 5 minutes before cutting into small fingers.

NUTRITIONAL ANALYSIS (PER BITE)

Energy	Protein	Carbohydrate	Fat	Fiber	Calcium	Iron	Sodium
38 kcal	3 g	1 g	2 g	–	26 mg	0.1 mg	86 mg

Makes 1¾ cups (425 mL)

Kitchen Tips

If your child does not have an allergy, eggs are a great source of protein.

The curry in this recipe is not overwhelming and adds a slightly different twist to an old favorite.

Egg Salad

5	hard-cooked eggs (see tip, page 174), finely chopped	5
½	small onion, finely chopped	½
¼ cup	mayonnaise	50 mL
Pinch	curry powder	Pinch
Pinch	freshly ground black pepper	Pinch

1. In a bowl, combine all ingredients and mix well. Use for sandwiches or serve filling on its own.

NUTRITIONAL ANALYSIS (PER ¼ CUP/50 ML)

Energy	Protein	Carbohydrate	Fat	Fiber	Calcium	Iron	Sodium
106 kcal	5 g	1 g	9 g	–	23 mg	1 mg	168 mg

Makes 16 squares

Many parents tell us that even the fussiest child can almost always be persuaded to eat a ham sandwich. This variation on the simple slice-of-ham type of sandwich adds a little more interest.

Ham Salad Sandwich

¾ cup	diced ham	175 mL
¼ cup	shredded Cheddar cheese	50 mL
1 tbsp	finely minced green onion	15 mL
2 tbsp	mayonnaise	25 mL
2 tbsp	butter or margarine	25 mL
8	slices whole wheat bread, crusts removed if desired	8

1. In a small bowl, stir together ham, cheese, onion and mayonnaise.

2. Thinly spread each bread slice with butter. Spread 4 slices with ¼ cup (50 mL) filling. Top with remaining slices. Cut each sandwich into 4 squares and serve.

NUTRITIONAL ANALYSIS (PER SQUARE)

Energy	Protein	Carbohydrate	Fat	Fiber	Calcium	Iron	Sodium
79 kcal	4 g	8 g	4 g	1 g	26 mg	1 mg	222 mg

Sloppy Joe Sauce

Kitchen Tip

This versatile sauce is a great source of iron for the whole family. It freezes well and can be quickly thawed and heated for an instant lunch or dinner.

1 lb	lean ground beef	500 g
1	onion, finely chopped	1
1	can (28 oz/796 mL) tomatoes, crushed	1
1 tbsp	vinegar	15 mL
1 tsp	brown sugar	5 mL
1 tsp	Worcestershire sauce	5 mL
1 tsp	prepared mustard	5 mL
1 tbsp	ketchup	15 mL
	Whole wheat hot dog or hamburger buns	

1. In a frying pan over medium-high heat, cook ground beef, breaking up meat with a spoon, until browned. Drain off fat. With a slotted spoon, transfer beef to a paper towel–lined plate or colander to drain.

2. Add onions to frying pan and sauté until soft. Return beef to pan, along with tomatoes, vinegar, brown sugar, Worcestershire sauce, mustard and ketchup. Simmer over low heat, stirring occasionally, for about 45 minutes or until thick.

3. Serve on hot dog or hamburger buns.

NUTRITIONAL ANALYSIS (PER ½ CUP/125 ML)

Energy	Protein	Carbohydrate	Fat	Fiber	Calcium	Iron	Sodium
110 kcal	10 g	8 g	5 g	1 g	37 mg	2 mg	234 mg

Tuna and Corn Patties

Just about everyone has a can of tuna or salmon in their kitchen cupboard. Either works well in these great-tasting patties.

Kitchen Tip

This recipe provides an excellent use for corn left over from Corn Chowder (see recipe, page 161).

Food Safety Tip

Make time in your schedule to regularly sanitize countertops, cutting boards and utensils with a mild solution of bleach and water. Gives the kitchen that extra-fresh scent!

1½ cups	packaged biscuit mix	375 mL
½ tsp	dried dill	2 mL
1	can (6½ oz/184 g) tuna, drained and flaked	1
1 cup	cream-style corn	250 mL
1 tbsp	finely chopped onion	15 mL
2	eggs	2
½ cup	whole milk	125 mL
2 tsp	vegetable oil, divided	10 mL

1. In a bowl, combine biscuit mix and dill. Set aside.
2. In another bowl, combine tuna, corn, onion, eggs and milk; stir to mix well. Stir in biscuit-dill mixture.
3. In a skillet, heat 1 tsp (5 mL) of the oil over medium-high heat. Using a ¼-cup (50 mL) measure for each patty, drop batter into skillet and cook for about 3 minutes or until bubbles break on surface; turn and cook second side until golden brown. Repeat procedure with remaining batter, adding more oil if needed.

NUTRITIONAL ANALYSIS (PER PATTY)

Energy	Protein	Carbohydrate	Fat	Fiber	Calcium	Iron	Sodium
123 kcal	5 g	15 g	5 g	1 g	48 mg	1 mg	319 mg

Makes 12 baby servings, or 4 adult servings

An easy oven luncheon for wintertime, or anytime, this custard combines carrots (some children's favorite vegetable) with eggs and cheese.

Kitchen Tip

Zucchini makes a good replacement for carrots in this recipe.

Carrot 'n' Cheese Crustless Quiche

Preheat oven to 300°F (150°C)
8-inch (2 L) square cake pan, greased

1 tbsp	butter or margarine	15 mL
½	small onion, finely chopped	½
1 cup	grated carrots (about 2 medium)	250 mL
½ tsp	salt	2 mL
½ tsp	curry powder (optional)	2 mL
4	eggs	4
⅔ cup	2% milk	150 mL
1 cup	shredded mozzarella cheese	250 mL
	Paprika	

1. In a skillet, heat butter over medium heat. Add onion and sauté for 5 minutes. Add carrots, salt and curry powder, if using; cook for 5 minutes or until golden brown. Remove from heat; let cool.

2. In a medium bowl, whisk together eggs and milk; stir into vegetable mixture. Pour into prepared baking pan. Bake in preheated oven for 20 minutes.

3. Remove quiche from oven. Top with cheese and sprinkle with paprika. Return to oven and bake for another 15 minutes or until custard is firm and cheese is melted. Cut into squares to serve.

NUTRITIONAL ANALYSIS (PER BABY SERVING)

Energy	Protein	Carbohydrate	Fat	Fiber	Calcium	Iron	Sodium
75 kcal	5 g	3 g	5 g	0.4 g	98 mg	0.2 mg	171 mg

Makes 1 serving

Leftovers — what to do with them? When it comes to cooked rice, just add them to eggs and do a fast scramble.

Rice 'n' Scrambled Egg

1 tsp	butter or margarine	5 mL
1	egg	1
¼ cup	cold cooked rice	50 mL
1 tbsp	2% milk	15 mL
Pinch	freshly ground black pepper	Pinch

1. In a small skillet, melt butter over medium-low heat.

2. In a bowl, stir together egg, rice and milk. Pour into skillet; cook, stirring frequently, for about 2 minutes or until egg is cooked to desired consistency. Season to taste with pepper.

NUTRITIONAL ANALYSIS

Energy	Protein	Carbohydrate	Fat	Fiber	Calcium	Iron	Sodium
158 kcal	8 g	10 g	9 g	0.1 g	51 mg	1 mg	97 mg

Makes 2 cups (500 mL)

This combination of cheese and vegetables is bound to entice children to eat their vegetables.

Vegetables with Cheese

1 cup	thinly sliced carrots	250 mL
1 cup	thinly sliced zucchini	250 mL
½ cup	shredded Cheddar cheese	125 mL
2 tbsp	milk	25 mL
½ tsp	dried basil	2 mL

1. In a small saucepan, combine carrots and zucchini with just enough water to cover. Bring to a boil; cook for 10 minutes or until tender. Drain. Stir in cheese, milk and basil. Return saucepan to low heat; cook until warmed through and cheese melts.

NUTRITIONAL ANALYSIS (PER ¼ CUP/50 ML)

Energy	Protein	Carbohydrate	Fat	Fiber	Calcium	Iron	Sodium
62 kcal	3 g	3 g	3 g	1 g	105 mg	0.2 mg	279 mg

Makes 8 baby servings, or 2 adult servings

Here's a healthy, vegetable-packed version of classic mac and cheese! Use any vegetables that appeal to your family. Little ones are always fascinated by macaroni's squishy texture.

Kitchen Tip

Use leftover cooked vegetables or frozen mixed vegetables, thawed.

Macaroni and Vegetables with Cheese

Preheat oven to 350°F (180°C)
3-cup (750 mL) casserole dish, greased

¾ cup	dry macaroni	175 mL
2 cups	water	500 mL
1½ cups	shredded medium Cheddar cheese, divided	375 mL
1 tbsp	butter or margarine	15 mL
½ cup	whole milk	125 mL
¾ cup	mixed cooked vegetables (such as carrots, peas, corn, broccoli and/or green beans)	175 mL
½ cup	coarse whole wheat bread crumbs	125 mL

1. In a medium saucepan, cook macaroni in boiling water according to package directions or until tender but firm. Drain. Add 1 cup (250 mL) of the cheese, butter, milk and vegetables. Stir until cheese is melted.

2. Spoon into prepared casserole dish; top with crumbs and remaining cheese. Bake in preheated oven for 25 minutes or until crumbs are brown and macaroni is hot.

NUTRITIONAL ANALYSIS (PER BABY SERVING)							
Energy	Protein	Carbohydrate	Fat	Fiber	Calcium	Iron	Sodium
183 kcal	8 g	15 g	9 g	1 g	191 mg	1 mg	209 mg

A colorful and interesting combination of foods, and a terrific meatless meal option, this casserole is well suited to any finger-eaters in your family, and it's quick and easy to make. Omit the kidney beans if you wish, but they do provide extra protein and fiber.

Kitchen Tips

Mixed vegetables are usually a combination of frozen peas, corn, green beans and carrots cut into small pieces.

Any kidney beans and tomato soup leftovers can be used another day to make chili.

Lunchtime Pasta and Bean Casserole

½ cup	shell pasta	125 mL
½ cup	frozen mixed vegetables (see tip)	125 mL
½ cup	canned kidney beans, rinsed and drained (optional)	125 mL
¼ cup	shredded mozzarella or Cheddar cheese	50 mL
¼ cup	reduced-sodium tomato soup	50 mL
¼ cup	milk	50 mL
⅛ tsp	salt	0.5 mL
⅛ tsp	freshly ground black pepper	0.5 mL

1. In a medium saucepan, cook pasta in boiling water for 5 minutes, until it is just beginning to soften. Add mixed vegetables. Return to a boil and cook until pasta is tender but firm. Drain well.
2. Add kidney beans, if using, and cheese; stir until cheese has melted. Stir in tomato soup and milk. Season to taste with salt and pepper.

NUTRITIONAL ANALYSIS (PER ½ CUP/125 ML)							
Energy	Protein	Carbohydrate	Fat	Fiber	Calcium	Iron	Sodium
134 kcal	7 g	22 g	2 g	3 g	84 mg	2 mg	195 mg

Makes 2 baby servings

Cook this up when little appetites can't wait another minute. For fastest preparation, keep cooked broccoli and cooked pasta on hand in the refrigerator. Broccoli's vitamins and minerals, and pasta's protein make this a nutritious meal.

Kitchen Tip

Use homemade or reduced-sodium stock to lower the sodium content of this recipe. If you don't have stock, use ½ tsp (2 mL) reduced-sodium liquid chicken or vegetable bouillon concentrate with enough added water to make ¼ cup (50 mL).

Variation

Other vegetables can replace (or be added to) broccoli. Try cooked carrots, peas, corn or mixed vegetables.

Broccoli with Pasta

1 tsp	olive oil	5 mL
2 tbsp	finely chopped onion	25 mL
¼ cup	chicken or vegetable stock (see tip)	50 mL
¼ cup	chopped cooked broccoli	50 mL
½ cup	cooked macaroni or other pasta	125 mL
1 tsp	grated Parmesan cheese	5 mL

1. In a small skillet, heat oil on medium heat. Add onion and cook for 3 minutes. Add broth, broccoli and pasta; cook, covered, until just heated through. Add cheese; toss and serve.

NUTRITIONAL ANALYSIS (PER BABY SERVING)

Energy	Protein	Carbohydrate	Fat	Fiber	Calcium	Iron	Sodium
95 kcal	3 g	13 g	3 g	1 g	22 mg	1 mg	63 mg

Makes 6½ cups (1.625 L)

So easy and fast to make, yet delicious and tasty. Adjust the amount of hot pepper sauce used to individual tastes — a good way to introduce kids to spicier foods.

Kitchen Tips

Start with the lesser quantity of hot pepper sauce for children who are not used to spicier food.

Use reduced-sodium soy sauce and homemade or reduced-sodium stock to lower the sodium content of this recipe.

Junior Hot-and-Sour Soup

6 cups	chicken stock	1.5 L
3 tbsp	soy sauce	45 mL
4 tsp	ground ginger	20 mL
1 tbsp	rice vinegar	15 mL
2 tsp	granulated sugar	10 mL
½ to 1 tsp	hot pepper sauce (see tip)	2 to 5 mL
1 tsp	sesame oil	5 mL
4 oz	silken tofu, diced	125 g
2	green onions, sliced	2

1. In a large saucepan, combine stock with soy sauce, ginger, vinegar, sugar, hot pepper sauce and sesame oil. Bring to a boil. Add tofu and green onions. Cook for 1 minute longer and serve.

NUTRITIONAL ANALYSIS (PER ½ CUP/125 ML)

Energy	Protein	Carbohydrate	Fat	Fiber	Calcium	Iron	Sodium
54 kcal	3 g	5 g	2 g	0.1 g	8 mg	0.4 mg	351 mg

In Spanish, queso *means cheese. Combine it with a tortilla, and you end up with a quesadilla. This dish is ideal for young ones — small enough to clutch easily, and the filling keeps the tortillas from falling apart.*

Mexican Quesadilla Sandwich

2	9-inch (22.5 cm) flour tortillas	2
½ tbsp	salsa or ketchup	7 mL
¼ cup	shredded Cheddar cheese	50 mL
¼ cup	canned beans in tomato sauce, mashed	50 mL

1. Place 1 tortilla on a microwave-safe plate lined with paper towels. Spread with salsa.

2. In a small bowl, combine cheese and beans. Spoon mixture evenly over tortilla. Press second tortilla over bean mixture.

3. Microwave at Medium-High for 2 minutes or until tortillas are warm and cheese has melted. (For a crisper tortilla, bake in a preheated 350°F (180°C) oven for 10 minutes.) With sharp knife, cut into 8 small pie-shaped pieces. Let cool before serving.

NUTRITIONAL ANALYSIS (PER WEDGE)

Energy	Protein	Carbohydrate	Fat	Fiber	Calcium	Iron	Sodium
56 kcal	2 g	7 g	2 g	1 g	43 mg	0.5 mg	123 mg

Makes 1 serving

Make a slice of ham and cheese into something different from "just another sandwich."

Variation

Replace ham with flaked tuna or salmon. Combine fish, cheese and mayonnaise. Spread on each bread slice and broil as directed in recipe.

Ham and Cheese Melt

Preheat broiler
Baking sheet

¼ cup	diced cooked ham	50 mL
¼ cup	shredded Cheddar cheese	50 mL
1 tsp	mayonnaise	5 mL
1	slice whole wheat or multigrain bread	1

1. In a bowl, combine ham, cheese and mayonnaise. Spread mixture on bread. Transfer bread to baking sheet. Broil just until cheese starts to melt. Remove from heat and let cool. Cut into small pieces before serving.

NUTRITIONAL ANALYSIS

Energy	Protein	Carbohydrate	Fat	Fiber	Calcium	Iron	Sodium
282 kcal	18 g	18 g	16 g	2 g	233 mg	2 mg	920 mg

Makes 8 wedges

Kitchen Tip

Be careful when microwaving food for young children. It can quickly become hot enough to burn their sensitive mouths.

Turkey Pita Wedges

1 cup	shredded Cheddar cheese	250 mL
1 cup	chopped cooked turkey or chicken	250 mL
½	red bell pepper, cored and thinly sliced	½
2	whole wheat pita breads, quartered	2

1. In a small bowl, combine cheese, turkey and red pepper. Stuff each pita quarter with turkey mixture. Microwave on High for 30 seconds or until the cheese melts. Repeat procedure with remaining quarters. Serve immediately.

NUTRITIONAL ANALYSIS (PER WEDGE)

Energy	Protein	Carbohydrate	Fat	Fiber	Calcium	Iron	Sodium
136 kcal	10 g	10 g	6 g	1 g	110 mg	1 mg	193 mg

Makes 8 pockets

Kitchen Tip

Instead of pita bread, serve filling on a bed of lettuce.

Broccoli and Chicken Pita Pockets

½	medium head broccoli, florets cut into bite-size pieces	½
1 cup	diced cooked chicken	250 mL
2 tbsp	diced celery	25 mL
2 tbsp	diced radish	25 mL
2½ tbsp	mayonnaise	32 mL
2 tbsp	plain yogurt	25 mL
½ tsp	Dijon mustard	2 mL
Pinch	dried rosemary, crushed	Pinch
Pinch	salt	Pinch
2	pita breads, quartered	2

1. In a large saucepan, blanch the broccoli in boiling water for 1 minute. Drain and rinse under cold water. Drain again.

2. In a large bowl, combine broccoli, chicken, celery and radish. Set aside.

3. In another large bowl, combine mayonnaise, yogurt, mustard, rosemary and salt. Stir in broccoli mixture. Cover and chill for 1 hour.

4. Spoon the chilled mixture into the pita pieces.

NUTRITIONAL ANALYSIS (PER POCKET)

Energy	Protein	Carbohydrate	Fat	Fiber	Calcium	Iron	Sodium
92 kcal	6 g	13 g	2 g	2 g	30 mg	1 mg	212 mg

Makes 1¼ cups (300 mL) filling

This smooth chickpea mixture makes a delicious filling for pita breads. Use miniature pitas for little people — they are easier for small hands to hold. The rather sticky filling holds the pita together, much like peanut butter.

Kitchen Tips

Try adding garnishes to the top of the filled pita — such as chopped tomato, green pepper and shredded lettuce.

Keep any leftover filling in the refrigerator for nutritious snacks. It will keep for several days.

Food Safety Tip

Be careful about spreading the filling too thick when serving to young children. Like peanut butter, it should be spread thinly to prevent choking.

Falafel-Style Pitas

1 tsp	olive oil	5 mL
½	small onion, finely chopped	½
1	clove garlic, minced	1
1 tbsp	sesame seeds	15 mL
1 cup	canned chickpeas, rinsed and drained	250 mL
½ cup	plain yogurt	125 mL
⅛ tsp	ground cumin	0.5 mL
⅛ tsp	salt	0.5 mL
⅛ tsp	freshly ground black pepper	0.5 mL
2½	whole wheat pita breads (or use miniature pitas)	2½
2 tbsp	shredded mild Cheddar cheese	25 mL

1. In a nonstick skillet, heat oil over medium heat. Add onion, garlic and sesame seeds; cook for 4 minutes or until onion is tender. Let cool slightly.
2. In a food processor, combine onion mixture, chickpeas, yogurt, cumin, salt and pepper; process until smooth.
3. Cut regular-sized pitas into halves. Spoon a small amount of mixture into each half and top with a little cheese. (If using miniature pitas, open one side and spoon about 1 tbsp/15 mL filling into each.)
4. Place each pita on a paper towel–lined microwave-safe plate; microwave at High for 10 seconds (for miniature pitas) or 30 seconds (for regular size), until cheese has just melted.

NUTRITIONAL ANALYSIS (PER ¼ PITA)

Energy	Protein	Carbohydrate	Fat	Fiber	Calcium	Iron	Sodium
97 kcal	4 g	15 g	2 g	3 g	64 mg	1.1 mg	120 mg

Makes 4 servings

These burritos are ready in minutes from the microwave oven — the perfect fast fix for a last-minute lunch or dinner.

Kitchen Tip

You may want to cut each burrito into smaller pieces for your toddler.

Vegetable Burritos

1	plum tomato, chopped	1
1	small carrot, peeled and thinly sliced	1
4	strips green pepper	4
½ cup	mashed black beans, divided	125 mL
2	8-inch (20 cm) flour tortillas	2
½ cup	shredded mozzarella or Cheddar cheese, divided	125 mL
⅛ tsp	dried basil	0.5 mL
⅛ tsp	dried oregano	0.5 mL

1. In a microwave-safe container, combine tomato, carrot and green pepper. Cover and microwave on High for 2 minutes or until vegetables are tender.

2. Spoon ¼ cup (50 mL) beans down the center of each tortilla; top with some of the vegetable mixture and ¼ cup (50 mL) cheese. Fold sides of tortillas into the center. Fold bottom over filling and roll up. Place on a microwave-safe dish. Microwave at Medium-High for 5 minutes or until burritos are warm. Let cool to a safe temperature before serving to children.

NUTRITIONAL ANALYSIS (PER ½ BURRITO)

Energy	Protein	Carbohydrate	Fat	Fiber	Calcium	Iron	Sodium
158 kcal	7 g	18 g	6 g	4 g	133 mg	1 mg	280 mg

Makes 12 baby servings, or 4 adult servings

Quiches are a great way to add protein, milk, and fruit or vegetables to a meal. This version is popular with both infants and adults.

Cheddar 'n' Apple Quiche

Preheat oven to 350°F (180°C)
9-inch (23 cm) pie plate

2 tbsp	butter or margarine	25 mL
1 tbsp	finely chopped onion	15 mL
1 cup	coarsely crushed cornflakes	250 mL
2	large apples, peeled, cored and sliced	2
3	eggs	3
1 cup	cottage cheese	250 mL
1 cup	shredded Cheddar cheese	250 mL
1/4 cup	2% milk	50 mL
1/2 tsp	salt	2 mL
1/8 tsp	freshly ground black pepper	0.5 mL
1/8 tsp	ground nutmeg	0.5 mL

1. In a nonstick skillet, melt butter over medium heat. Add onions and cook for 5 minutes or until tender. Stir in cornflakes. Press mixture into pie plate, forming a crust. Bake in preheated oven for 8 minutes.

2. Meanwhile, cook apples in 2 tbsp (25 mL) boiling water for 4 minutes or until barely tender; drain well. Arrange apples in crust.

3. In a blender or food processor, combine eggs, cottage cheese, Cheddar cheese, milk, salt and pepper; process until smooth. Pour into crust. Sprinkle with nutmeg.

4. Bake in preheated oven for 45 minutes or until a knife inserted in center comes out clean. Let stand for 10 minutes before cutting into wedges.

NUTRITIONAL ANALYSIS (PER BABY SERVING)

Energy	Protein	Carbohydrate	Fat	Fiber	Calcium	Iron	Sodium
118 kcal	7 g	6 g	7 g	0.4 g	94 mg	0.7 mg	273 mg

Makes 6 cups (1.5 L)

Kitchen Tips

Want a lower-fat version of this dish? In Step 2, omit the butter; heat the milk until hot (but not boiling) and add 2 oz (60 g) light cream cheese. Mix flour with grated Cheddar; gradually add it to the milk mixture, stirring until Cheddar cheese has melted and the sauce is thick. Continue with Step 3.

Look for whole wheat varieties of macaroni.

Macaroni and Cheese

Preheat oven to 375°F (190°C)
8-cup (2 L) casserole dish, lightly greased

2½ cups	dry macaroni	625 mL
3 tbsp	butter or margarine	45 mL
¼ cup	all-purpose flour	50 mL
2 cups	milk	500 mL
2 cups	grated old Cheddar cheese	500 mL
¼ tsp	dry mustard	2 mL
	Salt and freshly ground black pepper to taste	

Topping

½ cup	fine dry bread crumbs	125 mL
1 tbsp	butter or margarine, melted	15 mL
2 tbsp	grated old Cheddar cheese	25 mL
Pinch	paprika	Pinch

1. In a large saucepan, cook the macaroni according to package instructions or until tender but firm.
2. In another large saucepan, melt butter over medium heat. Add flour and cook, stirring, until it starts to bubble. Gradually add milk, stirring constantly, and cook until thickened. Add grated cheese; stir until melted. Stir in mustard; season to taste with salt and pepper.
3. Transfer drained macaroni to prepared casserole dish; pour sauce over. Stir just until mixed.
4. *Topping:* In a bowl, combine bread crumbs and melted butter; distribute evenly over macaroni. Sprinkle with 2 tbsp (25 mL) cheese and paprika.
5. Bake in preheated oven for 30 minutes or until mixture is heated through and topping is browned.

NUTRITIONAL ANALYSIS (PER ½ CUP/125 ML)							
Energy	Protein	Carbohydrate	Fat	Fiber	Calcium	Iron	Sodium
251 kcal	10 g	25 g	12 g	1 g	209 mg	1 mg	207 mg

Makes 3 servings

Kitchen Tip

Use whatever pizza toppings your kids like. Mozzarella can be replaced by whatever cheese you have in your refrigerator. Cheddar or marble cheese works just as well.

Pizza Omelet

Preheat broiler

3	eggs	3
2 tbsp	2% milk	25 mL
Pinch	salt	Pinch
Pinch	freshly ground black pepper	Pinch
Pinch	dried basil	Pinch
Pinch	dried oregano	Pinch
1 tbsp	butter or margarine	15 mL
2 tbsp	tomato sauce	25 mL
¼ cup	grated mozzarella cheese	50 mL
¼ cup	chopped vegetables (such as peppers, mushrooms, etc.)	50 mL

1. In a bowl, whisk together eggs, milk, salt, pepper, basil and oregano.

2. In a small skillet with an ovenproof handle, melt butter over medium heat. Add egg mixture and cook until underside is set. With a spatula, flip omelet and cook other side. Garnish with tomato sauce, cheese and vegetables. Place under preheated broiler and broil for 1 to 2 minutes, until cheese melts.

NUTRITIONAL ANALYSIS (PER SERVING)							
Energy	Protein	Carbohydrate	Fat	Fiber	Calcium	Iron	Sodium
146 kcal	9 g	2 g	22 g	0.3 g	109 mg	1 mg	267 mg

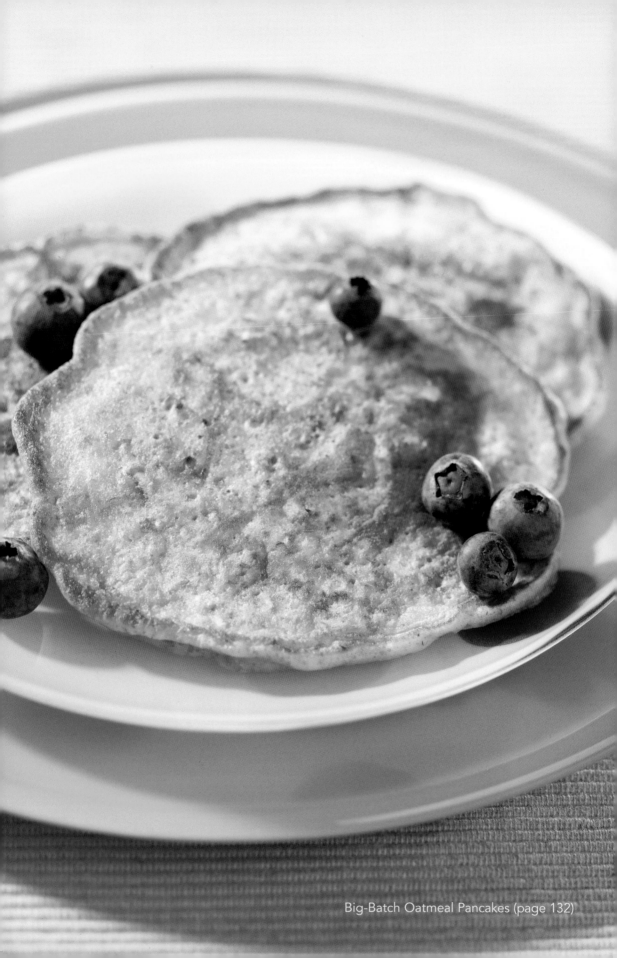

Big-Batch Oatmeal Pancakes (page 132)

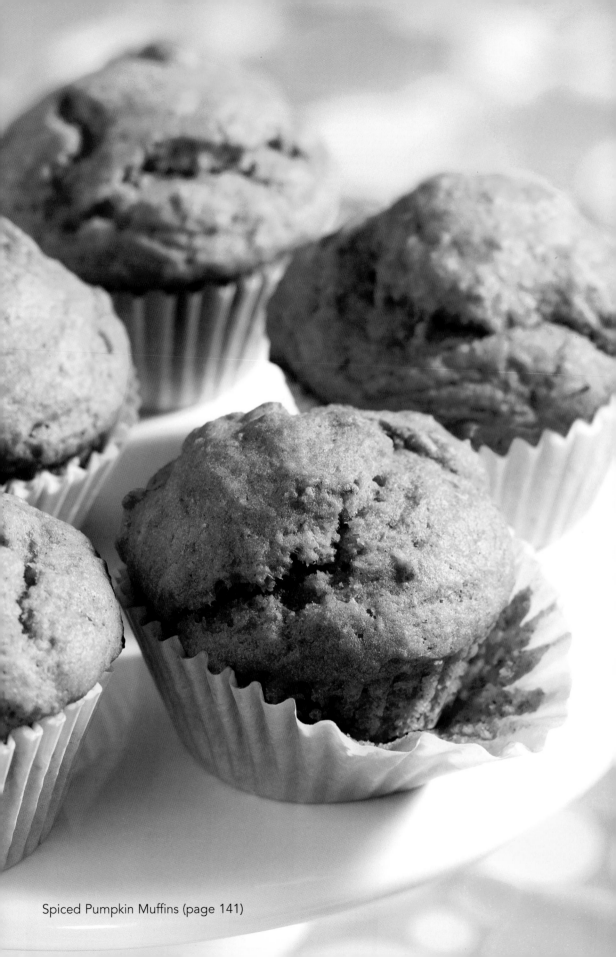

Spiced Pumpkin Muffins (page 141)

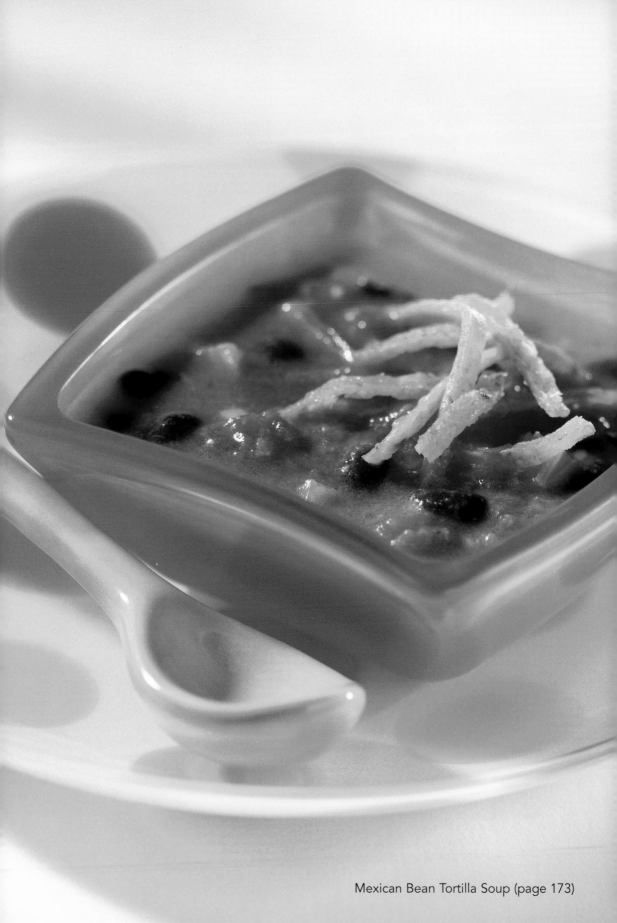

Mexican Bean Tortilla Soup (page 173)

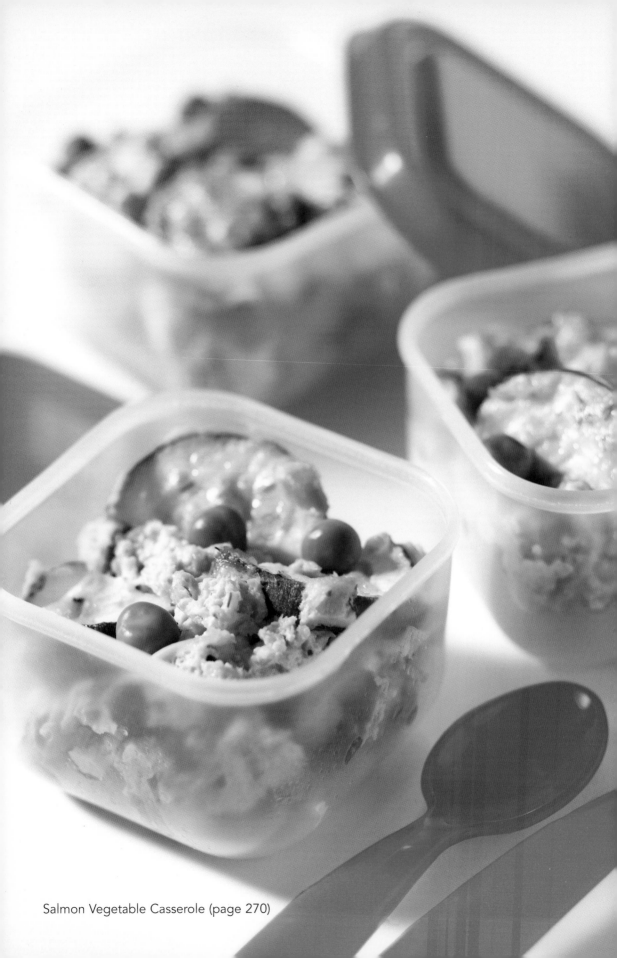

Salmon Vegetable Casserole (page 270)

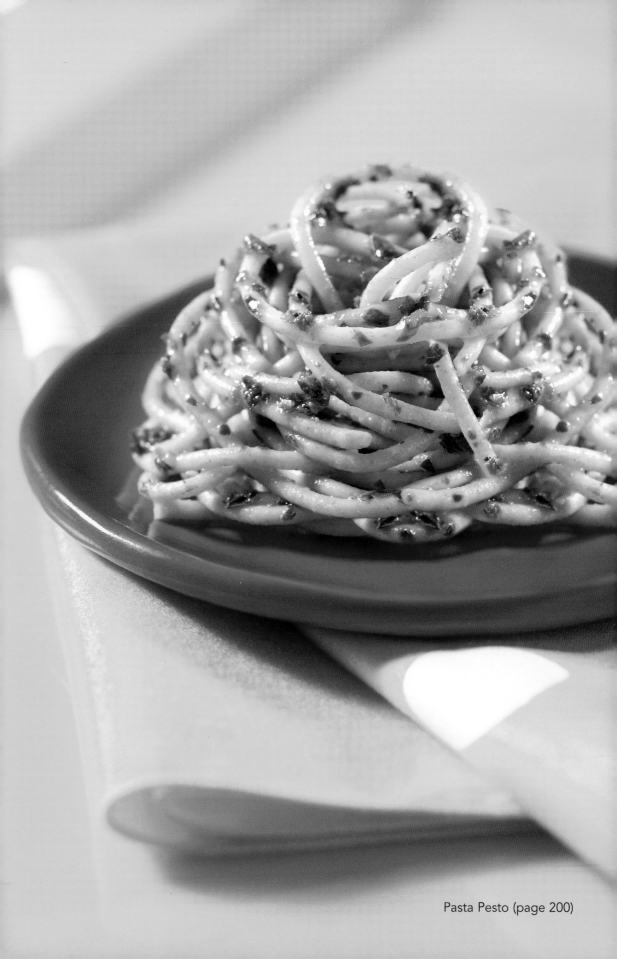

Pasta Pesto (page 200)

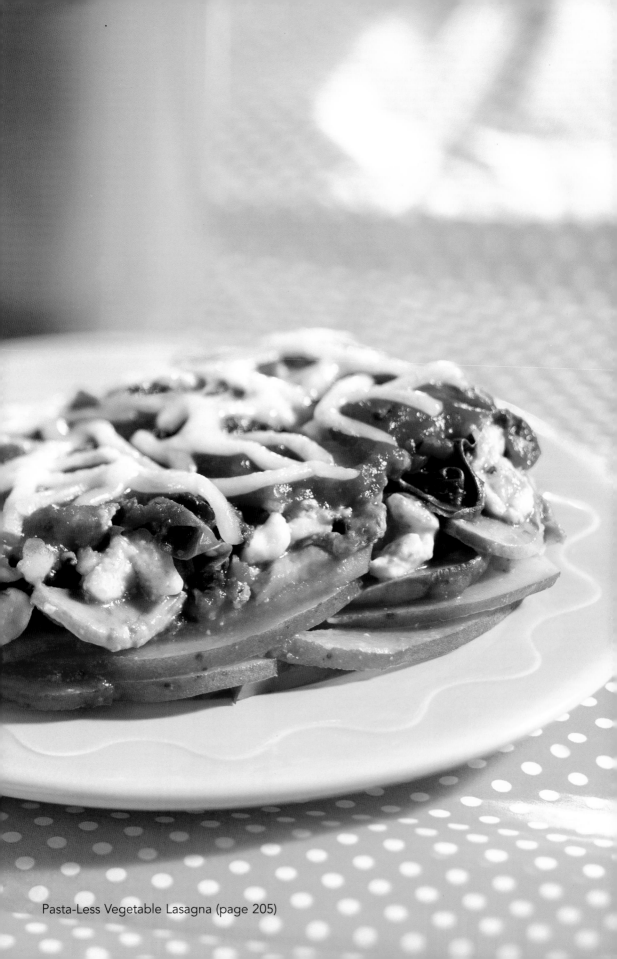

Pasta-Less Vegetable Lasagna (page 205)

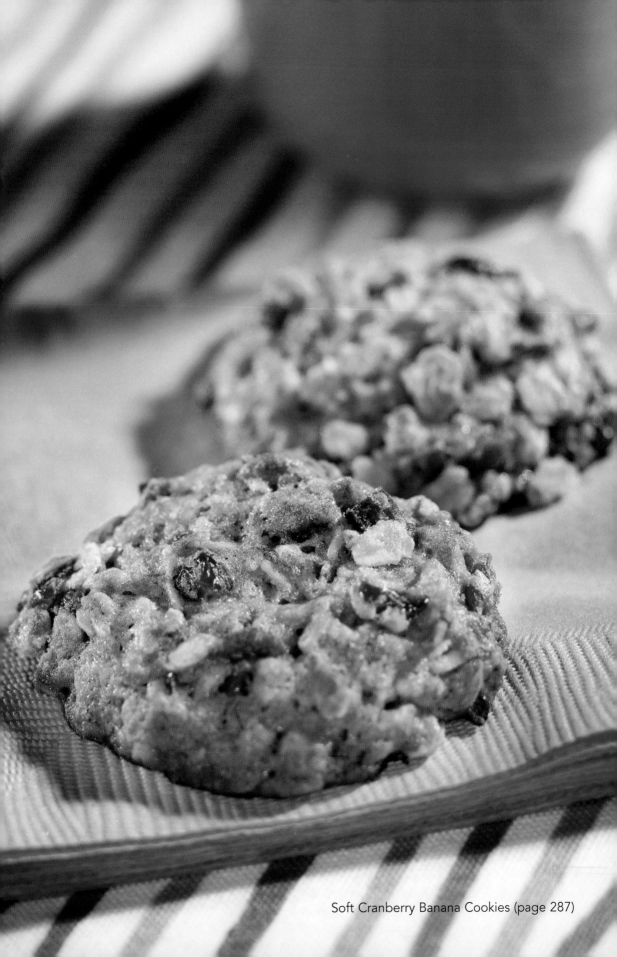

Soft Cranberry Banana Cookies (page 287)

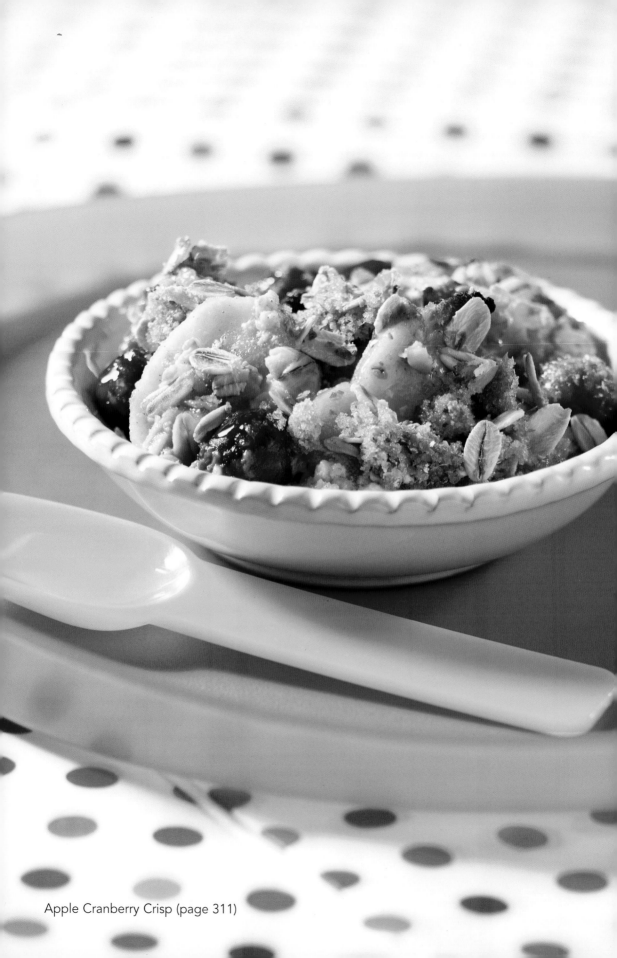

Apple Cranberry Crisp (page 311)

Marinated Vegetables

Crisp raw vegetables gain great flavor — and favor — when marinated in a light dressing of olive oil and vinegar. Junior diners will enjoy eating these veggies alone or with cubes of cheese. Parents may wish to place the vegetables on paper toweling to absorb excess marinade before serving to finger-eaters.

Kitchen Tip

If your child prefers vegetables partially cooked, just blanch them in a saucepan of boiling water for about 2 minutes, then plunge into cold water to stop the cooking.

Food Safety Tip

Refrigerate prepared vegetables or any leftovers within 2 hours after cooking.

1	medium carrot, sliced (see tip)	1
½ cup	frozen peas, thawed	125 mL
½ cup	sliced yellow beans	125 mL
½ cup	small broccoli florets	125 mL
½ cup	small cauliflower florets	125 mL
½ cup	tomato juice	125 mL
1 tbsp	olive oil	15 mL
1 tbsp	red wine vinegar	15 mL
½ tsp	dried basil	2 mL
½ tsp	dried oregano	2 mL
Pinch	salt	Pinch
Pinch	freshly ground black pepper	Pinch

1. Place carrot, peas, beans, broccoli and cauliflower in a plastic bag.

2. In a tightly sealed container, shake together tomato juice, oil, vinegar, basil, oregano, salt and pepper. Add dressing to vegetables; seal bag and shake to distribute evenly. Marinate in the refrigerator for several hours. Drain and serve. Vegetables will keep in the refrigerator for several days.

NUTRITIONAL ANALYSIS (PER ¼ CUP/50 ML)

Energy	Protein	Carbohydrate	Fat	Fiber	Calcium	Iron	Sodium
25 kcal	1 g	3 g	1 g	1 g	12 mg	0.3 mg	61 mg

Makes 4 cups (1 L)

Kitchen Tip

For an attractive presentation, garnish with sliced hard-cooked eggs and a pinch of paprika.

Potato Salad

6	potatoes (preferably a waxy variety), peeled and cut into pieces	6
¾ cup	mayonnaise	175 mL
1	small onion, chopped	1
2	radishes, chopped	2
1 tsp	prepared mustard	5 mL
¼ tsp	curry powder	1 mL
	Salt and freshly ground black pepper to taste	

1. In a large saucepan, boil potatoes in water to cover for 15 to 20 minutes, until they are just cooked. Drain and let cool. Cut into bite-size pieces.
2. In a large bowl, combine mayonnaise, onion, radishes, mustard, curry powder, salt and pepper. Add potatoes and toss to coat. Chill before serving

NUTRITIONAL ANALYSIS (PER ¼ CUP/50 ML)							
Energy	Protein	Carbohydrate	Fat	Fiber	Calcium	Iron	Sodium
98 kcal	1 g	15 g	4 g	1 g	8 mg	0.2 mg	86 mg

Food Safety Tip

Food served on skewers is considered unsafe for children under 4 years of age. Be sure to remove skewers from kebabs in this recipe.

Children's Cheese Kebabs

Preheat broiler

3	½-inch (1 cm) cubes Cheddar cheese	3
½	cherry tomatoes	3
½	slice whole wheat bread, buttered and cut into small squares	½
1	slice bacon, cooked	1

1. On a wooden or metal skewer, place alternating pieces of cheese, tomato, buttered bread and bacon. Place kebab on foil and cook under preheated broiler for 3 minutes, turning once. Remove skewer before serving.

NUTRITIONAL ANALYSIS

Energy	Protein	Carbohydrate	Fat	Fiber	Calcium	Iron	Sodium
196 kcal	11 g	8 g	13 g	1 g	198 mg	1 mg	482 mg

Makes 2 servings

Kitchen Tip

Use the toppings suggested here — or whatever your child likes best.

English Muffin Mini Pizzas

Preheat oven to 350°F (180°C)
Baking sheet

1	whole wheat English muffin, halved	1
¼ cup	spaghetti sauce	50 mL
¼ cup	shredded mozzarella cheese	50 mL
6	slices pepperoni	6
2	mushrooms, sliced	2

1. On each half of muffin, divide sauce and the cheese equally. Top each with 3 slices of pepperoni and 1 sliced mushroom. Bake in preheated oven for 10 to 15 minutes or until cheese has melted.

NUTRITIONAL ANALYSIS (PER SERVING)

Energy	Protein	Carbohydrate	Fat	Fiber	Calcium	Iron	Sodium
274 kcal	13 g	18 g	17 g	3 g	197 mg	1 mg	938 mg

Hungarian-Style Lentils

Makes 3 cups (750 mL)

Lentils are not typically soaked, but we tried soaking them and found it helped them cook quickly and become very tender without falling apart.

Kitchen Tip

Lentils can be made 1 day ahead and cooled completely, then chilled. Reheat to serving temperature the next day, adding extra water if needed.

1 cup	green lentils, rinsed	250 mL
2 cups	reduced-sodium chicken broth	500 mL
1	bay leaf	1
2 tbsp	canola oil	25 mL
1	small onion, finely chopped	1
1	large garlic clove, minced	1
2 tbsp	whole wheat flour	25 mL
1 tsp	paprika	5 mL
1 tbsp	red wine vinegar	15 mL
1 tbsp	freshly squeezed lemon juice	15 mL

1. In large saucepan, place lentils in enough cold water to cover; soak at room temperature for at least 8 hours or overnight. Drain and rinse well, then return to saucepan.

2. Add broth and bay leaf and bring to a boil over high heat. Reduce heat to medium-low and cook for 10 minutes or until lentils are tender.

3. Meanwhile in a nonstick skillet, heat oil over medium heat. Add onion and garlic; sauté for about 5 minutes or until beginning to brown. Whisk in flour; cook, stirring constantly, for 1 minute. Add paprika, vinegar and lemon juice; cook, stirring, for 1 minute longer. Stir into lentils and cook for 5 minutes or until mixture has thickened.

NUTRITIONAL ANALYSIS (PER ½ CUP/125 ML)							
Energy	Protein	Carbohydrate	Fat	Fiber	Calcium	Iron	Sodium
119 kcal	6 g	13 g	5 g	2 g	21 mg	1.7 mg	220 mg

Dinner

continued on next page

Dinner
(continued)

This recipe is an alternative to jarred "meat and rice" meals. It is easy to prepare your own, and leftovers can be frozen and kept for a later date. Either brown or white rice can be used, depending on what you have available.

Kitchen Tip

A ripe peach can be peeled and used raw in this recipe. For under-ripe peaches, simmer in a small amount of boiling water until tender.

Chicken and Rice Delight

½ cup	diced cooked boneless skinless chicken	125 mL
¼ cup	cooked brown rice	50 mL
1	peach, peeled and diced	1
2 tbsp	2% milk	25 mL

1. In a food processor or using a handheld blender, purée chicken, rice, peach and milk to desired texture.

NUTRITIONAL ANALYSIS (PER ¼ CUP/50 ML)

Energy	Protein	Carbohydrate	Fat	Fiber	Calcium	Iron	Sodium
86 kcal	12 g	6 g	1 g	1 g	18 mg	1 mg	24 mg

Puréed Baby Meat

| ½ cup | cooked meat (chicken, beef, etc.), cut into small pieces | 125 mL |
| ¼ cup | water or cooking liquid or milk | 50 mL |

1. In a food processor or blender, combine meat and water. Process for 1 to 2 minutes or until smooth. Serve immediately or freeze in an ice-cube tray for future use (see pages 51–52).

NUTRITIONAL ANALYSIS (PER SERVING) — *FOR CHICKEN* (4 OZ/125 G DRUMSTICK MEAT)

Energy	Protein	Carbohydrate	Fat	Fiber	Calcium	Iron	Sodium
67 kcal	9 g	–	3 g	–	5 mg	0.5 mg	26 mg

NUTRITIONAL ANALYSIS (PER SERVING) — *FOR BEEF*

Energy	Protein	Carbohydrate	Fat	Fiber	Calcium	Iron	Sodium
134 kcal	18 g	–	7 g	–	11 mg	2 mg	33 mg

NUTRITIONAL ANALYSIS (PER SERVING) — *FOR LAMB*

Energy	Protein	Carbohydrate	Fat	Fiber	Calcium	Iron	Sodium
133 kcal	14 g	–	8 g	–	6 mg	1 mg	25 mg

Makes 2 cups (500 mL)

Kitchen Tips

The pesto can be stored in an airtight container in the refrigerator for up to 3 days.

Look for enriched pasta made with chickpeas and lentils, which add protein, fiber and iron.

Pasta Pesto

Pesto

1	clove garlic	1
1 cup	lightly packed fresh basil leaves	250 mL
½ cup	pine nuts	125 mL
½ cup	olive oil	125 mL
2 cups	whole wheat or enriched pasta, cooked	500 mL
	Grated Parmesan cheese (optional)	

1. *Pesto:* In a food processor, process garlic, basil and pine nuts until chopped. With the motor running, gradually add olive oil through the feed tube and process until smooth. Makes 2 cups (500 mL).

2. Place 1 tbsp (15 mL) pesto sauce on each ½ cup (125 mL) pasta. Sprinkle lightly (1 tsp/5 mL) with Parmesan cheese, if desired (keep in mind that Parmesan adds sodium).

NUTRITIONAL ANALYSIS (PER ¼ CUP/50 ML)

Energy	Protein	Carbohydrate	Fat	Fiber	Calcium	Iron	Sodium
200 kcal	2 g	2 g	21 g	0.4 g	8 mg	1 mg	1 mg

Makes 2½ cups (625 mL)

This is a thinner, lower-fat version of the famous Greek tzatziki sauce!

Cucumber Yogurt Dip

2 cups	plain yogurt	500 mL
½	medium cucumber, peeled and finely chopped	½
1	clove garlic, minced	1
1 tsp	dried dill	5 mL

1. In a bowl combine yogurt, cucumber, garlic and dill. Refrigerate for at least 1 hour to let flavors blend. Serve on a pita or as a side dish with meat.

NUTRITIONAL ANALYSIS (PER ¼ CUP/50 ML)

Energy	Protein	Carbohydrate	Fat	Fiber	Calcium	Iron	Sodium
33 kcal	3 g	4 g	1 g	–	95 mg	–	35 mg

Sunshine Carrots

Makes 4 servings

The "sunshine" in these carrots refers to their bright orange glaze. Adding a pinch of sugar helps to mellow any bitterness, which makes the humble carrot even more attractive to small children.

4	medium carrots, peeled and cut diagonally into 1-inch (2.5 cm) thick slices	4
Pinch	granulated sugar	Pinch
½ tsp	cornstarch	2 mL
⅛ tsp	salt	0.5 mL
⅛ tsp	ground ginger	0.5 mL
2 tbsp	orange juice	25 mL
1 tbsp	butter or margarine	15 mL

1. In a saucepan, cook carrots in boiling water for 10 minutes or until tender. Drain.

2. Meanwhile, in a small saucepan, combine sugar, cornstarch, salt and ginger. Add orange juice and cook, stirring constantly, until mixture thickens. Boil for 1 minute. Stir in butter. Pour over carrots; toss evenly to coat.

NUTRITIONAL ANALYSIS (PER SERVING)							
Energy	Protein	Carbohydrate	Fat	Fiber	Calcium	Iron	Sodium
64 kcal	1 g	9 g	3 g	2 g	28 mg	0.3 mg	137 mg

Creamed Spinach

Here's a recipe that raises spinach to new heights of flavor. Many guests who have tasted this vegetable dish request the recipe — especially the mothers of toddlers! It's a great way to get them to eat their spinach.

Kitchen Tips

If you wish, omit the bacon and use 1 tbsp (15 mL) olive oil to sauté the onions and garlic.

The recipe may be made ahead and reheated at serving time.

2	slices bacon, finely chopped (see tip)	2
1	small onion, finely chopped	1
1	clove garlic, minced	1
2 tbsp	all-purpose flour	25 mL
½ tsp	paprika	2 mL
½ tsp	salt	2 mL
⅛ tsp	freshly ground black pepper	0.5 mL
1 cup	2% milk	250 mL
1	package (10 oz/300 g) frozen chopped spinach, thawed, excess liquid squeezed out	1

1. In a skillet over medium-high heat, sauté bacon and onion for 5 minutes. Add garlic and cook for 5 minutes or until onions are tender and bacon has become crisp. Remove from heat.
2. Stir in flour, paprika, salt and pepper; blend well. Return skillet to heat. Slowly add milk and cook, stirring frequently, until thickened. Stir in spinach, mix well and serve.

NUTRITIONAL ANALYSIS (PER ¼ CUP/50 ML)							
Energy	Protein	Carbohydrate	Fat	Fiber	Calcium	Iron	Sodium
48 kcal	3 g	5 g	2 g	1 g	86 mg	1 mg	216 mg

Makes 4 cups (1 L)

So delicious, you'll probably have to double the recipe! Be prepared to share it with others — who are bound to ask you for the recipe as soon as they taste this dish.

Kitchen Tip

You can make this dish using any number of different cheeses. If your child prefers stronger flavors, try old instead of medium Cheddar.

Spinach Cheese Bake

Preheat oven to 350°F (180°C)
Casserole dish

1 tbsp	butter or margarine	15 mL
2	eggs	2
¾ cup	whole milk	175 mL
¼ cup	all-purpose flour	50 mL
½ tsp	baking powder	2 mL
¼ tsp	salt	1 mL
⅛ tsp	ground nutmeg	0.5 mL
1	package (10 oz/284 g) fresh spinach, rough stems removed, chopped	1
2 cups	grated medium Cheddar cheese	500 mL

1. Place butter in casserole dish and set in oven for about 2 minutes or until it is just melted. Set aside.

2. In a large bowl, beat eggs lightly. Stir in milk. Add flour, baking powder, salt and nutmeg; beat until mixture is smooth. Stir in spinach. Add cheese.

3. Place in prepared casserole dish and bake in preheated oven for 30 to 35 minutes.

NUTRITIONAL ANALYSIS (PER ½ CUP/125 ML)							
Energy	Protein	Carbohydrate	Fat	Fiber	Calcium	Iron	Sodium
290 kcal	17 g	5 g	23 g	1 g	485 mg	1.7 mg	467 mg

Makes 3 cups (750 mL)

This traditional French vegetable dish is chock-full of vitamins and minerals. It's sure to please young ones, served hot, on a cold winter night.

Ratatouille

2 tbsp	vegetable oil	25 mL
1	clove garlic, minced	1
½ cup	sliced onion	125 mL
½ cup	diced green pepper	125 mL
2	small zucchini, peeled and sliced	2
½	eggplant, peeled and thinly sliced	½
2	tomatoes, peeled and diced	2
½ tsp	salt	2 mL
¼ tsp	freshly ground black pepper	1 mL
Pinch	granulated sugar	Pinch

1. In a heavy-bottomed saucepan, heat oil over medium-high heat. Add garlic and the onion; sauté until softened. Add green pepper and cook until soft. Gently stir in zucchini, eggplant and tomatoes. Reduce heat to low; cover and simmer, stirring occasionally, for about 45 minutes. Serve hot or cold.

NUTRITIONAL ANALYSIS (PER ¼ CUP/50 ML)							
Energy	Protein	Carbohydrate	Fat	Fiber	Calcium	Iron	Sodium
31 kcal	1 g	3 g	2 g	1 g	7 mg	0.2 mg	82 mg

*This delicious meatless
lasagna is layered with fresh
vegetables and tomato
sauce — and yes, it features
potatoes rather than pasta.*

Pasta-Less Vegetable Lasagna

Preheat oven to 350°F (180°C)
13- by 9-inch (3 L) baking dish, greased

1	package (10 oz/284 g) fresh spinach, trimmed	1
2	medium potatoes (unpeeled), sliced	2
1 cup	sliced mushrooms (about 6 small)	250 mL
1½ cups	shredded mozzarella cheese, divided	375 mL
1 cup	cottage cheese	250 mL
1	can (14 oz/398 mL) reduced-sodium tomato sauce	1
1	clove garlic, minced	1
1 tsp	dried basil (or 2 tsp/10 mL chopped fresh)	5 mL
	Freshly ground black pepper	

1. In a steamer basket or large sieve set over a pot of boiling water, steam spinach over medium heat for 3 minutes or until wilted. Drain well, squeeze dry and chop.

2. In prepared baking dish, layer potatoes, mushrooms, 1 cup (250 mL) of the mozzarella cheese, cottage cheese and spinach.

3. In a bowl, combine tomato sauce, garlic, basil and pepper to taste. Pour over vegetables. Cover with foil and bake in preheated oven for 40 minutes or until potatoes are tender. Remove foil and sprinkle with remaining mozzarella cheese for the last 5 minutes of baking time.

NUTRITIONAL ANALYSIS (PER BABY SERVING)							
Energy	Protein	Carbohydrate	Fat	Fiber	Calcium	Iron	Sodium
84 kcal	6 g	15 g	1 g	3 g	76 mg	2 mg	168 mg

Makes 8 baby servings, or 4 adult servings

Kitchen Tips

Use whatever variety of squash you like — acorn, buttercup or butternut will work equally well.

Squash is a great source of vitamin A.

Variation

Make a flavorful topping by combining 2 tbsp (25 mL) brown sugar, 1 tbsp (15 mL) butter or margarine, 1½ tsp (7 mL) all-purpose flour and ½ tsp (2 mL) salt. Spread over squash and apples before baking.

Baked Squash

Preheat oven to 350°F (180°C)
Shallow baking dish, greased

| 1 lb | squash, peeled and sliced | 500 g |
| 1 | large baking apple, peeled, cored and cut into ½-inch (1 cm) rings | 1 |

1. Arrange squash in prepared baking dish. Top with the apple rings. Bake in preheated oven for 1 hour or until tender.

NUTRITIONAL ANALYSIS (PER BABY SERVING)

Energy	Protein	Carbohydrate	Fat	Fiber	Calcium	Iron	Sodium
41 kcal	1 g	11 g	0.1 g	2 g	31 mg	0.5 mg	2 mg

Makes 4 baby servings, or 1 to 2 adult servings

These are a healthy baked alternative to traditional french fries.

Kitchen Tips

For infants who may not be able to chew it well, remove skin before serving.

Sweet potatoes are a great source of vitamin A.

Sweet Potato Fries

Preheat oven to 350°F (180°C)
Baking sheet, lined with parchment paper

| 1 | sweet potato (unpeeled), well scrubbed | 1 |
| 1 tbsp | olive oil | 15 mL |

1. Cut sweet potato into ½-inch (1 cm) cubes. In a medium bowl, toss sweet potato with oil. Spread out on prepared baking sheet. Bake in preheated oven for 50 minutes.

NUTRITIONAL ANALYSIS (PER BABY SERVING)

Energy	Protein	Carbohydrate	Fat	Fiber	Calcium	Iron	Sodium
49 kcal	0.5 g	7 g	2 g	1 g	10 mg	0.2 mg	10 mg

Makes 4 logs

With their crunchy coating of cornflake crumbs, these logs make a nice change from plain old mashed potatoes. Children like them not only for their flavor, but for their shape, which is more interesting and less imposing than a glob of ordinary mashed.

Kitchen Tip

Instead of cooking potatoes for this recipe, you can use leftover cooked potatoes. Or you can cook extra potatoes and use them for another day's potato logs.

Potato Logs

Preheat oven to 450°F (230°C)
Baking sheet, greased

3	large potatoes, peeled and cubed	3
2 tbsp	butter or margarine	25 mL
1	small onion, finely chopped	1
¼ cup	whole milk	50 mL
1	egg, beaten	1
¼ tsp	ground nutmeg	1 mL
¼ tsp	salt	1 mL
¼ tsp	freshly ground black pepper	1 mL
¾ cup	crushed corn flakes cereal	175 mL

1. In a medium saucepan, cook potatoes in boiling water for 15 minutes or until tender. Drain well. Dry drained potatoes over low heat while shaking pan. Mash potatoes well. Stir in butter, onion, milk, egg, nutmeg, salt and pepper. Beat with an electric mixer until smooth.

2. When mixture is cool enough to handle, shape into small logs. Roll in crushed crumbs and place on prepared baking sheet. Bake in preheated oven for 15 minutes or until browned, turning halfway through baking time.

NUTRITIONAL ANALYSIS (PER LOG)							
Energy	Protein	Carbohydrate	Fat	Fiber	Calcium	Iron	Sodium
200 kcal	5 g	31 g	7 g	2 g	35 mg	1 mg	214 mg

Super Simple Hash Browns

Preheat oven to 350°F (180°C)
8-cup (2 L) casserole dish

1	bag (1 lb/454 g) frozen hash brown potatoes	1
½ cup	sour cream	125 mL
1½ cups	grated Cheddar cheese	375 mL
1	can (10 oz/284 mL) reduced-sodium cream of mushroom soup	1
1 tbsp	butter or margarine	15 mL

1. In a large bowl, combine hash browns, sour cream, cheese, soup and butter; mix well. Transfer mixture to casserole dish. Bake for about 1½ hours or until golden brown.

NUTRITIONAL ANALYSIS (PER ¼ CUP/50 ML)

Energy	Protein	Carbohydrate	Fat	Fiber	Calcium	Iron	Sodium
114 kcal	2 g	5 g	10 g	0.3 g	61 mg	0.4 mg	162 mg

Kitchen Tip

Potato skins are a great source of fiber.

Garlic Mashed Potato

1	potato (new or red), well scrubbed	1
1	clove garlic	1
1 tsp	butter or margarine	5 mL
2 tbsp	2% milk	25 mL

1. Leaving skin on, cut potato into chunks.
2. In a small saucepan, boil potato and garlic for 15 to 20 minutes or until potato is soft. Drain. Add butter and milk. Mash.

NUTRITIONAL ANALYSIS (PER SERVING)

Energy	Protein	Carbohydrate	Fat	Fiber	Calcium	Iron	Sodium
98 kcal	2 g	18 g	2 g	1 g	25 mg	0.3 mg	24 mg

This dish is always a family favorite, especially served with ham or roast pork.

Variation

Add ½ cup (125 mL) shredded Cheddar cheese between potato layers.

Scalloped Potatoes

Preheat oven to 350°F (180°C)
4-cup (1 L) casserole dish, greased

3 cups	thinly sliced peeled potatoes	750 mL
1	medium onion, chopped	1
2 tbsp	all-purpose flour	25 mL
3 tbsp	butter or margarine	45 mL
1¼ cups	whole milk	300 mL
½ tsp	salt	2 mL
¼ tsp	freshly ground black pepper	1 mL
¼ tsp	paprika	1 mL

1. In prepared casserole dish, alternate layers of potato slices, onions and flour.

2. In a small saucepan, heat butter and milk over low heat until melted; stir in salt and pepper. Pour over layers. Sprinkle with paprika. Bake in preheated oven for 50 minutes or until tender.

NUTRITIONAL ANALYSIS (PER BABY SERVING)

Energy	Protein	Carbohydrate	Fat	Fiber	Calcium	Iron	Sodium
74 kcal	2 g	8 g	4 g	0.5 g	34 mg	0.2 mg	113 mg

This dish is a favorite with the young set, who all seem to love mashed potatoes. Anytime you have leftover mashed potatoes, use them in this recipe.

Kitchen Tip

Sour cream is a good replacement for milk.

Mashed Potato Casserole

Preheat oven to 400°F (200°C)
4-cup (1 L) casserole dish, greased

3	large potatoes, peeled and cubed	3
¼ cup	2% milk (see tip)	50 mL
¼ tsp	ground nutmeg	1 mL
¼ tsp	salt	1 mL
¼ tsp	freshly ground black pepper	1 mL
2 tbsp	butter or margarine	25 mL
½	small onion, finely chopped	½
¼ cup	dry bread crumbs	50 mL
1 tbsp	melted butter or margarine	15 mL

1. In a large saucepan, cook potatoes in boiling water for 20 minutes or until tender. Drain well; dry potatoes over low heat. Mash potatoes. Stir in milk, nutmeg, salt and pepper.

2. In a small skillet, melt the 2 tbsp (25 mL) butter. Add onion and sauté for 5 minutes or until softened. Stir into potatoes.

3. Spoon potatoes into prepared casserole dish. Combine bread crumbs with the 1 tbsp (15 mL) melted butter. Sprinkle over potatoes. Bake in a preheated oven for 20 minutes or until heated through and crumbs are golden brown.

NUTRITIONAL ANALYSIS (PER BABY SERVING)

Energy	Protein	Carbohydrate	Fat	Fiber	Calcium	Iron	Sodium
106 kcal	2 g	15 g	4 g	1 g	20 mg	0.4 mg	115 mg

Makes 3 cups (750 mL)

Risotto Tips

Arborio rice is much easier to find in supermarkets today, thanks to the growing popularity of risotto.

There are several easy but important steps in cooking risotto.

* Keep the broth hot.

* Allow all the liquid to be absorbed before more stock is added. This results in rice with a creamy texture, while the grains remain separate and firm.

* Contrary to popular belief, it is unnecessary to stir risotto constantly. All that's required is an occasional stir as you pass by the stove, keeping the mixture at a slow boil.

* For a traditional flavor for adults, add ¼ cup (50 mL) white wine in Step 2 as a replacement for the same amount of stock. It should be added before any broth to increase the flavor of the dish.

Variations

While rice is cooking, sauté assorted chopped vegetables in oil until soft, then stir them into the cooked risotto just before serving. Try mushrooms, red or yellow bell peppers or zucchini.

Other foods you can add to risotto include cooked vegetables, shellfish, chicken, beef or sausage, as well as other cheeses and herbs.

Classic Creamy Risotto

2 tsp	olive oil	10 mL
2 tsp	butter or margarine	10 mL
¼ cup	finely chopped onion	50 mL
1	clove garlic, minced	1
1 cup	Arborio rice (see tip)	250 mL
3 cups	hot chicken or vegetable stock	750 mL
¼ cup	freshly grated Parmesan cheese	50 mL
⅛ tsp	freshly ground black pepper	0.5 mL
⅛ tsp	ground nutmeg	0.5 mL

1. In a large saucepan, heat oil and butter over medium heat. Add onion and garlic; cook for 5 minutes or until tender. Stir in rice and cook for 3 minutes, being careful not to let it brown.
2. Add hot stock, ½ cup (125 mL) at a time. Cook mixture, stirring occasionally, until broth is almost absorbed. Continue additions of stock, cooking and stirring occasionally, until mixture becomes creamy and rice is tender. (The total cooking time should be about 20 minutes). Remove from heat. Stir in cheese, pepper and nutmeg. Taste and adjust seasonings.

NUTRITIONAL ANALYSIS (PER ¼ CUP/50 ML)

Energy	Protein	Carbohydrate	Fat	Fiber	Calcium	Iron	Sodium
74 kcal	3 g	10 g	2 g	1 g	25 mg	0.2 mg	239 mg

Makes 3 cups (750 mL)

Barley stands in for rice in this clever version of risotto. The only difference is, you do not need to stand and stir slowly as you add broth. Instead, you can let it simmer away while you prepare the rest of the meal.

Barley Risotto with Vegetables

1 tbsp	canola or olive oil	15 mL
1	onion, finely chopped	1
1	clove garlic, minced	1
1	carrot, shredded	1
¼ cup	chopped red bell pepper	50 mL
½ cup	pearl barley	125 mL
2 cups	reduced-sodium chicken broth	500 mL
Pinch	freshly ground black pepper	Pinch

1. In a saucepan, heat oil over medium heat. Add onion and garlic; sauté for 5 minutes or until soft. Add carrot and red pepper; sauté for 3 minutes. Add barley and sauté for 1 minute.
2. Add broth and bring to a boil. Reduce heat to low, cover and simmer for 40 minutes or until barley is tender. Season with pepper.

NUTRITIONAL ANALYSIS (PER ½ CUP / 125 ML)

Energy	Protein	Carbohydrate	Fat	Fiber	Calcium	Iron	Sodium
103 kcal	2 g	18 g	3 g	2 g	24 mg	0.5 mg	268 mg

Makes 8 baby servings, or 3 adult servings

When you have leftover cooked rice, here is a fine use for it the next day, as either a lunch or a dinner dish.

Kitchen Tip

To cook dried red lentils, add to boiling water and return to boil; reduce heat to low, cover and cook for 10 minutes or until tender. Drain. One-half cup (125 mL) dried lentils will yield about 1 cup (250 mL) cooked.

Baked Lentils 'n' Rice

Preheat oven to 350°F (180°C)
9-inch (2.5 L) square baking dish

2	eggs, beaten	2
1 cup	cooked brown rice	250 mL
1 cup	cooked red lentils (see tip)	250 mL
1 cup	shredded Cheddar cheese, divided	250 mL
1	green onion, chopped	1
½ cup	finely shredded carrot	125 mL
¼ cup	2% milk	50 mL
Pinch	freshly ground black pepper	Pinch
2	tomatoes, diced	2

1. In a bowl, combine eggs, rice, lentils, ¾ cup (175 mL) of the cheese, onion, carrot, milk and pepper. Spoon into prepared baking dish.

2. Bake in preheated oven for 30 minutes or until set. Top with diced tomatoes and remaining cheese and bake for 5 minutes or until cheese is melted. To serve, cut into squares.

NUTRITIONAL ANALYSIS (PER BABY SERVING)

Energy	Protein	Carbohydrate	Fat	Fiber	Calcium	Iron	Sodium
162 kcal	9 g	17 g	7 g	3 g	130 mg	1 mg	116 mg

Makes 6 cups (1.5 L)

Kitchen Tips

This dish is a great source of iron and protein.

Freeze in small portions for quick use later on.

Baked Beans

Preheat oven to 300°F (150°C)
Deep baking dish

12 oz	dried navy beans	375 g
2 tbsp	molasses	25 mL
2 tbsp	packed brown sugar	25 mL
1	can (14 oz/398 mL) tomatoes	1
1 tsp	dry mustard	5 mL
½ tsp	freshly ground black pepper	2 mL
½	onion, chopped	½
¼ tsp	salt	1 mL

1. In a large saucepan, soak beans in 3 times the quantity of water for 12 hours or overnight. Drain and rinse. Add fresh water to cover and bring to a boil. Reduce heat to low; cover and simmer for 1 hour. Transfer beans to baking dish.
2. Stir in molasses, brown sugar, tomatoes, mustard, pepper, onion and salt. Bake, covered, in preheated oven for 3 hours, adding water several times as needed to keep the beans moist.

NUTRITIONAL ANALYSIS (PER ¼ CUP/50 ML)							
Energy	Protein	Carbohydrate	Fat	Fiber	Calcium	Iron	Sodium
78 kcal	4 g	14 g	1 g	1 g	17 mg	1 mg	58 mg

Makes 12 baby servings, or 4 adult servings

Quiche is so delicious and versatile, it should be part of every family cook's repertoire. This one is particularly healthy, with the traditional pastry replaced by a bread crumb crust. Any small pieces left after dinner can be used as a snack. It is a good way to add cottage cheese to a child's diet.

Kitchen Tip

If you prefer, make this quiche in a square baking pan; cut into small squares to serve as appetizers.

Cheese and Vegetable Quiche

Preheat oven to 350°F (180°C)
9-inch (23 cm) pie plate, greased

1	slice whole wheat bread	1
2 tbsp	melted butter or margarine, divided	25 mL
1 cup	chopped spinach	250 mL
1 cup	chopped mushrooms	250 mL
½	red bell pepper, chopped	½
½ tsp	dried basil	2 mL
½ tsp	dried oregano	2 mL
¼ tsp	salt	1 mL
¼ tsp	freshly ground black pepper	1 mL
1 cup	cottage cheese	250 mL
4	eggs, beaten	4
⅔ cup	2% milk	150 mL
¼ cup	shredded Cheddar cheese	50 mL

1. Crumble bread into fine crumbs; toss with 1 tbsp (15 mL) of the melted butter. Sprinkle bread crumbs into prepared pie plate.

2. In a large skillet, heat remaining butter over medium-high heat. Add spinach, mushrooms and red pepper; cook, stirring occasionally, for 10 minutes or until vegetables are softened. Add basil, oregano, salt and pepper. Stir in cottage cheese. Spoon into pie plate.

3. In a small bowl, whisk together eggs, milk and cheese. Pour over vegetable mixture. Bake in preheated oven for 45 minutes or until puffy and set in center. Let stand for 10 minutes before cutting.

NUTRITIONAL ANALYSIS (PER BABY SERVING)

Energy	Protein	Carbohydrate	Fat	Fiber	Calcium	Iron	Sodium
82 kcal	6 g	3 g	5 g	1 g	83 mg	0.7 mg	201 mg

Makes 6 baby servings, or 2 adult servings

The cottage cheese in this pie provides protein and calcium, and the many vegetables add color and fiber.

Vegetable Cottage Cheese Quiche

Preheat oven to 350°F (180°C)
9-inch (23 cm) deep-dish pie plate, greased

4	eggs, lightly beaten	4
1	container (1 lb/500 g) cottage cheese	1
½ cup	plain yogurt	125 mL
¼ cup	whole wheat flour	50 mL
¼ tsp	salt	1 mL
⅛ tsp	freshly ground black pepper	0.5 mL
1 cup	fresh whole wheat bread crumbs	250 mL
1 cup	finely chopped mixed vegetables (carrot, zucchini, onion and mushroom)	250 mL
2	tomatoes, cut into thin wedges	2
Pinch	dried oregano	Pinch
Pinch	dried basil	Pinch

1. In a bowl, combine eggs, cottage cheese, yogurt, flour, salt and pepper.

2. In another bowl, stir ⅓ cup (75 mL) egg mixture into bread crumbs; press into bottom and sides of prepared pie plate.

3. Add mixed vegetables to remaining egg mixture; pour over crumbs, smoothing top. Bake in preheated oven for 35 minutes or until puffy and set in center.

4. Arrange tomato wedges around outer edge of pie and sprinkle with oregano and basil. Bake for 5 minutes longer or until tomatoes are warm. Let stand for 10 minutes before cutting into wedges.

NUTRITIONAL ANALYSIS (PER BABY SERVING)

Energy	Protein	Carbohydrate	Fat	Fiber	Calcium	Iron	Sodium
248 kcal	19 g	28 g	7 g	3 g	159 mg	2.1 mg	591 mg

Tofu takes on the flavors of its accompanying vegetables in this crustless quiche.

Kitchen Tips

The optional tomato provides added color to this dish.

Firm tofu will also work in this recipe, but the silken variety will give it a smoother texture.

Yummy Tofu Quiche

Preheat oven to 350°F (180°C)
8-inch (20 cm) pie plate, greased

2	eggs	2
1 cup	cubed drained silken tofu	250 mL
1 tbsp	all-purpose flour	15 mL
2 tsp	lemon juice or 2% milk	10 mL
⅛ tsp	ground nutmeg	0.5 mL
⅛ tsp	salt	0.5 mL
⅛ tsp	freshly ground black pepper	0.5 mL
½ cup	finely chopped frozen mixed vegetables, thawed	125 mL
1 tbsp	butter or margarine, melted	15 mL
½ cup	fresh whole wheat bread crumbs	125 mL
2 tbsp	grated Parmesan cheese	25 mL
1	medium tomato (optional), cut into wedges	1

1. In a food processor or blender, combine eggs and tofu; process until smooth. Add flour, juice and seasonings; blend to combine. Transfer to bowl; stir in chopped vegetables.
2. In a bowl, combine melted butter and bread crumbs. Press into bottom of prepared pan. Pour tofu mixture over bread crumbs. Sprinkle with cheese. Bake in preheated oven for 35 minutes or until set in center. Arrange tomato wedges, if using, around outer edge; bake for 5 minutes longer to warm tomatoes.
3. Cut quiche into 4 wedges for adults, 12 for babies.

NUTRITIONAL ANALYSIS (PER BABY SERVING)							
Energy	Protein	Carbohydrate	Fat	Fiber	Calcium	Iron	Sodium
55 kcal	3 g	5 g	3 g	1 g	26 mg	0.5 mg	78 mg

Makes 6 baby servings, or 4 adult servings

Children will love this vibrantly flavored dish. Be sure to select firm water-packed tofu, which stands up well to stir-frying. With stir-frying, vegetables are often tender-crisp, but little ones may like theirs more tender, so just cook them a little longer than the recipe suggests. Serve over cooked brown rice, if desired.

Kitchen Tip

To reduce the sodium content of this recipe, replace the soy sauce with homemade vegetable broth.

Vegetarian Stir-Fry

Shallow baking pan, lined with foil

½ cup	reduced-sodium soy sauce	125 mL
1	large clove garlic, crushed	1
1 tsp	sesame oil	5 mL
1	package (12 oz/350 g) firm tofu, cut into ½-inch (1 cm) slices	1
1 tbsp	reduced-sodium soy sauce	15 mL
½ tsp	granulated sugar	2 mL
¼ tsp	freshly ground black pepper	1 mL
1 tbsp	canola oil	15 mL
3	green onions, sliced diagonally	3
1	clove garlic, sliced	1
½	red bell pepper, cut into thin strips	½
½	yellow bell pepper, cut into thin strips	½
1 cup	trimmed snow peas	250 mL
8	mushrooms, sliced	8

1. In a bowl, combine the ½ cup (125 mL) soy sauce, crushed garlic, sesame oil and tofu; toss to coat tofu. Cover and let stand at room temperature for 1 hour or refrigerate for up to 4 hours. Arrange in a single layer in prepared baking pan.

2. Preheat oven to 375°F (190°C). Bake tofu for 35 minutes. Using tongs, transfer tofu to a bowl and discard marinade. Set tofu aside.

3. In a small bowl, combine the 1 tbsp (15 mL) soy sauce, sugar and pepper.

4. In a wok or large nonstick skillet, heat canola oil over medium-high heat. Add onions and sliced garlic; stir-fry for 2 minutes. Add bell peppers; stir-fry for 2 minutes. Add peas, mushrooms and 2 tbsp (25 mL) water; cover and cook for 3 minutes or until tender. Add tofu and soy sauce mixture; toss gently to combine. Cover and cook for 2 minutes or until heated through.

NUTRITIONAL ANALYSIS (PER BABY SERVING)

Energy	Protein	Carbohydrate	Fat	Fiber	Calcium	Iron	Sodium
118 kcal	8 g	10 g	6 g	2 g	97 mg	2 mg	768 mg

Thai Vegetable Sauce

Asian foods are increasing in popularity and may even become your child's favorite. Choose your favorite fish fillets or chicken breasts and cook as desired, then serve with prepared Thai Vegetable Sauce.

⅓ cup	finely chopped carrot	75 mL
⅓ cup	finely chopped celery	75 mL
⅓ cup	finely chopped red bell pepper	75 mL
¼ cup	finely chopped onion	50 mL
⅓ cup	reduced-sodium chicken broth	75 mL
¼ cup	reduced-sodium soy sauce	50 mL
¼ cup	rice vinegar	50 mL
2 tbsp	ketchup	25 mL
1 tbsp	granulated sugar	15 mL

1. In a small saucepan, combine carrot, celery, red pepper, onion, chicken broth, soy sauce, vinegar, ketchup and sugar. Bring to a boil over high heat. Reduce heat to low, cover and simmer for 10 minutes or until vegetables are just tender. Let cool slightly and serve, or refrigerate in an airtight container for up to 5 days.

NUTRITIONAL ANALYSIS (PER ½ CUP/125 ML)

Energy	Protein	Carbohydrate	Fat	Fiber	Calcium	Iron	Sodium
85 kcal	3 g	20 g	0.5 g	2 g	33 mg	1 mg	1029 mg

Great Spaghetti Sauce

Makes 7 cups (1.75 L)

Kitchen Tips

Freeze in this sauce in batches to have on hand for a quick pasta meal.

Serve over your child's favorite pasta. Good choices include rotini or gemilli (spiral pasta).

1 tbsp	vegetable oil	15 mL
1 lb	lean ground beef	500 g
2¾ cups	prepared tomato sauce	675 mL
1	can (19 oz/540 mL) whole tomatoes with Italian seasoning	1
1 tbsp	garlic powder	15 mL
1 tbsp	dried basil	15 mL

1. In a large skillet, heat oil over high heat. Add beef and cook until brown and cooked through. Drain fat. Reduce heat to medium. Add tomato sauce, tomatoes, garlic powder and basil; cook, uncovered, for 10 to 15 minutes.

NUTRITIONAL ANALYSIS (PER ¼ CUP/50 ML)

Energy	Protein	Carbohydrate	Fat	Fiber	Calcium	Iron	Sodium
49 kcal	4 g	3 g	2 g	1 g	15 mg	1 mg	185 mg

Makes 4 cups (1 L)

Kitchen Tips

Use fontina, mozzarella and Parmesan cheeses for the kids, then add gorgonzola (or another cheese) for adult portions.

Use homemade or reduced-sodium stock to lower the sodium content of this recipe.

Four-Cheese Pasta with Vegetables

3 tbsp	butter or margarine	45 mL
1½ tbsp	all-purpose flour	22 mL
¼ tsp	ground nutmeg	1 mL
⅛ tsp	salt	0.5 mL
⅛ tsp	freshly ground black pepper	0.5 mL
¾ cup	light (5%) cream	175 mL
¾ cup	vegetable stock	175 mL
⅓ cup	shredded fontina cheese	75 mL
⅓ cup	shredded mozzarella cheese	75 mL
⅓ cup	grated Parmesan cheese	75 mL
¼ cup	crumbled gorgonzola or blue cheese (see tip)	50 mL
½ lb	dry medium shell pasta or rotini	250 g
1 cup	finely chopped cooked vegetables	250 mL

1. In a saucepan, melt butter over low heat. Whisk in flour, nutmeg, salt and pepper; cook for 1 minute. Whisk in cream and vegetable stock; cook, whisking constantly, for 5 minutes or until mixture is smooth and thickened. Add fontina, mozzarella and Parmesan cheeses; stir until cheese is melted.
2. Meanwhile, in a large amount of boiling water, cook pasta according to package directions until tender but firm. Drain. Add cheese sauce and cooked vegetables; toss well to combine.
3. Serve children's portions, then add gorgonzola; cover for a few minutes until gorgonzola is melted. Stir well and serve.

NUTRITIONAL ANALYSIS (PER ½ CUP/125 ML)

Energy	Protein	Carbohydrate	Fat	Fiber	Calcium	Iron	Sodium
252 kcal	9 g	27 g	12 g	2 g	163 mg	1 mg	347 mg

Tortellini is probably the most child-friendly of pastas — easy for little fingers to pick up without the need for a fork or spoon. Messy, but fun!

Cheese Tortellini with Mixed Vegetables

1 cup	tomato sauce	250 mL
1	small clove garlic, minced (optional)	1
½ tsp	dried basil	2 mL
½ tsp	dried oregano	2 mL
⅛ tsp	granulated sugar	0.5 mL
⅛ tsp	salt	0.5 mL
⅛ tsp	freshly ground black pepper	0.5 mL
2 cups	frozen cheese tortellini	500 mL
1 cup	frozen mixed vegetables	250 mL
2 tbsp	grated Parmesan cheese	25 mL

1. In a saucepan, combine tomato sauce, garlic (if using), basil, oregano, sugar, salt and pepper. Bring to a boil. Reduce heat to low and simmer, covered and stirring occasionally, for 10 minutes.

2. Meanwhile, bring a large saucepan of water to a boil. Add tortellini, return to a boil and cook according to package directions. During the last 5 minutes of cooking, add mixed vegetables; continue to cook until vegetables are tender. Drain well.

3. Toss drained tortellini with tomato sauce and serve sprinkled with cheese.

NUTRITIONAL ANALYSIS (PER ½ CUP/125 ML)							
Energy	Protein	Carbohydrate	Fat	Fiber	Calcium	Iron	Sodium
154 kcal	7 g	25 g	3 g	2 g	92 mg	1 mg	428 mg

Makes 20 baby servings, or 6 adult servings

Variations

Cottage cheese can replace ricotta, if desired.

If you like using oat bran, substitute an equal amount for the bread crumbs.

Spinach Cannelloni

Preheat oven to 350°F (180°C)
13- by 9-inch (3 L) baking pan, greased

1	package (10 oz/300 g) frozen chopped spinach, thawed	1
1 tbsp	olive oil	15 mL
⅓ cup	finely chopped onion	75 mL
1	clove garlic, minced	1
8	mushrooms, chopped	8
1 cup	grated Parmesan cheese, divided	250 mL
1 cup	ricotta cheese (see tip)	250 mL
¾ cup	whole wheat bread crumbs (see tip)	175 mL
1 tbsp	freshly squeezed lemon juice	15 mL
Pinch	freshly ground black pepper	Pinch
20	oven-ready cannelloni shells	20
2 cups	mild salsa, divided	500 mL

1. Squeeze excess liquid from spinach and discard liquid.

2. In a nonstick skillet, heat oil over medium heat. Add onion and garlic; sauté for 3 minutes or until tender. Add mushrooms and sauté for 5 minutes; transfer to a bowl.

3. Add spinach, ¾ cup (175 mL) Parmesan cheese, ricotta, bread crumbs, lemon juice and pepper to onion mixture and stir until blended. Loosely pack into each cannelloni shell.

4. Spread ¾ cup (175 mL) salsa evenly over bottom of prepared baking pan. Arrange filled shells over salsa. Spoon remaining salsa over shells and sprinkle with remaining Parmesan cheese. Bake in preheated oven for 40 minutes or until noodles are tender and filling is heated through.

NUTRITIONAL ANALYSIS (PER BABY SERVING)

Energy	Protein	Carbohydrate	Fat	Fiber	Calcium	Iron	Sodium
164 kcal	8 g	23 g	5 g	2 g	114 mg	1.7 mg	283 mg

Makes 9 cups (2.25 L)

Kitchen Tip

This is a quick and easy meal. Use whatever kind of noodles you like.

Fiesta Tomato Surprise

1 lb	lean ground beef	500 g
1 lb	dry rotini or other spiral pasta	500 g
2	cans (each 10 oz/284 mL) sodium-reduced tomato soup	2
½	soup can of water	½
1 tsp	dried basil	5 mL
½ tsp	dried oregano	2 mL
1 tbsp	grated Parmesan cheese	15 mL

1. In a large skillet, cook ground beef over medium-high heat until browned. Remove from heat and drain excess fat.

2. Meanwhile, in a large pot of boiling water, cook noodles according to package directions or until tender but firm. Drain. Add cooked beef, soup, water, basil and oregano. Heat for 5 minutes or until warmed through. Serve garnished with Parmesan cheese.

NUTRITIONAL ANALYSIS (PER ½ CUP/125 ML)

Energy	Protein	Carbohydrate	Fat	Fiber	Calcium	Iron	Sodium
170 kcal	9 g	26 g	3 g	1 g	16 mg	1 mg	202 mg

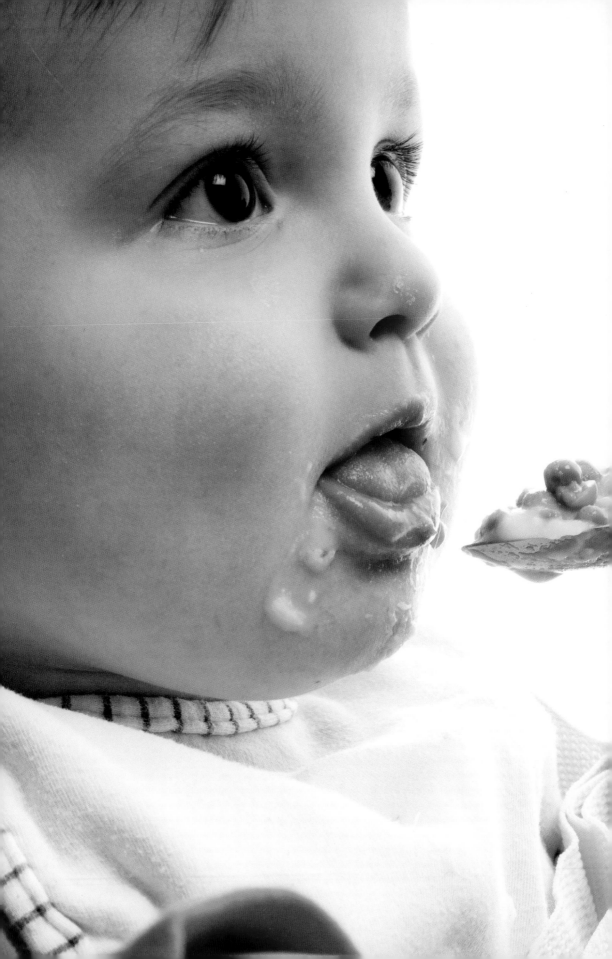

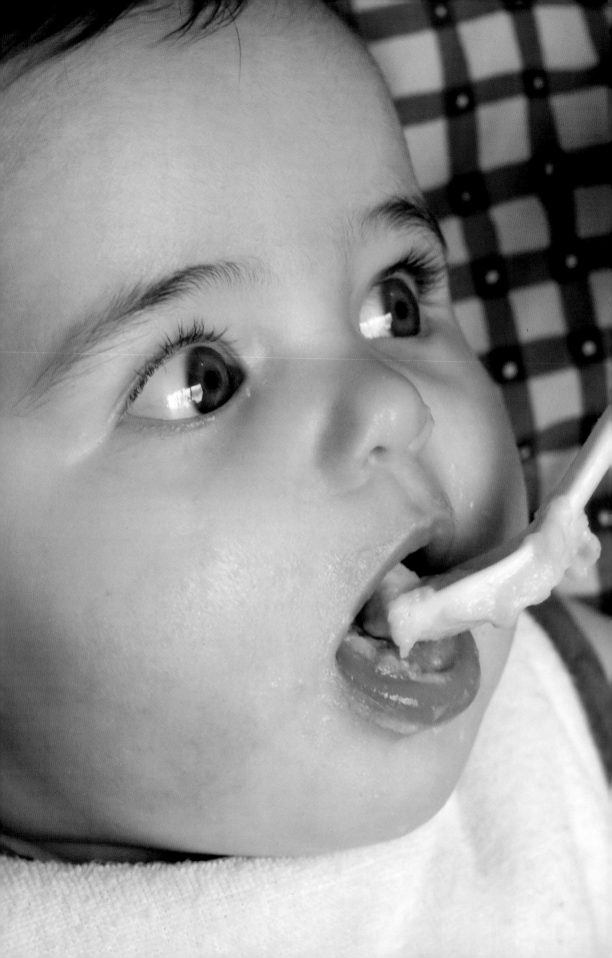

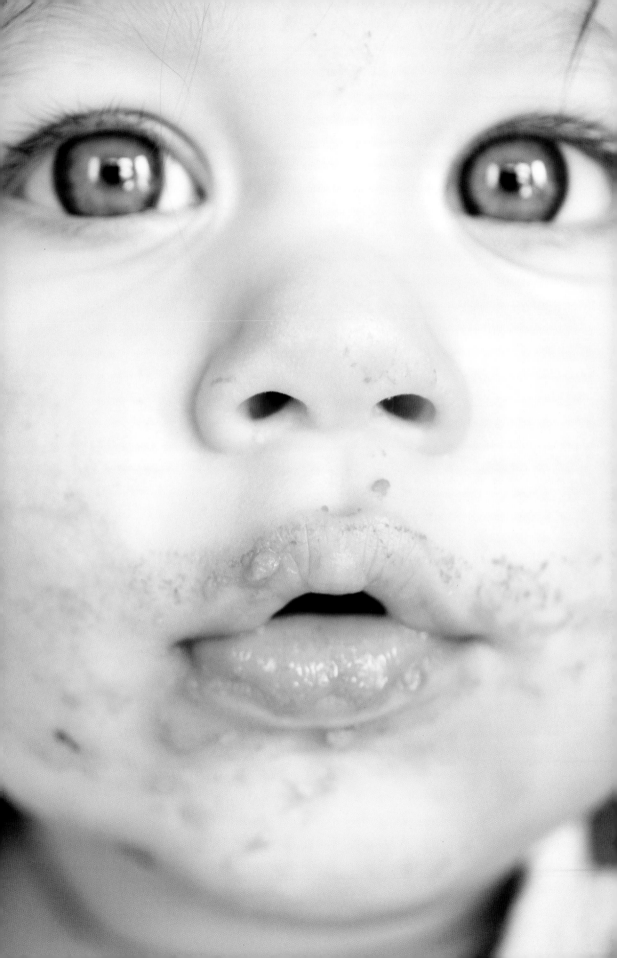

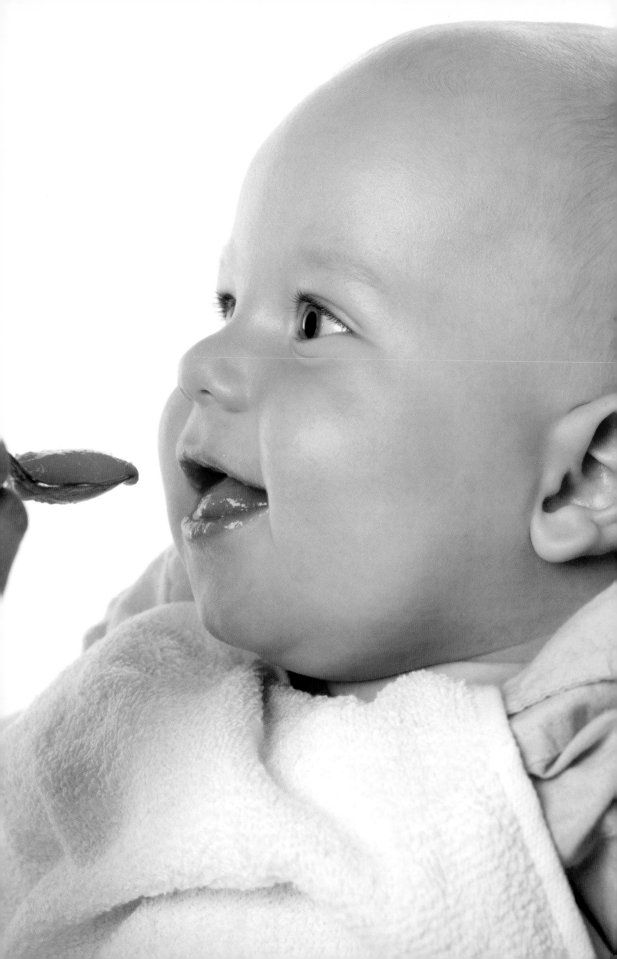

Everyone knows the Italian version of lasagna. But in this recipe we add a new twist with Mexican flavors, which children particularly seem to enjoy.

Kitchen Tips

Make sure that infant portions have noodles cut into small bites, and are allowed to cool before serving.

This version of lasagna lacks the usual cottage cheese, since it's not part of Mexican cuisine. You can add it back, if you wish: Use 1 cup (250 mL), divided between layers of noodles.

Food Safety Tip

Always use separate cutting boards for meats, poultry, fruits and vegetables, and breads. Clean cutting boards in the dishwasher or scrub with hot water and detergent after each use.

Mexican Lasagna

Preheat oven to 350°F (180°C)
11- by 7-inch (2 L) baking pan, greased

1 tsp	vegetable oil	5 mL
1 lb	lean ground beef	500 g
½ cup	finely chopped onion	125 mL
½ cup	finely chopped green pepper	125 mL
1	can (7½ oz/213 mL) tomato sauce	1
½ cup	water	125 mL
1 to 2 tsp	chili powder	5 to 10 mL
½ tsp	salt	2 mL
½ tsp	dried oregano	2 mL
½ tsp	garlic powder	2 mL
6	cooked lasagna noodles	6
2 cups	shredded Monterey Jack cheese	500 mL

1. In a large nonstick skillet, heat oil over medium heat. Add ground beef and cook for 10 minutes or until no longer pink; drain fat. Stir in onion and green pepper; cook for 5 minutes longer or until vegetables are tender. Add tomato sauce, water, chili powder, salt, oregano and garlic powder; cook for about 10 minutes.

2. Arrange 3 noodles in bottom of prepared pan. Spoon half of sauce and half of cheese over noodles. Repeat layers.

3. Bake in preheated oven for 25 minutes or until cheese melts and casserole is bubbling. Remove from oven and let stand for 10 minutes before cutting.

NUTRITIONAL ANALYSIS (PER BABY SERVING)							
Energy	Protein	Carbohydrate	Fat	Fiber	Calcium	Iron	Sodium
203 kcal	14 g	11 g	12 g	1 g	216 mg	1.5 mg	297 mg

Makes 20 baby servings, or 8 adult servings

Here's a recipe that kids love. Serve over rice or pasta, or serve with bread that children can use for dipping.

Kitchen Tip

This recipe is a great source of iron. It freezes well, too.

Easy Meatballs

2 lbs	lean ground beef	1 kg
2	eggs	2
½ tsp	salt	2 mL
½ tsp	freshly ground black pepper	2 mL
½ cup	water	125 mL
½ cup	dry bread crumbs	125 mL
1 tbsp	lemon juice	15 mL
½ cup	granulated sugar	125 mL
2 cups	water	500 mL
2½ cups	tomato juice	625 mL
3	stalks celery, diced	3
1	small onion, diced	1
1	can (2¾ oz/80 mL) tomato paste	1

1. In a large bowl, combine ground beef, eggs, salt, pepper, ½ cup (125 mL) water and bread crumbs. Mix well. With your hands, roll meat mixture into 1-inch (2.5 cm) meatballs. Set aside.

2. In a large saucepan over medium-high heat, combine lemon juice, sugar, 2 cups (500 mL) water, tomato juice, celery and onion; cook, covered, for 30 minutes. Reduce heat to simmer. Add meatballs and tomato paste; cook, uncovered, for 2 hours.

NUTRITIONAL ANALYSIS (PER BABY SERVING)

Energy	Protein	Carbohydrate	Fat	Fiber	Calcium	Iron	Sodium
127 kcal	10 g	10 g	5 g	1 g	20 mg	1 mg	199 mg

Makes 22 meatballs

Soft meat in a nicely herbed sauce make this a child's favorite.

Kitchen Tips

This dish is a good source of iron. It also freezes well.

Serve over pasta, such as linguine (cut up for children), or with rice.

Use homemade or reduced-sodium stock to lower the sodium content of this recipe.

Meatballs and Mushrooms

2 tsp	vegetable oil or olive oil	10 mL
2 cups	sliced mushrooms	500 mL
2 tsp	chopped fresh dill or basil (or 1 tsp/5 mL dried)	10 mL
¼ tsp	salt	1 mL
¼ tsp	freshly ground black pepper	1 mL
⅔ cup	evaporated milk, divided	150 mL
¼ cup	crushed corn flakes cereal	50 mL
¼ cup	finely chopped onion	50 mL
¼ tsp	ground allspice	1 mL
¼ tsp	ground nutmeg	1 mL
19 oz	lean ground beef	575 g
4 tsp	all-purpose flour	20 mL
⅔ cup	beef stock	150 mL

1. In a large skillet, heat oil over medium-high heat. Add mushrooms, dill and a pinch of the salt and pepper; sauté for 8 to 10 minutes or until brown. Transfer to a bowl and set aside.
2. In another bowl, combine 2 tbsp (25 mL) of the milk with cereal crumbs, onion, allspice, nutmeg and the remaining salt and pepper. Add beef; mix well. With your hands, shape into meatballs, about 1 inch (2.5 cm) in diameter.
3. Return skillet to heat and add meatballs; cook for 8 to 10 minutes or until they are brown. Add reserved mushrooms. Stir in flour. Add stock and remaining milk. Bring to a boil. Simmer, stirring, for another 5 minutes or until thickened.

NUTRITIONAL ANALYSIS (PER MEATBALL)							
Energy	Protein	Carbohydrate	Fat	Fiber	Calcium	Iron	Sodium
61 kcal	6 g	2 g	3 g	0.1 g	25 mg	1 mg	62 mg

Makes 12 slices

The ketchup topping makes a tangy crust that your children will love.

Kitchen Tip

Drain any excess oil from the meatloaf halfway through cooking.

Easy Meatloaf

Preheat oven to 350°F (180°C)
9- by 5-inch (2 L) loaf pan, greased

1 lb	lean or extra-lean ground beef	500 g
1	egg	1
½ tsp	salt	2 mL
¼ tsp	freshly ground black pepper	1 mL
½	onion, chopped	½
¼ cup	dry bread crumbs	50 mL
¼ cup	ketchup	50 mL
1 tsp	steak sauce	5 mL
	Additional ketchup for topping	

1. In a large bowl, combine beef, egg, salt and pepper, onion, bread crumbs, ¼ cup (50 mL) ketchup and steak sauce. Mix well and transfer to prepared loaf pan. Cover top with additional ketchup. Bake for 1 hour or until juices run clear.

NUTRITIONAL ANALYSIS (PER SLICE)							
Energy	Protein	Carbohydrate	Fat	Fiber	Calcium	Iron	Sodium
91 kcal	9 g	3 g	5 g	0.2 g	11 mg	1 mg	98 mg

Makes 24 baby servings, or 6 adult servings

Here's a soft-textured one-dish meal that your family will love.

Kitchen Tip

You'll need about 4 medium potatoes to make 2 cups (500 mL) mashed.

Variation

Replace the corn with 1½ cups (375 mL) mixed frozen vegetables.

Shepherd's Pie

Preheat oven to 375°F (190°C)
13- by 9-inch (3 L) baking dish

1½ lbs	lean ground beef	750 g
2 tbsp	chopped onion	25 mL
¼ tsp	salt	1 mL
¼ tsp	mixed dried herbs (parsley, thyme, sage)	1 mL
1¼ cups	gravy or bouillon	300 mL
1	can (10 oz/284 mL) reduced-sodium corn kernels	1
2 cups	mashed potatoes	500 mL
¼ cup	grated Cheddar cheese (optional)	50 mL

1. In a large skillet, over medium-high heat, brown beef. Add onion and cook for 3 minutes or until softened. Stir in salt, herbs, gravy and corn.

2. Pour beef mixture into baking dish and cover with mashed potatoes. Bake in preheated oven for 30 to 35 minutes or until potatoes are browned. If desired, top with cheese and bake for another 5 minutes.

NUTRITIONAL ANALYSIS (PER BABY SERVING)							
Energy	Protein	Carbohydrate	Fat	Fiber	Calcium	Iron	Sodium
93 kcal	7 g	8 g	4 g	1 g	15 mg	1 mg	141 mg

Makes 12 baby servings, or 4 adult servings

This old-fashioned meal will be a big winner, especially on cold winter nights.

Kitchen Tips

This recipe freezes really well before baking. When baking from frozen, bake for 2 hours at 350°F (180°C). If desired, broil for the last 2 to 5 minutes to brown the top.

Use homemade or reduced-sodium stock to lower the sodium content of this recipe.

Variation

Substitute leftover cooked turkey for the chicken.

Chicken Pot Pie

Preheat oven to 400°F (200°C)
9-inch (23 cm) pie plate

2 tbsp	butter or margarine	25 mL
⅓ cup	all-purpose flour	75 mL
1½ cups	chicken stock	375 mL
1½ cups	2% milk	375 mL
2 cups	cubed cooked chicken	500 mL
1 cup	diced cooked turnips	250 mL
1 cup	diced cooked carrots	250 mL
1 cup	frozen peas, thawed	250 mL
¼ tsp	dried thyme	2 mL
Pinch	cayenne pepper	Pinch
¼ tsp	freshly ground black pepper	2 mL
1 tsp	salt (omit if using canned chicken broth or bouillon)	5 mL
1	pie shell (unbaked)	1

1. In a large saucepan, melt butter over medium heat. Whisk in flour, stock and milk. Bring to a boil, whisking constantly. Reduce heat to low and simmer for 5 minutes or until smooth and thickened. Stir in chicken, turnips, carrots, peas, thyme, cayenne pepper, black pepper and salt.
2. Pour mixture into pie plate. Top with pie shell, crimp the edges and poke holes in the top to let steam escape. Bake in preheated oven for 20 minutes; reduce heat to 350°F (180°C) and bake for another 40 minutes or until pastry is browned. Let stand for 10 to 15 minutes before serving.

NUTRITIONAL ANALYSIS (PER BABY SERVING)

Energy	Protein	Carbohydrate	Fat	Fiber	Calcium	Iron	Sodium
177 kcal	14 g	14 g	7 g	2 g	63 mg	1 mg	331 mg

Makes 8 servings

Kitchen Tip

This dish is a very good source of iron. Young children enjoy it because the thighs are soft and never dry.

Chicken Thighs with Herbs

Preheat oven to 375°F (190°C)
Casserole or baking dish, greased

3 tbsp	mayonnaise	45 mL
2 tbsp	Dijon mustard	25 mL
1 tbsp	lemon juice	15 mL
1 tsp	dried rosemary, crushed	5 mL
1 tsp	dried basil	5 mL
1 tsp	dried thyme	5 mL
1 tsp	dried savory	5 mL
2 tsp	grated Parmesan cheese	10 mL
2 cups	crushed corn flakes cereal	500 mL
¼ tsp	freshly ground black pepper	1 mL
8	boneless skinless chicken thighs	8

1. In a small bowl, combine mayonnaise, mustard, lemon juice, herbs and Parmesan cheese.

2. In a medium bowl, mix corn flakes with pepper.

3. Dip chicken thighs one at a time into the mayonnaise/herb mixture, then into cereal mixture, making sure each is well coated. Place thighs in prepared baking dish and bake for 35 to 40 minutes or until juices run clear when pierced with a fork.

NUTRITIONAL ANALYSIS (PER SERVING)							
Energy	Protein	Carbohydrate	Fat	Fiber	Calcium	Iron	Sodium
136 kcal	14 g	8 g	5 g	0.3 g	19 mg	2 mg	203 mg

Makes 4 servings

Adding Mediterranean flavors to succulent salmon gives a delightful twist to this favorite fish. Baking the salmon in broth ensures that the fish remains moist — which makes it easier (and more enjoyable) for children to eat.

Kitchen Tips

If you don't have fresh salmon, you can use frozen fillets.

Use homemade or reduced-sodium stock to lower the sodium content of this recipe.

Baked Mediterranean Salmon Fillets

Preheat oven to 400°F (200°C)
8-inch (2 L) square baking pan, greased

1 lb	salmon fillets (about 4)	500 g
¼ tsp	dried oregano	1 mL
¼ tsp	dried thyme	1 mL
½	lemon, thinly sliced	½
1	large tomato, sliced	1
½	green bell pepper, diced	½
¼ cup	finely chopped onion	50 mL
½ cup	chicken stock	125 mL
1 tbsp	lemon juice	15 mL
	Chopped fresh parsley (optional)	

1. Arrange fish fillets in prepared baking pan. Sprinkle with oregano and thyme. Place lemon and tomato slices, green pepper and onion over fish.
2. In a small bowl, combine chicken stock and lemon juice; pour over vegetables and fish. Cover and bake in preheated oven for 20 minutes or until fish flakes easily with a fork at its thickest part. If desired, garnish with parsley before serving.

NUTRITIONAL ANALYSIS (PER SERVING)							
Energy	Protein	Carbohydrate	Fat	Fiber	Calcium	Iron	Sodium
238 kcal	28 g	5 g	11 g	1 g	19 mg	1 mg	110 mg

Makes 12 baby servings, or 4 adult servings

Keep this basic marinade on hand for spur-of-the-minute fish preparation!

Kitchen Tip

The marinade can be stored in an airtight container in the refrigerator for up to 1 week.

Lemon-Grilled Salmon with Herbs

Preheat broiler or barbecue grill to medium-high
Broiler pan, greased, or greased barbecue rack

Marinade

½ cup	freshly squeezed lemon juice	125 mL
¼ cup	olive or canola oil	50 mL
1	small onion, finely chopped	1
1	clove garlic, minced	1
2 tbsp	chopped fresh dill (or 2 tsp/10 mL dried)	25 mL
Pinch	freshly ground black pepper	Pinch
4	salmon steaks or skinless fillets (each about 4 oz/125 g)	4

1. *Marinade:* In a small bowl, combine lemon juice, oil, onion, garlic, dill and pepper.
2. Place salmon in a shallow dish and pour marinade over. Cover and refrigerate for up to 4 hours, turning once.
3. Remove salmon from marinade, discarding marinade. Place on broiler pan or barbecue rack. Broil about 4 inches (10 cm) from heat or grill for 10 minutes per 1 inch (2.5 cm) thickness or until salmon flakes easily with a fork.

NUTRITIONAL ANALYSIS (PER BABY SERVING)							
Energy	Protein	Carbohydrate	Fat	Fiber	Calcium	Iron	Sodium
86 kcal	6 g	1 g	6 g	0.1 g	7 mg	0.5 mg	15 mg

Makes 8 baby servings, or 4 adult servings

Soufflés are an easy main dish for the cook to prepare and for guests or family to enjoy.

Kitchen Tips

Extra milk may be needed to soften bread. Add up to 2 tbsp (25 mL) more if required.

Extra seasonings may be added for the more adventurous family. Try celery seed or dried or fresh basil, dill or thyme.

Salmon Soufflé

Preheat oven to 375°F (190°C)
4-cup (1 L) casserole dish, greased

1	can (7½ oz/213 g) salmon	1
¼ cup	2% milk	50 mL
1	slice whole wheat bread, crust removed	1
3	eggs, separated	3
Pinch	freshly ground black pepper	Pinch
	Cucumber slices	
	Whole wheat toast triangles	

1. Drain liquid from salmon into a small saucepan. Add milk to liquid and heat gently over medium heat until warm.
2. Remove skin from salmon, if desired. In a bowl, mash salmon well with a fork, breaking bones into very small pieces; set aside.
3. Place bread in a shallow bowl. Pour milk mixture over bread and let stand in a warm location to soften bread, about 10 minutes. Stir bread mixture well with a fork. Stir in salmon, egg yolks and pepper until smooth.
4. In another bowl, using an electric mixer, beat egg whites until stiff. Gently fold into salmon mixture. Spoon mixture into prepared casserole dish.
5. Bake in preheated oven for about 20 minutes or until puffed and golden and set in center. Serve with cucumber slices and toast triangles.

NUTRITIONAL ANALYSIS (PER BABY SERVING)							
Energy	Protein	Carbohydrate	Fat	Fiber	Calcium	Iron	Sodium
72 kcal	6 g	2 g	4 g	0.3 g	63 mg	0.5 mg	125 mg

Kitchen Tip

Try the salmon and potato mixture on its own — it's tasty and particularly appealing to younger children who still like their food a little mushy. Makes great use of leftover mashed potatoes.

Simple Salmon Cakes

Preheat oven to 375°F (190°C)
Baking sheet, well greased

2	cans (each 7½ oz/213 g) salmon, bones and skin removed, drained and flaked	2
1½ cups	mashed potatoes (about 3 medium)	375 mL
2	eggs, separated	2
2 tbsp	all-purpose flour	25 mL
Pinch	salt	Pinch
½ cup	dry bread crumbs	125 mL

1. In a bowl, combine salmon and potato. Blend in egg yolks. With your hands, form mixture into flat cakes. Dust each cake with a mixture of flour and salt. Brush cakes with egg white. Coat with bread crumbs and bake in preheated oven for 15 minutes or until golden brown.

NUTRITIONAL ANALYSIS (PER CAKE)

Energy	Protein	Carbohydrate	Fat	Fiber	Calcium	Iron	Sodium
89 kcal	8 g	10 g	2 g	1 g	86 mg	1 mg	156 mg

Makes 8 baby servings, or 4 adult servings

Kitchen Tip

You can also make your own garlic sauce: Mix together 1 clove garlic, crushed, and 2 tbsp (25 mL) each of packed brown sugar, sodium-reduced soy sauce, rice vinegar and olive oil. Store any extra in an airtight container in the refrigerator for up to 3 days.

Simply Tasty Trout

Preheat oven to 400°F (200°C)
Clay or glass baking dish

1 lb	trout fillets	500 g
1 tbsp	olive oil	15 mL
3 tbsp	honey garlic sauce or teriyaki sauce	45 mL

1. Place trout, skin side down, on baking dish. Drizzle with oil and honey garlic sauce.

2. Bake in preheated oven for 10 to 12 minutes or until fish flakes easily with a fork.

NUTRITIONAL ANALYSIS (PER BABY SERVING)

Energy	Protein	Carbohydrate	Fat	Fiber	Calcium	Iron	Sodium
114 kcal	13 g	1 g	6 g	–	29 mg	1 mg	324 mg

Makes 16 baby servings, or 4 adult servings

This soft vegetable and pasta combination is a real treat for young children.

Tuna Noodle Casserole

Preheat oven to 350°F (180°C)
Casserole dish

1 lb	rotini or other pasta	500 g
2 tbsp	vegetable oil	25 mL
1	medium onion, chopped	1
1 or 2	cloves garlic, chopped	1 or 2
1	green pepper, diced	1
2 cups	sliced mushrooms	500 mL
2	cans (each 6½ oz/184 g) tuna, drained	2
⅔ cup	sliced pitted green olives (optional)	150 mL
1½ cups	condensed cream of mushroom soup	375 mL
¼ cup	grated Parmesan cheese	50 mL

1. In a large saucepan of boiling water, cook pasta according to package directions or until tender but firm.

2. In a large skillet, heat oil over medium heat. Add onions, garlic, green pepper and mushrooms; cook for 5 to 7 minutes or until vegetables begin to soften. Add tuna and sliced olives; cook for about 1 minute.

3. Transfer pasta to casserole dish. Add vegetable-tuna mixture and toss together. Pour soup over and top with Parmesan cheese. Bake in preheated oven for 1 hour.

NUTRITIONAL ANALYSIS (PER BABY SERVING)

Energy	Protein	Carbohydrate	Fat	Fiber	Calcium	Iron	Sodium
100 kcal	6 g	10 g	4 g	0.6 g	27 mg	0.6 mg	178 mg

Makes 8 baby servings, or 4 adult servings

This all-time favorite uses a white milk sauce rather than canned soup. Add any vegetable your family enjoys.

Tuna 'n' Egg Noodle Casserole

Preheat oven to 375°F (190°C)
4-cup (1 L) casserole dish, greased

1½ cups	egg noodles	375 mL
1	can (6½ oz/184 g) water-packed flaked tuna, drained	1
½ cup	frozen peas, carrots or mixed vegetables	125 mL
1 tbsp	butter or margarine	15 mL
1 tbsp	whole wheat flour	15 mL
½ cup	2% milk	125 mL
Pinch	freshly ground black pepper	Pinch
⅓ cup	shredded mild Cheddar cheese	75 mL

1. In a large pot of boiling water, cook noodles according to package directions. Drain well. In prepared casserole dish, combine noodles, tuna and peas. Set aside.

2. In a small saucepan, melt butter over medium heat. Whisk in flour and cook, stirring, for about 1 minute or until bubbly. Gradually whisk in milk and pepper. Cook, stirring constantly, for about 3 minutes or until thickened. Pour over noodle mixture, stirring to combine. Sprinkle with cheese.

3. Bake in preheated oven for 20 minutes or until hot and bubbly.

NUTRITIONAL ANALYSIS (PER BABY SERVING)							
Energy	Protein	Carbohydrate	Fat	Fiber	Calcium	Iron	Sodium
109 kcal	7 g	11 g	4 g	1 g	59 mg	1 mg	99 mg

Makes 16 baby servings, or 4 adult servings

Don't be discouraged by the number of steps in this recipe — it is really very simple to prepare!

Kitchen Tips

This is a delicious fish recipe that freezes well.

If you really love the flavor of fish, double the quantity called for in the recipe. The rest of the ingredients remain the same.

Fresh or frozen fish will work equally well here; just adjust the poaching time.

Poaching is a method of cooking food gently in a liquid just below the boiling point. Use enough liquid just to cover the food.

Sole and Spinach Casserole

Preheat broiler
Casserole dish

14 oz	fillets of sole or other white fish	400 g
Seasoned Spinach		
1½ cups	spinach, trimmed and washed, but not dried	375 mL
1 tsp	reduced-sodium soy sauce	5 mL
1 tsp	butter or margarine	5 mL
½ tsp	salt	2 mL
¼ tsp	freshly ground black pepper	1 mL
1 tbsp	all-purpose flour	15 mL
White Sauce		
1 tbsp	butter or margarine	15 mL
1½ tbsp	all-purpose flour	22 mL
1 cup	whole milk	250 mL
½ tsp	salt	2 mL
½ tsp	freshly ground black pepper	2 mL
Mushrooms		
1 tsp	olive oil	5 mL
2 cups	sliced mushrooms	500 mL
¼ cup	grated Parmesan cheese	50 mL

1. In a skillet or poacher or steamer, poach sole until it flakes with a fork. (See tips.) Drain.
2. *Seasoned Spinach:* In a large saucepan over high heat, cook spinach (with no more water than is clinging to the leaves) until soft. Add soy sauce, butter, salt and pepper. Sprinkle 1 tbsp (15 mL) flour over spinach and stir thoroughly to absorb any excess liquid. Coarsely chop spinach.
3. *White Sauce:* In a medium saucepan over low heat, melt 1 tbsp (15 mL) butter. Stir in 1½ tbsp (22 mL) flour; cook, stirring, for 3 to 5 minutes. Slowly whisk in milk; cook, whisking constantly, until sauce is thickened and smooth. Add salt and pepper.

4. *Mushrooms:* In a skillet over medium-high heat, heat olive oil. Add mushrooms and cook for about 5 minutes or until softened. Set aside.

5. Spread seasoned spinach in a layer on bottom of casserole dish. Arrange poached sole fillets on top of spinach. Sprinkle mushrooms over sole. Pour white sauce over. Sprinkle with Parmesan cheese. Broil until white sauce starts to bubble.

NUTRITIONAL ANALYSIS (PER BABY SERVING)

Energy	Protein	Carbohydrate	Fat	Fiber	Calcium	Iron	Sodium
64 kcal	8 g	2 g	3 g	0.3 g	44 mg	0.4 mg	194 mg

12 to 18 months

Makes 10 baby servings, or 4 adult servings

Beloved even by finicky eaters, this recipe can be prepared in advance and cooked before serving.

Kitchen Tip

This recipe freezes well after baking.

Fish, Tomato and Spinach Casserole

Preheat oven to 350°F (180°C)
11-cup (2.75 L) casserole dish

1	package (10 oz/284 g) fresh spinach, washed, coarse stems removed	1
2 cups	tomato sauce	500 mL
14 to 24 oz	frozen cod or sole, thawed	398 to 680 g
2 cups	grated mozzarella or white Cheddar cheese	500 mL

1. In a saucepan over medium-high heat, cook wet spinach leaves for 5 to 8 minutes until just limp. Drain, squeeze out remaining moisture and chop coarsely.

2. Pour half of tomato sauce into casserole dish. Create layers of fish, then spinach, then cheese, using half of each of these ingredients. Repeat layers with remainder of ingredients, starting with tomato sauce and ending with cheese.

3. Bake in preheated oven for 45 minutes or until bubbling.

NUTRITIONAL ANALYSIS (PER BABY SERVING)

Energy	Protein	Carbohydrate	Fat	Fiber	Calcium	Iron	Sodium
145 kcal	14 g	4 g	8 g	1 g	182 mg	1 mg	450 mg

Makes 1 cup (250 mL)

Kids will love this tangy dressing. It can be used on salads, as a vegetable dip, or as a dipping sauce for baked fish or fish sticks.

Honey Salad Dressing

¾ cup	mayonnaise	175 mL
1½ tbsp	red wine vinegar	22 mL
1½ tbsp	liquid honey	22 mL
1	clove garlic, crushed	1
2 tsp	Dijon mustard	10 mL
1 tsp	Worcestershire sauce	5 mL
¼ tsp	hot pepper sauce	1 mL
¼ tsp	salt	1 mL
¼ tsp	freshly ground black pepper	1 mL

1. In a bowl, whisk together all ingredients until thoroughly blended. Use to dress salad or as a dip for vegetables.

NUTRITIONAL ANALYSIS (PER 1 TBSP/15 ML)

Energy	Protein	Carbohydrate	Fat	Fiber	Calcium	Iron	Sodium
50 kcal	0.2 g	4 g	4 g	–	4 mg	0.1 mg	120 mg

Makes 4½ cups (1.125 L)

This tasty, sweet rice salad is a great accompaniment to just about any meat or fish.

Kitchen Tip

For increased flavor and nutrients, use half brown rice and half white rice.

Variations

Replace half the diced celery with diced red or green pepper.

Add 1 tsp (5mL) curry powder to the dressing for a different taste

Rice Salad

3 cups	cooked white rice	750 mL
½ cup	diced celery	125 mL
½ cup	chopped onion	125 mL
10 oz	peas (canned or frozen), drained	300 g
¼ cup	vegetable oil	50 mL
2 tbsp	granulated sugar	25 mL
2 tbsp	reduced-sodium soy sauce	25 mL
1½ tbsp	rice vinegar	22 mL

1. In a large bowl, combine rice, celery, onion and peas.

2. In a small bowl, whisk together oil, sugar, soy sauce and vinegar. Pour dressing over rice. Toss and let stand for at least 1 hour before serving.

NUTRITIONAL ANALYSIS (PER ¼ CUP/50 ML)

Energy	Protein	Carbohydrate	Fat	Fiber	Calcium	Iron	Sodium
75 kcal	1 g	11 g	3 g	1 g	12 mg	0.3 mg	59 mg

Makes 3 servings

Serve this tasty salad when peaches are in season and at their best. A whole wheat roll or toast finishes the meal.

Serving Tip

Children will probably love the peach and chicken mixture, but certainly try them on some romaine lettuce as well.

Food Safety Tip

Always check the label for the "best before " date or the "packaged on" date when purchasing chicken. When you get home, immediately freeze any chicken you do not intend to use within 1 to 3 days. Enclose the packages in plastic freezer bags or overwrap them with heavy-duty foil.

Maximum storage times for chicken in the refrigerator
40°F (4°C): 1 day for ground chicken; 2 to 3 days for whole chicken or chicken pieces; and 3 to 4 days for cooked chicken.

Maximum storage times for chicken in the freezer
0°F (-18°C): 2 to 3 months for ground chicken; 6 months for chicken pieces; 12 months for a whole chicken; and 2 to 3 months for cooked chicken.

Chicken and Peach Salad

2	cooked boneless skinless chicken breasts, cut into slivers	2
2	ripe peaches, peeled and sliced	2
2	green onions, sliced	2
2 tbsp	orange juice	25 mL
2 tbsp	mayonnaise	25 mL
1 tbsp	red wine vinegar	15 mL
	Romaine lettuce	
1 to 2 tbsp	chopped fresh basil (optional)	15 to 25 mL

1. In a bowl combine chicken, peaches and green onions.

2. In a small container with a tight-fitting lid, shake together juice, mayonnaise and vinegar. Pour dressing over chicken mixture; toss lightly to coat. Cover and refrigerate for 30 minutes or longer.

3. Tear lettuce into small pieces and arrange in a serving bowl. Top with chicken mixture; sprinkle with basil, if using, and serve.

NUTRITIONAL ANALYSIS (PER SERVING)

Energy	Protein	Carbohydrate	Fat	Fiber	Calcium	Iron	Sodium
156 kcal	18 g	9 g	5 g	1 g	8 mg	1 mg	102 mg

Makes 4 cups (1 L)

This salad offers a delicious mix of flavors that surprises everyone — even those that don't usually eat chickpeas!

Kitchen Tip

For a change of flavor, use Dijon or dried mustard.

Chickpea and Red Pepper Salad

2	cans (each 19 oz/540 mL) chickpeas, rinsed and drained	2
2	red bell peppers, finely chopped	2
3	green onions, chopped	3

Dressing

2 tbsp	balsamic vinegar	25 mL
2 tbsp	vegetable oil	25 mL
2 tsp	prepared mustard	10 mL
1 tsp	dried basil	5 mL

1. In a bowl, combine chickpeas with red peppers and green onions.

2. *Dressing:* In a small bowl, whisk together vinegar, oil, mustard and basil. Drizzle over salad and toss.

NUTRITIONAL ANALYSIS (PER ¼ CUP/50 ML)

Energy	Protein	Carbohydrate	Fat	Fiber	Calcium	Iron	Sodium
127 kcal	6 g	19 g	3 g	5 g	37 mg	2 mg	15 mg

Makes 3½ cups (875 mL)

Kitchen Tips

If feta is too strong for your child, you may want to try a milder cheese, such as Cheddar.

Serve this dish with bread. It's also delicious over pasta.

Zucchini and Feta Sauté

¼ cup	butter or margarine	50 mL
½ cup	chopped onions	125 mL
½ tsp	salt	2 mL
½ tsp	dried basil	2 mL
⅛ tsp	garlic powder	0.5 mL
3 cups	shredded unpeeled zucchini	750 mL
1 cup	diced tomatoes	250 mL
1 cup	crumbled feta cheese	250 mL
¼ cup	Parmesan cheese	50 mL

1. In a large skillet, melt the butter over medium heat. Stir in onions, salt, basil and garlic powder; cook, uncovered, for 5 minutes or until onions are soft. Add zucchini and cook, stirring occasionally, for 2 to 3 minutes.

2. Sprinkle tomatoes and cheeses over the zucchini. Cover and cook for another 2 minutes.

NUTRITIONAL ANALYSIS (PER ½ CUP/125 ML)

Energy	Protein	Carbohydrate	Fat	Fiber	Calcium	Iron	Sodium
139 kcal	5 g	5 g	11 g	1 g	155 mg	0.4 mg	469 mg

Makes 3 servings

These roast potato wedges are as crisp as French fries. They're just right for dipping into things like ketchup, salsa or a creamy Red Pepper Dip (see recipe, page 277). They are also excellent served on their own as an accompaniment to a dinner entrée. Try the same thing with carrots, zucchini or sweet potatoes.

Kitchen Tip

Packaged herb blends can be found in the seasonings section of most supermarkets. Or make your own.

Oven-Roasted Potato Wedges

Preheat oven to 400°F (200°C)
Nonstick baking sheet

1 lb	baking potatoes, scrubbed and cut into wedges	500 g
2 tbsp	vegetable oil	25 mL
1 tbsp	garlic and herb blend (see tip)	15 mL

1. In a large bowl, toss potatoes with oil and seasonings. Spread in a single layer on baking sheet. Bake in preheated oven for 40 minutes, turning halfway through cooking time, until potatoes are crisp on the outside and tender on the inside.

NUTRITIONAL ANALYSIS (PER SERVING)							
Energy	Protein	Carbohydrate	Fat	Fiber	Calcium	Iron	Sodium
199 kcal	4 g	30 g	8 g	3 g	21 mg	1 mg	10 mg

The perfect recipe for when you have only 10 minutes to prepare dinner. Eggs, one of "nature's true convenience foods," are a principal ingredient. It also tastes good, appeals to children and is nutritious.

Speedy Skillet Supper

2 tbsp	butter or margarine	25 mL
½ cup	finely chopped onion	125 mL
½ cup	finely chopped green or red bell pepper	125 mL
5	eggs	5
3 tbsp	2% milk	45 mL
½ tsp	dried basil	2 mL
½ tsp	salt	2 mL
½	package (8 oz/250 g) light cream cheese, cubed	½
1	medium tomato, chopped	1
½ cup	diced cooked ham	125 mL
	Whole wheat toast	

1. In a skillet, melt butter over medium-high heat. Add onion and green pepper; sauté for 5 minutes or until tender. Reduce heat to medium-low.

2. Meanwhile, in a small bowl, whisk together eggs, milk and seasonings. Stir in cheese and tomato.

3. Pour egg mixture and ham into skillet; cook over low heat, stirring occasionally, for 5 minutes or until eggs are cooked but still moist. Serve over toast.

NUTRITIONAL ANALYSIS (PER SERVING)							
Energy	Protein	Carbohydrate	Fat	Fiber	Calcium	Iron	Sodium
288 kcal	13 g	22 g	17 g	4 g	90 mg	3 mg	905 mg

Makes 3 servings

Tofu's bland taste gives it the ability to take on the flavor of foods with which it is cooked. In this recipe, tofu cubes adopt the Asian tastes of its marinade — soy, garlic and ginger. While tofu is a mainstay of vegetarian diets, non-vegetarians will find it surprisingly tasty when prepared in this manner. However, if you still find tofu just a little too earnest, replace it with cubes of chicken. Beginning self-feeders find the cubes easy to eat.

Kitchen Tips

Use more or less garlic, according to taste.

If using wooden skewers, remember to soak them in water for at least 30 minutes before use. This will prevent the wood from burning on the grill.

Remove skewers before serving; they are unsafe for children under the age of 4 years.

If you substitute chicken for tofu, boil the marinade for 5 minutes before using it to brush on chicken while it is being grilled. Or discard marinade if not using.

Asian Barbecued Tofu Cubes

Preheat grill to medium

8 oz	firm tofu, cubed	250 g
1 to 2 tbsp	reduced-sodium soy sauce	15 to 25 mL
½	small garlic clove, crushed (see tip)	½
1 tsp	minced gingerroot	5 mL
1 tsp	lemon juice	5 mL
1 tsp	olive oil	5 mL
	Metal or wooden skewers (see tip)	

1. Place tofu cubes in a small, sealable plastic bag.

2. In a small bowl, combine soy sauce, garlic, ginger, lemon juice and oil. Pour over tofu, seal bag and refrigerate for several hours.

3. Remove cubes from marinade and thread on skewers. Reserve marinade (you may need to boil it; see tip). Grill skewers on preheated barbecue for 10 minutes or until crisp. Baste frequently with reserved marinade.

NUTRITIONAL ANALYSIS (PER SERVING)

Energy	Protein	Carbohydrate	Fat	Fiber	Calcium	Iron	Sodium
138 kcal	13 g	4 g	9 g	2 g	571 mg	2 mg	175 mg

Makes 12 baby servings, or 4 adult servings

This vegetarian-style burger will satisfy young taste buds while supplying protein. Shape them into the size best suited for each of your family members' appetites.

Kitchen Tip

Should you prefer to make "bean balls" rather than patties, shape bean mixture into balls (size them based on your family members' appetites) and cook, turning to brown all sides, for 3 to 4 minutes or until golden brown and heated through. These can then be dipped in the Yogurt Sauce. Messy but tasty!

Bulgur Bean Burgers

1 cup	water	250 mL
½ cup	bulgur	125 mL
1	can (19 oz/540 mL) reduced-sodium black beans, drained and rinsed	1
2 tbsp	plain yogurt	25 mL
¼ tsp	ground allspice	1 mL
¼ tsp	ground cinnamon	1 mL
¼ tsp	ground cumin	1 mL
	Whole wheat buns	
	Sliced tomato and shredded lettuce	

Yogurt Sauce

⅔ cup	plain yogurt	150 mL
½ cup	finely shredded carrot	125 mL
½ cup	finely shredded cucumber	125 mL

1. In a small saucepan, bring water to a boil over high heat. Add bulgur, cover, reduce heat to low and cook for 10 minutes or until water is absorbed and bulgur is tender. Set aside.
2. In bowl, mash beans with yogurt until almost smooth. Stir in bulgur, allspice, cinnamon and cumin. Pack mixture into ½-cup (125 mL) dry measures or desired size. Place each on a plate, pressing to flatten. Cover and refrigerate for at least 30 minutes or for up to 2 days.
3. Spray each side of bean patties with nonstick cooking spray.
4. Heat a nonstick skillet over medium heat. Add patties, in batches as necessary, and cook, turning once, for about 8 minutes or until golden brown and heated through.
5. *Yogurt Sauce:* In a small bowl, combine yogurt, carrot and cucumber.
6. Place each patty on a bun; top with yogurt sauce, tomato and lettuce.

NUTRITIONAL ANALYSIS (PER BABY SERVING)							
Energy	Protein	Carbohydrate	Fat	Fiber	Calcium	Iron	Sodium
78 kcal	5 g	14 g	0.5 g	4 g	42 mg	1 mg	16 mg

Makes 8 servings

This pizza starts with a store-bought shell. Add an interesting herb-cheese mixture, scatter vegetables and more cheese on top and into the oven. Deliciously easy!

Kitchen Tips

Feel free to substitute carrots with other vegetables, such as blanched broccoli florets, diced zucchini, sliced mushrooms or chopped green or yellow bell peppers.

Jars of roasted red peppers are available in supermarkets. They will keep for months in the refrigerator.

Vegetable Pizza

Preheat oven to 450°F (230°C)
Baking sheet

1 tbsp	olive oil	15 mL
1½ cups	shredded carrots (see tip)	375 mL
¼ cup	chopped fresh parsley	50 mL
2	cloves garlic, minced	2
2 tbsp	red wine vinegar or balsamic vinegar	25 mL
1 tsp	dried oregano	5 mL
½ tsp	dried basil	2 mL
3 cups	shredded mozzarella cheese, divided	750 mL
1	12-inch (30 cm) pizza shell	1
2 tbsp	diced roasted red pepper (see tip)	25 mL

1. In a skillet, heat oil over medium heat. Add carrots and stir to coat. Sprinkle with 2 tbsp (25 mL) water; cover and cook for 5 minutes. Set aside.

2. Meanwhile, combine parsley, garlic, vinegar, oregano and basil. Combine with 2 cups (500 mL) of the cheese. Place crust on baking sheet. Spread with herb-cheese mixture. Scatter carrots and red pepper over. Top with remaining cheese. Bake in preheated oven for 15 minutes or until golden brown and cheese is melted.

NUTRITIONAL ANALYSIS (PER SERVING)							
Energy	Protein	Carbohydrate	Fat	Fiber	Calcium	Iron	Sodium
399 kcal	31 g	22 g	20 g	2 g	662 mg	2 mg	697 mg

Makes 6 cups (1.5 L)

Kitchen Tip

Fusilli and rotini worked well for this dish, but any kind of pasta will do.

Pasta Primavera

3 cups	fusilli or rotini	750 mL
3½ cups	mixed vegetables (fresh or frozen, thawed)	875 mL
1	can (14 oz/398 mL) evaporated milk	1
1 cup	shredded old Cheddar cheese	250 mL
½ cup	grated Parmesan cheese	125 mL
4	slices ham, cut into thin strips	4
	Salt and freshly ground black pepper to taste	

1. In a large pot of boiling water, cook pasta according to package directions or until tender but firm. Add vegetables and cook for 5 minutes. Drain. Return pasta and vegetables to the pot.

2. Over medium-high heat, gently add the evaporated milk, Cheddar cheese, Parmesan cheese and ham. Cook, stirring, until cheese has melted and sauce thickens. Season to taste with salt and pepper.

NUTRITIONAL ANALYSIS (PER ½ CUP/125 ML)

Energy	Protein	Carbohydrate	Fat	Fiber	Calcium	Iron	Sodium
206 kcal	12 g	27 g	6 g	2 g	231 mg	1 mg	239 mg

Makes 4 cups (1 L)

Our version of this classic pasta dish is very quick and easy to prepare. Almost a meal in itself, you only need to add a salad or cooked vegetable!

Kitchen Tip

Clean mushrooms just before using. Never immerse mushrooms in water; they'll absorb the water and become mushy. It's best just to wipe with a damp paper towel. Trim a small amount from stem ends and you're ready to go.

Creamy Fettuccine Mushroom Alfredo

3 tbsp	olive oil	45 mL
2 cups	sliced mushrooms (see tip)	500 mL
1	clove garlic, minced	1
½ cup	light (5%) cream	125 mL
½	package (8 oz/250 g) light cream cheese, cubed	½
½ tsp	dried tarragon	2 mL
½ tsp	dried thyme	2 mL
8 oz	fettuccine	250 g
	Grated Parmesan cheese	

1. In a large skillet, heat oil over medium-high heat. Add mushrooms and garlic; sauté, stirring constantly, for 5 minutes. Reduce heat. Add cream, cream cheese, tarragon and thyme; stir until smooth and cheese has melted.

2. Meanwhile, in a large saucepan, cook fettuccine in boiling water according to package directions. Drain well and return to saucepan. Stir in mushroom sauce. Sprinkle generously with cheese.

NUTRITIONAL ANALYSIS (PER ½ CUP/125 ML)

Energy	Protein	Carbohydrate	Fat	Fiber	Calcium	Iron	Sodium
88 kcal	2 g	5 g	7 g	0.4 g	21 mg	0.4 mg	9 mg

Makes 3½ cups (875 mL)

Children enjoy this good-for-you vegetarian chili for the simple reason that it tastes great. So will their parents. Served with cooked brown or white rice or toast, it is a complete-protein meal.

Kitchen Tips

Leftover chickpeas can be used to make Hummus (see recipe, page 277).

Use red lentils in this recipe. They cook down to a nice mushy consistency that's ideal for chili.

Add chili powder after you have removed the children's portion.

Use homemade or reduced-sodium stock to lower the sodium content of this recipe.

Vegetarian Chili

1 cup	tomato juice	250 mL
1 cup	vegetable or beef stock	250 mL
1 cup	canned chickpeas, drained and rinsed	250 mL
1	medium potato, diced	1
¼ cup	red lentils, washed (see tip)	50 mL
1	medium carrot, chopped	1
½	small onion, chopped	½
½ cup	finely chopped green pepper	125 mL
1	clove garlic, minced	1
1 tbsp	chili powder (see tip)	15 mL
¼ tsp	salt	1 mL
¼ tsp	freshly ground black pepper	1 mL

1. In a saucepan, combine tomato juice, stock, chickpeas, potato, lentils, carrot, onion, green pepper and garlic. Cover and bring to a boil. Reduce heat and simmer, covered, for about 20 minutes or until vegetables and lentils are tender. Stir frequently, since the mixture has a tendency to stick as it thickens.

2. Taste and adjust flavor by adding chili powder, salt and pepper; cook for another 5 minutes and serve.

NUTRITIONAL ANALYSIS (PER ½ CUP/125 ML)

Energy	Protein	Carbohydrate	Fat	Fiber	Calcium	Iron	Sodium
100 kcal	5 g	19 g	1 g	4 g	30 mg	2 mg	324 mg

Makes 6½ cups (1.625 L)

This chili is delicious served with grated Cheddar cheese and a dollop of sour cream on top, with some bread for dipping.

Kitchen Tip

Feel free to add whatever vegetables are handy in your kitchen. Try sautéed green and red peppers or mushrooms — or whatever your kids enjoy. Be careful if freezing this dish; once frozen and thawed, it can become quite spicy.

Chili Con Carne

2 tbsp	vegetable oil	25 mL
½ cup	finely chopped onions	125 mL
1 lb	lean or extra-lean ground beef	500 g
1	can (28 oz/796 mL) kidney beans, rinsed and drained	1
1	can (28 oz/796 mL) tomatoes	1
7 oz	tomato sauce or canned condensed tomato soup	210 mL
½ to 1 tsp	granulated sugar	2 to 5 mL
½ tsp	chili powder	2 mL
½ tsp	salt	2 mL
Pinch	cayenne pepper	Pinch

1. In a large saucepan, heat oil over medium-high heat. Add onions and sauté until tender and translucent. Add ground beef and continue to cook until brown. Add beans, tomatoes, tomato sauce, sugar, chili powder, salt and cayenne pepper. Bring to a boil; reduce heat and simmer for 45 minutes.

NUTRITIONAL ANALYSIS (PER ½ CUP/125 ML)

Energy	Protein	Carbohydrate	Fat	Fiber	Calcium	Iron	Sodium
201 kcal	12 g	16 g	11 g	8 g	68 mg	5 mg	341 mg

Makes 9 cups (2.25 L)

Kitchen Tip

Use homemade or reduced-sodium stock to lower the sodium content of this recipe.

Beef and Vegetable Stew

2 tbsp	all-purpose flour	25 mL
¼ tsp	salt	1 mL
Pinch	freshly ground black pepper	Pinch
1¼ lbs	stewing beef, cut into bite-size cubes	625 g
2 tbsp	butter or margarine	25 mL
1	onion, chopped	1
2⅔ cups	beef stock	650 mL
3	carrots, peeled and sliced	3
3	stalks celery, chopped	3
1 cup	sliced mushrooms	250 mL
1	can (28 oz/796 mL) chopped tomatoes	1

1. In a small bowl, stir together flour, salt and pepper. Dredge beef in flour. Shake off any excess and transfer to a plate.

2. In a large saucepan, melt butter over medium-high heat. Add beef and onion; cook for about 2 minutes or until meat is browned and onion has softened. Stir in stock slowly and bring to a boil; cook, stirring constantly, until thick. Add carrots, celery, mushrooms and tomatoes; cover and let simmer for 2 to 2½ hours.

NUTRITIONAL ANALYSIS (PER ½ CUP/125 ML)							
Energy	Protein	Carbohydrate	Fat	Fiber	Calcium	Iron	Sodium
71 kcal	7 g	5 g	2 g	1 g	27 mg	1 mg	157 mg

Makes 16 baby servings, or 4 adult servings

You can prepare this easy recipe ahead of time (for example, while the baby naps), then simply reheat and serve over freshly cooked noodles.

Kitchen Tips

Any kind of boneless beef you would like to use will work. Slicing the beef into thin strips will help the beef to cook faster and will make it easier for your children to enjoy.

To decrease the fat content, reduce the butter to 2 to 3 tbsp (25 to 45 mL).

Beef Stroganoff

¼ cup	butter or margarine, divided	50 mL
2	small onions, chopped	2
10	mushrooms, sliced	10
1 lb	stir-fry beef strips	500 g
3	tomatoes, peeled and diced	3
½ tsp	freshly ground black pepper	2 mL
1 cup	sour cream	250 mL
2 cups	hot cooked noodles (such as broad egg noodles)	500 mL

1. In a large skillet, melt 1 tbsp (15 mL) of the butter over medium-high heat. Add onions and sauté until softened, about 5 minutes. Remove onions to a bowl and set aside.
2. Add mushroom slices and cook for 4 to 5 minutes, until they release their liquid. Remove and set aside.
3. Add remaining butter to skillet. Increase heat to high. Add beef and cook for 3 to 5 minutes, until browned. Drain off excess fat. Return vegetables to skillet and add tomatoes. Season with pepper. Stir in sour cream. Heat just until mixture begins to simmer. Serve over noodles.

NUTRITIONAL ANALYSIS (PER BABY SERVING)

Energy	Protein	Carbohydrate	Fat	Fiber	Calcium	Iron	Sodium
118 kcal	7 g	8 g	7 g	1 g	24 mg	1 mg	38 mg

Makes 16 baby servings, or 8 adult servings

This excellent make-ahead casserole is economical to prepare and freezes well for later use. Make it in one casserole dish for a crowd or large family. Noodles and cheese make this dish attractive to younger family members. It also sticks together for easy eating.

Kitchen Tips

If you use spaghetti sauce instead of plain tomato sauce, you may not need to add the basil and oregano unless extra spice is desired.

Cooked beef mixture may be prepared to the end of Step 1 and frozen, or used at once in the casserole recipe.

If eating one casserole, which is sufficient for 4, cover and freeze the second one for later use.

Cooked vegetables may be added if desired.

Beef Sour Cream Noodle Bake

Preheat oven to 350°F (180°C)
Two 4-cup (1 L) casserole dishes, greased

1 lb	lean or extra-lean ground beef	500 g
1	medium onion, finely chopped	1
2	cloves garlic, minced	2
1 cup	tomato sauce or spaghetti sauce	250 mL
1 tsp	dried basil (see tip)	5 mL
1 tsp	dried oregano (see tip)	5 mL
¼ tsp	salt	1 mL
¼ tsp	freshly ground black pepper	1 mL
2 cups	dry broad egg noodles	500 mL
1 cup	2% cottage cheese	250 mL
1 cup	sour cream	250 mL
¾ cup	shredded mozzarella or mild Cheddar cheese	175 mL

1. In a large nonstick skillet, cook beef, onion and garlic until beef is no longer pink; drain excess fat. Add tomato sauce and seasonings. Bring to a boil. Reduce heat to low and cook for 5 minutes.

2. Meanwhile, in a large saucepan, cook noodles in boiling water according to package directions or until tender but firm. Drain. Add cottage cheese and sour cream; stir to combine.

3. Spoon one-quarter of noodle mixture into prepared casserole dishes. Cover each with one-quarter of ground beef mixture; repeat layers. Divide cheese over top of each casserole. Bake, uncovered, for 35 minutes or until thoroughly heated.

NUTRITIONAL ANALYSIS (PER BABY SERVING)

Energy	Protein	Carbohydrate	Fat	Fiber	Calcium	Iron	Sodium
140 kcal	11 g	8 g	7 g	0.5 g	79 mg	1.1 mg	226 mg

Makes 5 cups (1.25 L)

This classic dish from a generation ago was really nothing more than a fancy way to get rid of leftovers. Well, nothing has changed. This recipe turns leftover cooked vegetables and meats into a tasty family meal, just like your mother's.

Kitchen Tip
Use grated Parmesan or any melting cheese for this dish.

À la King Supper

¼ cup	butter or margarine	50 mL
1	medium onion, finely chopped	1
6	large mushrooms, sliced	6
3 tbsp	all-purpose flour	45 mL
2 cups	2% milk	500 mL
2 cups	cooked vegetables	500 mL
2 cups	diced cooked meat	500 mL
½ cup	shredded cheese (see tip)	125 mL
	Hot buttered whole wheat toast or whole wheat English muffins, cooked brown rice or baked potatoes	

1. In a large saucepan, melt butter over medium-high heat. Add onion and mushrooms; cook for 5 minutes or until softened.
2. Remove pan from heat. Stir in flour, then milk. Return to heat and cook, stirring constantly, until smooth and thickened. Add vegetables, meat and cheese. Stir until cheese melts and mixture is heated.
3. Serve over toast, muffin halves, rice or potatoes.

NUTRITIONAL ANALYSIS (PER ½ CUP/125 ML, NOT INCLUDING BREAD, RICE OR POTATO)

Energy	Protein	Carbohydrate	Fat	Fiber	Calcium	Iron	Sodium
170 kcal	14 g	11 g	8 g	1 g	136 mg	1 mg	165 mg

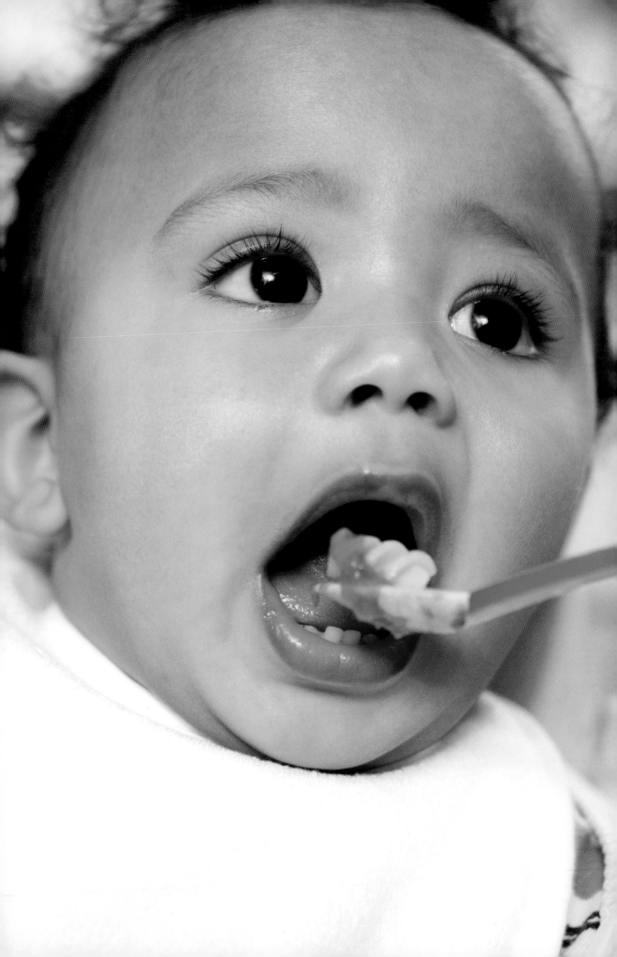

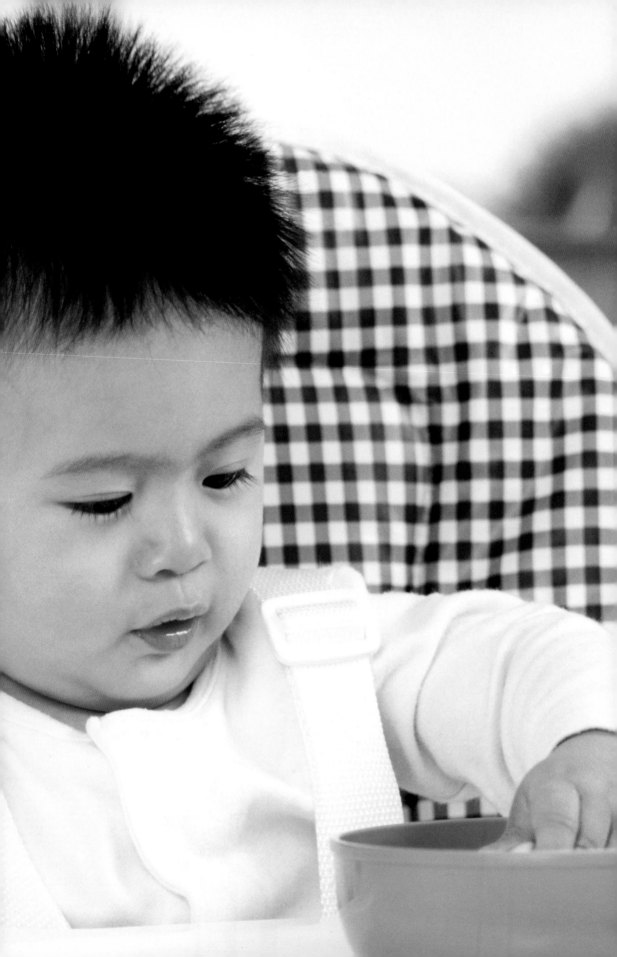

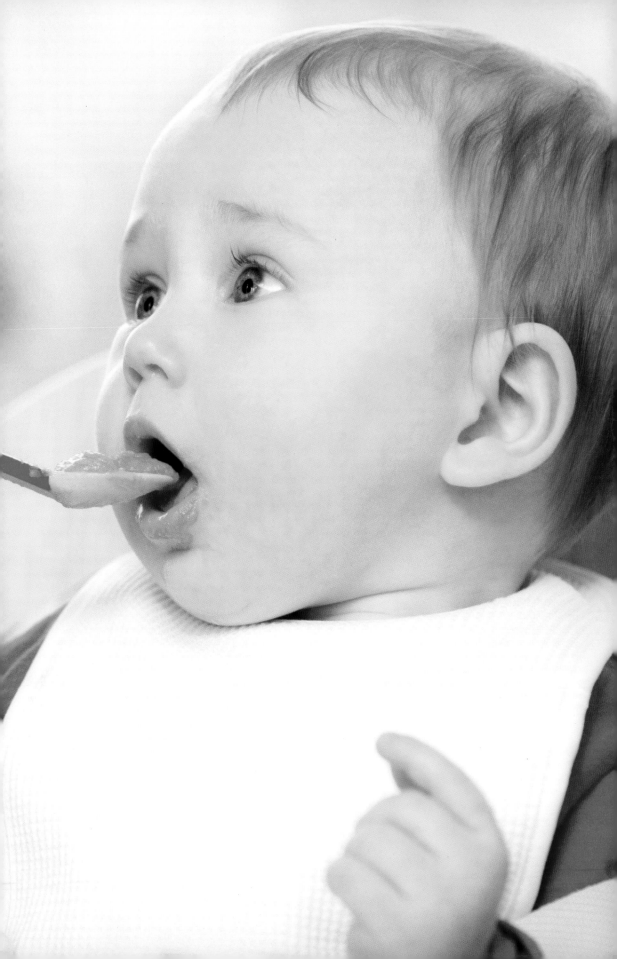

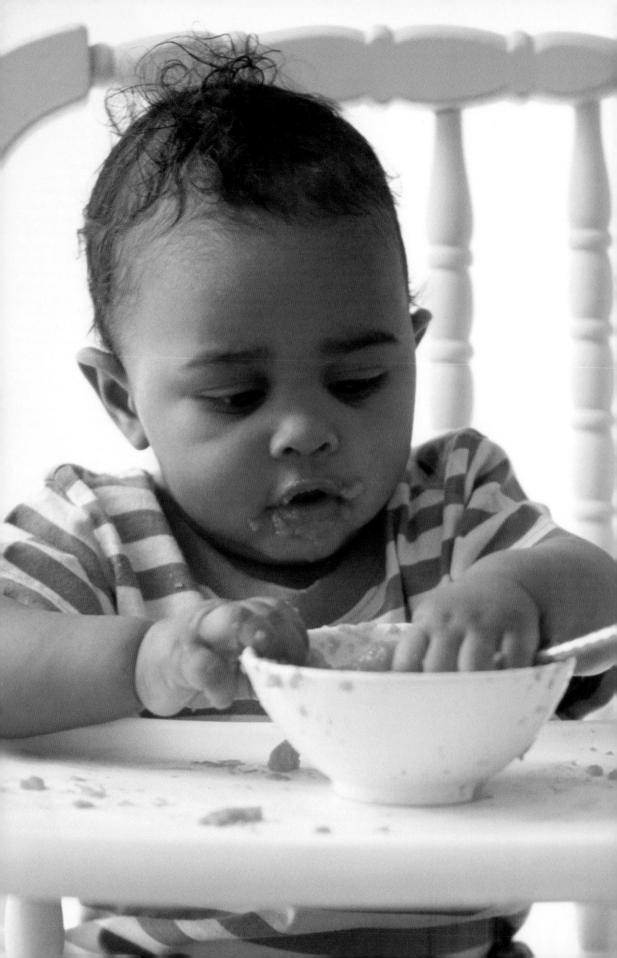

Makes 6 cups (1.5 L)

Stew always gives a wonderful lift to the day. We've noticed that most young family members enjoy stew as much as their older relatives.

Kitchen Tip

Stews freeze well, so why not double the recipe?

Pork Stew with Vegetables

2 tsp	vegetable oil	10 mL
1 lb	lean pork shoulder, trimmed of all visible fat and cut into small cubes	500 g
1	medium onion, finely chopped	1
1	medium cooking apple, cored and chopped	1
2	medium tomatoes, chopped	2
¼ cup	apple juice	50 mL
¼ cup	water	50 mL
¼ tsp	ground cinnamon	1 mL
¼ tsp	curry powder	1 mL
¼ tsp	salt	1 mL
1	bay leaf	1
2	large potatoes, diced	2

1. In a large skillet, heat oil over medium-high heat. Add pork and onion; cook for about 10 minutes or until golden. Add apple, tomatoes, apple juice, water, cinnamon, curry powder, salt and bay leaf. Cover, reduce heat and simmer for about 1 hour or until pork is tender.

2. Meanwhile, in a small saucepan, bring water to a boil. Add potatoes and cook for 15 minutes or until tender. Mash or serve in pieces.

3. Remove bay leaf from stew before serving over potato.

NUTRITIONAL ANALYSIS (PER ½ CUP/125 ML)							
Energy	Protein	Carbohydrate	Fat	Fiber	Calcium	Iron	Sodium
102 kcal	9 g	9 g	4 g	1 g	16 mg	0.4 mg	60 mg

Makes 6 cups (1.5 L)

Busy parents love stews because once the preparation is complete, cooking continues without any further work. And they are great for children. It's easy to adjust portions for their smaller appetites and the individual pieces of the stew are easy for them to handle.

Food Safety Tip

Take care that juices from any meats or poultry do not drip onto other foods. Keep raw meats and poultry separate from cooked meats or cold cuts in the refrigerator. This will prevent cross-contamination.

Homestyle Oven Pork and Barley Stew

Preheat oven to 375°F (190°C)
Large roasting pan

¼ cup	all-purpose flour	50 mL
½ tsp	salt	2 mL
½ tsp	dried thyme	2 mL
1¼ lbs	lean pork shoulder, trimmed of all visible fat and cut into cubes	625 g
2 tbsp	vegetable oil	25 mL
1 cup	apple juice	250 mL
½ cup	pearl barley	125 mL
4	carrots, peeled and cut into pieces	4
2	onions, cut into wedges	2
2	cloves garlic, finely chopped	2
3	strips orange zest	3
1	bay leaf	1
1 cup	water (approximate)	250 mL

1. In a plastic bag, combine flour, salt and thyme. Add pork cubes and toss to coat. Remove pork; reserve excess flour.

2. Add oil to large roasting pan. Stir in floured pork. Bake, uncovered, in preheated oven for 20 minutes; stir once.

3. Reduce oven temperature to 350°F (180°C). In a bowl, stir together apple juice and reserved flour; pour over meat. Add barley, carrots, onions, garlic, orange zest and bay leaf. Bake, covered, for 45 minutes or until pork and barley are tender. (Stir occasionally to check thickness of sauce; add water as mixture thickens.)

4. Remove orange zest and bay leaf before serving.

NUTRITIONAL ANALYSIS (PER ½ CUP/125 ML)							
Energy	Protein	Carbohydrate	Fat	Fiber	Calcium	Iron	Sodium
135 kcal	7 g	15 g	5 g	2 g	22 mg	1 mg	118 mg

Makes 4 servings

Lean and tender pork chops are cooked in a pineapple-herb sauce, which keeps them moist and flavorful.

Pork Chops in Creamy Herb Sauce

1 tbsp	vegetable oil	15 mL
4	boneless lean pork chops	4
1	small onion, sliced	1
½ cup	pineapple juice	125 mL
½ tsp	dried tarragon	2 mL
½ tsp	dried thyme	2 mL
1	large apple, cut into eighths	1
½ cup	sour cream	125 mL
1 tbsp	all-purpose flour	15 mL

1. In a skillet just large enough to hold chops, heat oil over medium-high heat. Brown chops on each side. Remove to a warm plate. Add onion and sauté for 3 minutes. Add pineapple juice, tarragon and thyme.
2. Return chops to skillet. Bring to a boil. Reduce heat, cover and cook for 15 minutes or until meat is tender. Add apple during last 5 minutes of cooking.
3. Remove meat, apple and onion to a warm platter. Boil remaining liquid to reduce slightly.
4. In a small bowl, whisk together sour cream and flour. Stir into boiling liquid, stirring constantly until thickened. Pour sauce over chops and serve. Cut infant's portion into small pieces.

NUTRITIONAL ANALYSIS (PER SERVING)							
Energy	Protein	Carbohydrate	Fat	Fiber	Calcium	Iron	Sodium
243 kcal	18 g	12 g	14 g	1 g	62 mg	1 mg	50 mg

Herbed Chicken

Kitchen Tips

If you can't find any fresh marjoram, substitute 2 tsp (10 mL) dried.

Use homemade or reduced-sodium stock to lower the sodium content of this recipe.

4	boneless skinless chicken breasts, cut into 1½-inch (4 cm) strips	4
¼ tsp	salt	1 mL
¼ tsp	freshly ground black pepper	1 mL
2 tbsp	olive oil	25 mL
3 tbsp	butter or margarine, divided	45 mL
1	onion, chopped	1
1 tbsp	all-purpose flour	15 mL
2 cups	chicken stock	500 mL
2 tbsp	lemon juice	25 mL
8 oz	mushrooms, quartered	250 g
2 tbsp	chopped fresh marjoram	25 mL
3	cloves garlic, crushed	3

1. Sprinkle chicken with salt and pepper. In a large frying pan, heat oil and 2 tbsp (25 mL) of the butter over medium heat. Add chicken and cook for about 4 to 5 minutes. Remove chicken to a warmed plate and set aside.

2. Reduce heat to medium. Melt remaining butter in pan. Add onion and cook for 2 minutes. Sprinkle with flour and cook, stirring constantly, for another 2 minutes. Stir in chicken stock and lemon juice. Return to medium-high heat. Add mushrooms, marjoram and garlic; cook for about 15 minutes or until sauce has been reduced to about 1 cup (250 mL). Return chicken to pan and heat through. Serve over steamed rice or noodles.

NUTRITIONAL ANALYSIS (PER ½ CUP/125 ML)							
Energy	Protein	Carbohydrate	Fat	Fiber	Calcium	Iron	Sodium
165 kcal	16 g	5 g	9 g	0.4 g	12 mg	1 mg	217 mg

*Try this zesty way to prepare
chicken. It's also delicious as
leftovers — if there are any!*

Kitchen Tip
Use homemade or reduced-
sodium stock to lower the
sodium content of this recipe.

Lemon Chicken

3 tbsp	all-purpose flour	45 mL
½ tsp	salt	2 mL
¼ tsp	freshly ground black pepper	1 mL
2 tbsp	olive oil	25 mL
4	boneless skinless chicken breasts	4
1 tbsp	butter or margarine	15 mL
1	onion, finely chopped	1
1 cup	chicken stock	250 mL
3 tbsp	lemon juice	45 mL
½ tsp	ground thyme	2 mL

1. In a plastic bag, combine flour, salt and pepper. Add chicken and shake in bag to coat lightly. Remove the chicken and reserve the excess flour.

2. In a large skillet, heat oil over medium heat. Add chicken and brown both sides for about 5 minutes each. Transfer to a warm plate.

3. Melt butter in skillet. Add onion and cook for 3 to 4 minutes or until softened. Add excess flour and cook for 1 minute. Add chicken stock, lemon juice and thyme. Bring to a boil, stirring constantly.

4. Return chicken to pan. Reduce heat to medium-low and cook for 7 to 8 minutes or until chicken is tender and no longer pink inside.

NUTRITIONAL ANALYSIS (PER BABY SERVING)

Energy	Protein	Carbohydrate	Fat	Fiber	Calcium	Iron	Sodium
64 kcal	7 g	2 g	3 g	0.1 g	2 mg	0.3 mg	105 mg

**Makes 24 baby servings,
or 6 adult servings**

Kitchen Tip

The sauce is best if made the day before. It's delicious served with rice or pasta.

Chicken-So-Good

Preheat oven to 350°F (180°C)
Large casserole dish

6	boneless skinless chicken breasts	6
½ cup	all-purpose flour	125 mL
½ tsp	salt	2 mL
¼ tsp	freshly ground black pepper	1 mL
2	eggs, slightly beaten	2
1½ cups	crushed Special K cereal	375 mL
⅓ cup	vegetable oil	75 mL
Sauce		
¼ cup	vegetable oil	50 mL
2	medium onions, minced	2
2	cloves garlic, minced	2
1½	green peppers, diced	1½
1 cup	sliced mushrooms	250 mL
1 tsp	salt	5 mL
½ tsp	freshly ground black pepper	2 mL
1 tsp	dried oregano	5 mL
2 tsp	Worcestershire sauce	10 mL
¼ tsp	hot pepper sauce	1 mL
1	1 can (2¾ oz/80 mL) tomato paste	1
1	1 can (28 oz/796 mL) tomato sauce	1
½ cup	water	125 mL
1 tbsp	lemon juice	15 mL
1 tsp	granulated sugar	5 mL

1. Place chicken between sheets of wax paper and pound until quite thin. In a bowl, combine flour, salt and pepper. Dip chicken in flour mixture, then in eggs. Coat with cereal crumbs.

2. In a large skillet, heat ⅓ cup (75 mL) oil over medium-high heat. Add chicken and sauté on both sides for about 10 minutes. Transfer chicken to casserole dish.

3. *Sauce:* Add ¼ cup (50 mL) oil to skillet. Add onions, garlic, green peppers and mushrooms; sauté for about 5 minutes. Add salt, pepper, oregano, Worcestershire sauce, hot pepper sauce, tomato paste and sauce, water, lemon juice and sugar. Cover and simmer for approximately 30 minutes. Add more water if sauce appears too thick.

4. Pour sauce over chicken in casserole dish. Bake in preheated oven for 35 minutes.

NUTRITIONAL ANALYSIS (PER BABY SERVING)

Energy	Protein	Carbohydrate	Fat	Fiber	Calcium	Iron	Sodium
114 kcal	7 g	9 g	6 g	1 g	15 mg	1 mg	352 mg

Over 18 months

Makes 16 baby servings, or 4 adult servings

This as an absolute must-try recipe. It is incredibly quick and easy to make. Your whole family will enjoy this and it tastes great the next day.

Kitchen Tips

Add other vegetables — such as sliced zucchini or green or red bell peppers — for additional flavor and color.

Use homemade or reduced-sodium stock to lower the sodium content of this recipe.

Chicken and Vegetables

Preheat oven to 400°F (200°C)
Casserole dish, greased

1 lb	carrots, peeled and sliced	500 g
2	sweet potatoes, sliced	2
¾ cup	chicken stock, divided	175 mL
½ tsp	salt	2 mL
½ tsp	freshly ground black pepper	2 mL
4	boneless skinless chicken breasts	4
4 tbsp	Dijon mustard	60 mL
½ tsp	dried thyme	2 mL

1. Place carrots on bottom of casserole dish. Arrange sweet potatoes on top of carrots. Pour half of the stock over vegetables. Cover with foil and bake in preheated oven for 20 minutes.

2. Reduce heat to 375°F (190°C). Stir vegetables and nestle chicken among vegetables. Add salt and pepper to remaining stock. Add mustard and thyme. Pour over chicken mixture and bake for 45 minutes, until chicken is no longer pink inside.

NUTRITIONAL ANALYSIS (PER BABY SERVING)

Energy	Protein	Carbohydrate	Fat	Fiber	Calcium	Iron	Sodium
70 kcal	6 g	10 g	1 g	2 g	23 mg	1 mg	218 mg

Makes 2 cups (500 mL)

The infants who tested this stir-fry showed great interest in its color as well as its flavor. Their parents liked it too!

Kitchen Tips

Cooked white or brown rice is the perfect complement to this fast stir-fry recipe. The rice will cook in about 15 minutes, so start it just before starting to cook the stir-fry.

Use reduced-sodium soy sauce to lower the sodium content of this recipe.

Food Safety Tip

If you are using frozen chicken breasts, the safest way to thaw them (or any other frozen meats) is in the refrigerator. Allow 6 to 9 hours per lb (14 to 20 hours per kg). Leave chicken in its freezer wrapper on a tray or plate on the bottom shelf. Never let meat thaw at room temperature. If you do, bacteria can grow on the surface of the meat, even while the inside remains frozen.

Chicken Stir-Fry

1 tbsp	hoisin sauce	15 mL
1 tbsp	soy sauce	15 mL
2 tsp	rice vinegar or white vinegar	10 mL
½ tsp	sesame oil	2 mL
½	red bell pepper, cut into large chunks	½
6	medium mushrooms, cut into large chunks	6
1 cup	small broccoli florets	250 mL
1 tbsp	vegetable oil	15 mL
2	boneless skinless chicken breasts, cut into chunks	2
2 cups	bean sprouts	500 mL

1. In a bowl, combine hoisin and soy sauce, vinegar and sesame oil. Add red pepper, mushrooms and broccoli; toss to coat. Set aside.

2. In a wok or large nonstick skillet, heat oil over medium-high heat. Add chicken and cook, stirring constantly, for 3 minutes or until no longer pink. Add vegetable mixture; cover and steam for 5 minutes. Stir in bean sprouts; cover and steam for 2 minutes.

NUTRITIONAL ANALYSIS (PER ½ CUP/125 ML)							
Energy	Protein	Carbohydrate	Fat	Fiber	Calcium	Iron	Sodium
142 kcal	17 g	8 g	5 g	2.5 g	24 mg	1.2 mg	248 mg

Kitchen Tips

Delicious when served over rice with a favorite vegetable!

Fish sauce is available in Asian markets or in the Asian food section of large supermarkets.

Thai Chicken

Preheat oven to 375°F (190°C)
Baking dish

1 tbsp	olive oil	15 mL
4	boneless skinless chicken breasts	4
2 tbsp	dried coriander	25 mL
2 tbsp	dried basil	25 mL
1 tbsp	dried mint	15 mL
1 tbsp	lemon juice	15 mL
2 tbsp	vegetable oil	25 mL
1 tbsp	granulated sugar	15 mL
2 tbsp	fish sauce	25 mL
3	garlic cloves, minced	3
1 tsp	grated lemon zest	5 mL
2	green onions, chopped	2

1. In a large skillet, heat oil over high heat. Add chicken and cook until browned. Set aside.

2. In a large bowl, combine coriander, basil, mint, lemon juice, oil, sugar, fish sauce, garlic, lemon zest and green onions.

3. Place chicken in marinade; refrigerate for at least 1 hour or overnight.

4. Remove chicken from marinade and place in baking dish. Bake in preheated oven for 20 minutes or until cooked through.

NUTRITIONAL ANALYSIS (PER BABY SERVING)

Energy	Protein	Carbohydrate	Fat	Fiber	Calcium	Iron	Sodium
72 kcal	7 g	2 g	4 g	0.3 g	17 mg	0.5 mg	28 mg

Makes 16 baby servings, or 4 adult servings

The sauce adds a sweet, pungent taste to chicken served over rice. It's a taste that many children adore and, of course, so do their elders.

Food Safety Tip

Keep raw poultry (as well as other raw meats) away from other foods during storage and preparation. As well, keep separate cutting boards for raw meats and vegetables.

Baked Sweet 'n' Sour Chicken

Preheat oven to 350°F (180°C)
Rectangular casserole dish, greased

4	boneless skinless chicken breasts	4
1/2 cup	tomato sauce	125 mL
1/2	small onion, finely chopped	1/2
3 tbsp	brown sugar	45 mL
2 tbsp	cider vinegar	25 mL
1/2 cup	crushed pineapple, with juice	125 mL
1	clove garlic, mashed	1
	Cooked rice	
	Chopped fresh parsley	

1. Place chicken breasts in prepared casserole dish.

2. In a small bowl, combine tomato sauce, onion, sugar, vinegar, pineapple (with juice) and garlic; spoon over chicken. Bake in preheated oven for 45 minutes or until chicken is no longer pink and juices run clear.

3. Serve chicken and sauce over cooked rice sprinkled with parsley.

NUTRITIONAL ANALYSIS (PER BABY SERVING)							
Energy	Protein	Carbohydrate	Fat	Fiber	Calcium	Iron	Sodium
50 kcal	7 g	5 g	0.4 g	0.2 g	5 mg	0.3 mg	63 mg

Makes 16 baby servings, or 4 adult servings

Kitchen Tips

For an authentic finish to this dish, and where there is no danger of allergy, sprinkle 4 tbsp (60 mL) chopped unsalted peanuts over dish just before serving.

Fish sauce is available in Asian markets or in the Asian food section of large supermarkets.

Use homemade or reduced-sodium stock to lower the sodium content of this recipe.

Chicken Pad Thai

7 oz	wide rice stick noodles	210 g
⅔ cup	chicken stock	150 mL
⅓ cup	ketchup	75 mL
¼ cup	fish sauce (see tip)	50 mL
2 tbsp	each granulated sugar and cornstarch	25 mL
2 tbsp	lime juice	25 mL
1 tsp	hot pepper sauce	5 mL
4 tsp	vegetable oil, divided	20 mL
2	eggs, beaten	2
1 lb	boneless skinless chicken breasts, cut into thin strips	500 g
4	carrots, julienned	4
1	red bell pepper, thinly sliced	1
2	garlic cloves, minced	2
1 tbsp	minced gingerroot	15 mL
2 cups	bean sprouts	500 mL
2	green onions, chopped	2

1. In a large pot, soak noodles in warm water to cover for 30 minutes. Drain.

2. In a bowl, combine stock, ketchup, fish sauce, sugar, cornstarch, lime juice and hot pepper sauce. Set aside.

3. In a large nonstick skillet or wok, heat 2 tsp (10 mL) of the oil over medium-high heat. Add eggs and scramble for about 2 to 3 minutes. Transfer to a plate.

4. Heat remaining oil in same pan. Add chicken and stir-fry until browned; transfer to a plate. Add carrots, red pepper, garlic and ginger; stir-fry for 5 minutes. Add noodles and stir-fry for 2 minutes.

5. Return chicken to wok. Stir in reserved sauce and cook for about 5 minutes or until chicken is thoroughly cooked. Toss in egg mixture, bean sprouts and green onions; cook until warmed throughout.

NUTRITIONAL ANALYSIS (PER BABY SERVING)							
Energy	Protein	Carbohydrate	Fat	Fiber	Calcium	Iron	Sodium
133 kcal	9 g	18 g	3 g	1 g	18 mg	0.6 mg	141 mg

Makes 48 meatballs

This recipe eliminates all the time normally required to form round meatballs. Here we simply pat the ground chicken into a pan and cut it into squares after cooking. Squares can be cut to child or adult sizes.

Kitchen Tips

Ground beef can replace chicken.

Freeze any leftover squares in the pan. Place pan in a plastic freezer bag for longer storage. At serving time, reheat in a microwave oven.

To make soft bread crumbs, pull fresh bread into small pieces. One slice should be sufficient for this recipe.

Food Safety Tips

When defrosting ground meats or poultry in the microwave oven, remove outside portions as they thaw. This keeps the outside from starting to cook before the inside thaws. Any meats or poultry defrosted in the microwave should be cooked immediately.

If you will not be using ground meat or poultry within 1 day, freeze it.

Square Chicken Meatballs

Preheat oven to 400°F (200°C)
8-inch (2 L) square baking pan, greased

1 lb	lean ground chicken (see tip)	500 g
1 cup	finely chopped mushrooms	250 mL
2 tbsp	finely chopped onion	25 mL
¾ cup	soft bread crumbs (see tip)	175 mL
½ tsp	dried basil	2 mL
½ tsp	dried thyme	2 mL
⅛ tsp	salt	0.5 mL
⅛ tsp	freshly ground black pepper	0.5 mL

1. In a bowl, combine chicken, mushrooms, onion, bread, crumbs, basil, thyme, salt and pepper. Pat mixture into prepared pan. Mark into small squares.
2. Bake in preheated oven for 20 minutes or until chicken is well done and juices run clear. Remove and cut into squares.

NUTRITIONAL ANALYSIS (PER MEATBALL)

Energy	Protein	Carbohydrate	Fat	Fiber	Calcium	Iron	Sodium
20 kcal	2 g	1 g	1 g	0.1 g	4 mg	0.2 mg	16 mg

Makes 6 burgers

Kitchen Tip

Salsa helps to keep the lean turkey from drying out. It also adds flavor that your children will love. Moms and Dads can use a medium/hot salsa or a dash of hot pepper sauce if they prefer a little spice.

Turkey Burgers

1 lb	ground turkey or chicken	500 g
¼ cup	mild salsa	50 mL
1	egg	1
3 to 4 tsp	dry bread crumbs	15 to 20 mL

1. In a bowl, combine turkey, salsa, egg and bread crumbs. Form into 6 balls and flatten into patties. Grill for 15 to 20 minutes or until cooked through.

NUTRITIONAL ANALYSIS (PER BURGER)

Energy	Protein	Carbohydrate	Fat	Fiber	Calcium	Iron	Sodium
143 kcal	16 g	1 g	8 g	0.2 g	20 mg	1 mg	152 mg

Makes 16 baby servings, or 6 adult servings

This is a delicious fish recipe that freezes well — a great combo of cheese, spinach and fish.

Crispy Fish

Preheat oven to 350°F (180°C)

½	lemon	½
½ cup	olive oil	125 mL
1	large clove garlic, minced	1
2 tbsp	dried basil	25 mL
2 cups	dry bread crumbs	500 mL
½ cup	grated Parmesan cheese	125 mL
¼ tsp	freshly ground black pepper	1 mL
1½ lbs	fillets of sole or other fish, defrosted	750 g

1. In a food processor, purée lemon and oil. Pour into a skillet and heat over medium heat for 2 minutes. Add garlic and basil; sauté for 2 minutes. Add bread crumbs and sauté for 3 to 4 minutes or until dry. Transfer to a bowl. Stir in Parmesan cheese and pepper.

2. Place fish in a greased casserole dish. Spread topping over fish. Cover and bake in preheated oven for 20 minutes or until fish flakes easily with a fork.

NUTRITIONAL ANALYSIS (PER BABY SERVING)

Energy	Protein	Carbohydrate	Fat	Fiber	Calcium	Iron	Sodium
179 kcal	12 g	10 g	9 g	1 g	80 mg	1 mg	194 mg

A meal in a dish! And a great way to add extra vegetables for everyone in the family.

Salmon Vegetable Casserole

Preheat oven to 350°F (180°C)
4-cup (1 L) casserole dish, greased

1	can (7½ oz/213 g) salmon, drained and skin removed	1
2	eggs, beaten	2
1	small zucchini, thinly sliced	1
1 cup	shredded mozzarella cheese	250 mL
½ cup	frozen green peas, thawed	125 mL
2 tbsp	plain yogurt	25 mL
2 tbsp	mayonnaise	25 mL
2 tbsp	finely chopped onion	25 mL
¼ tsp	dried dill	1 mL
Pinch	freshly ground black pepper	Pinch

1. In a bowl, mash salmon well with a fork, mashing bones into very small pieces. Add eggs, zucchini, cheese, peas, yogurt, mayonnaise, onion, dill and pepper. Stir to combine.

2. Spoon mixture into prepared casserole dish. Bake in preheated oven for 35 minutes or until heated through and set in center.

NUTRITIONAL ANALYSIS (PER BABY SERVING)							
Energy	Protein	Carbohydrate	Fat	Fiber	Calcium	Iron	Sodium
159 kcal	15 g	5 g	9 g	1 g	230 mg	1 mg	358 mg

Snacks

Makes about ½ cup (125 mL)

Many dips call for sour cream or yogurt. This one uses silken tofu, which has a wonderfully smooth texture that children love. The younger infant may want to eat it off a spoon, while older children may enjoy dipping chunks of fresh fruit into the mixture.

Variation

If desired, the tofu can be replaced with plain yogurt.

Lemon Tofu Dip

½ cup	silken tofu, drained	125 mL
2 to 3 tsp	granulated sugar	10 to 15 mL
½ tsp	grated lemon zest	2 mL
1 tbsp	freshly squeezed lemon juice	15 mL

1. In a food processor or small bowl, process or beat tofu, sugar to taste, lemon zest and juice until smooth.
2. Serve immediately or transfer to an airtight container and store in the refrigerator for up to 5 days.

NUTRITIONAL ANALYSIS (PER 2 TBSP/25 ML)

Energy	Protein	Carbohydrate	Fat	Fiber	Calcium	Iron	Sodium
24 kcal	1 g	3 g	1 g	0.1 g	9 mg	0.2 mg	1 mg

Makes 4 cups (1 L)

Kitchen Tips

For this recipe to work, all bowls, pots and utensils must be very clean.

Serve yogurt over fruit or enjoy on its own.

Homemade Yogurt

Kitchen thermometer

| 4 cups | 2% milk | 1 L |
| ½ cup | plain yogurt | 125 mL |

1. In a large heavy saucepan, heat milk slowly, stirring occasionally, until it reaches 180°F (82°C). Transfer to a clean bowl. Let milk cool to 113°F (45°C).
2. In a small cup, mix yogurt with ¼ cup (50 mL) of the warm milk. Stir back into warmed milk. Cover bowl and wrap in tea towels to ensure mixture cools as slowly as possible. Let sit undisturbed for a minimum of 5 hours, then refrigerate. Keeps refrigerated for up to 1 week.

NUTRITIONAL ANALYSIS (PER ¼ CUP/50 ML)

Energy	Protein	Carbohydrate	Fat	Fiber	Calcium	Iron	Sodium
37 kcal	2 g	4 g	1 g	–	90 mg	–	32 mg

Makes 1 cup (250 mL)

Kitchen Tips

This soft cheese makes a great dip. Combine with French onion soup mix and serve with veggies.

If you don't have cheesecloth, a coffee filter will also work.

Yogurt Cheese

2 cups	plain yogurt	500 mL

1. Line a sieve with cheesecloth. Add yogurt and let drain for approximately 30 minutes.
2. Tie a knot in the top of cheesecloth with a wooden spoon. Suspend over a large bowl and keep overnight in the refrigerator.
3. Untie cheesecloth and remove cheese. Keep chilled until ready to serve.

NUTRITIONAL ANALYSIS (PER ¼ CUP/50 ML)

Energy	Protein	Carbohydrate	Fat	Fiber	Calcium	Iron	Sodium
79 kcal	7 g	9 g	2 g	–	229 mg	0.1 mg	88 mg

Makes 12 slices

Serving Suggestion

This bread is great with curried beef or chicken for lunch or dinner, or with jam and cream cheese for breakfast.

Chapati (Indian Bread)

1½ cups	whole wheat flour	375 mL
¾ cup	all-purpose flour	175 mL
¼ tsp	salt	1 mL
1 cup	water	250 mL
	Vegetable oil for frying	

1. In a bowl, combine whole wheat flour, all-purpose flour and salt. Add water in small amounts, mixing until the dough comes together in a ball. Knead dough for 5 minutes; let rest under a damp tea towel for about 30 minutes.
2. Divide dough into 12 pieces. Knead each piece briefly. Roll into flat circles about 5 inches (12.5 cm) in diameter.
3. In a large frying pan, heat oil over medium-high heat. Add chapati and cook one side, turning when bread puffs up. Cook other side and transfer to a plate.

NUTRITIONAL ANALYSIS (PER SLICE)

Energy	Protein	Carbohydrate	Fat	Fiber	Calcium	Iron	Sodium
82 kcal	3 g	17 g	0.4 g	2 g	7 mg	1 mg	41 mg

Banana Oat Bran Mini Muffins

Makes 48 mini muffins

This is a terrific recipe for toddlers and their parents who would like a little fiber boost. It's not too sweet, and is really quick to prepare, making these muffins an excellent on-the-go breakfast or snack choice. They also freeze well, which means they are always fresh when you eat them!

Kitchen Tips

Natural wheat bran and oat bran can be found in most large grocery stores. They are usually kept in the hot cereal aisle.

No mini muffin tin? No problem — these can be baked in a regular muffin tin. Makes 12 regular-sized muffins. Increase the baking time to about 20 minutes.

Preheat oven to 400°F (200°C)
24-cup mini muffin tin, lightly greased

¾ cup	oat bran	175 mL
½ cup	quick-cooking rolled oats	125 mL
½ cup	natural wheat bran	125 mL
½ cup	whole wheat flour	125 mL
½ cup	all-purpose flour	125 mL
½ cup	lightly packed brown sugar	125 mL
1 tbsp	baking powder	15 mL
½ tsp	baking soda	2 mL
½ tsp	ground cinnamon	2 mL
Pinch	salt	Pinch
2	eggs, lightly beaten	2
1 cup	mashed ripe bananas (about 3)	250 mL
½ cup	2% milk	125 mL
½ cup	butter, melted	125 mL

1. In a large bowl, combine oat bran, rolled oats, wheat bran, whole wheat flour, all-purpose flour, brown sugar, baking powder, baking soda, cinnamon and salt.
2. In another bowl, combine eggs, bananas, milk and melted butter. Add to dry ingredients and stir until just combined.
3. Spoon batter into prepared muffin cups; set remaining batter aside. Bake for 8 minutes or until a toothpick inserted in the center of a muffin comes out clean. Let cool in pan for 5 minutes, then remove to a wire rack to cool completely. Grease muffin tin again and repeat with remaining batter.

NUTRITIONAL ANALYSIS (PER MINI MUFFIN)

Energy	Protein	Carbohydrate	Fat	Fiber	Calcium	Iron	Sodium
57 kcal	1 g	8 g	3 g	1 g	19 mg	0.4 mg	50 mg

Makes 2½ cups (625 mL)

This dip is a delicious way to boost fiber, iron and calcium intake.

Avocado Chickpea Dip

1	large avocado, sliced	1
1	can (19 oz/540 mL) chickpeas, rinsed and drained	1
¼ cup	salsa	50 mL
1 tsp	freshly squeezed lemon juice	5 mL
	Whole-grain pita bread or whole-grain crackers	

1. In a food processor or blender, purée avocado, chickpeas, salsa and lemon juice until smooth. Transfer to a bowl and serve as a dip with pita bread or crackers.

NUTRITIONAL ANALYSIS (PER 2 TBSP/25 ML)

Energy	Protein	Carbohydrate	Fat	Fiber	Calcium	Iron	Sodium
51 kcal	2 g	6 g	3 g	2 g	11 mg	1 mg	22 mg

Makes 2⅓ cups (575 mL)

Few can resist this nutritious and eye-pleasing dip (and the fun of dipping). In time, they may even decide they like their spinach "straight up." Use vegetables or corn tortilla chips as dippers.

Kitchen Tip

Return any remaining dip to the refrigerator for up to 4 days.

Spinach Dip

1	package (10 oz/300 g) frozen chopped spinach, thawed, excess liquid squeezed out	1
1 cup	cottage cheese	250 mL
1	small clove garlic	1
1 cup	sour cream	250 mL
Dash	hot pepper sauce	Dash
⅛ tsp	salt	0.5 mL

1. In a food processor, combine spinach, cottage cheese and garlic; pulse until fairly smooth. Add sour cream, hot pepper sauce and salt; process to blend.

2. Transfer dip to a bowl; cover and refrigerate for several hours or overnight to let flavors develop.

NUTRITIONAL ANALYSIS (PER 1 TBSP/15 ML)

Energy	Protein	Carbohydrate	Fat	Fiber	Calcium	Iron	Sodium
18 kcal	1 g	1 g	1 g	0.3 g	27 mg	0.4 mg	43 mg

Citrus Yogurt Fruit Dip

Fussy little appetites can be enticed into trying new fruits with this yogurt dip. Children enjoy the fun of dipping — and this is about as nutritious as a snack can get.

Kitchen Tips

For a slightly sweeter — although higher-fat — version of this dip, substitute sour cream for yogurt.

This recipe is easily doubled.

¼ cup	plain yogurt (see tip)	50 mL
1 tsp	frozen orange juice concentrate, thawed	5 mL
Pinch	granulated sugar	Pinch
Pinch	ground ginger	Pinch
Pinch	ground nutmeg	Pinch
	Fruit, such as banana chunks, orange or mandarin segments, seedless grapes cut in half, cantaloupe or honeydew chunks, apple or pear slices, strawberry slices	

1. In a small bowl, combine yogurt, orange juice, sugar, ginger and nutmeg; stir well. For best flavor, chill for a short time in the refrigerator. Serve with fruit pieces for dipping.

NUTRITIONAL ANALYSIS (PER 1 TBSP/15 ML)

Energy	Protein	Carbohydrate	Fat	Fiber	Calcium	Iron	Sodium
12 kcal	1 g	2 g	0.3 g	0.1 g	23 mg	–	9 mg

Tangy Salsa

Kitchen Tips

Avocado adds calories and is a great source of monounsaturated fat.

Stores refrigerated for 2 to 3 days.

4	tomatoes, chopped and seeded	4
½	onion, chopped	½
½ cup	chopped peeled avocado	125 mL
¼ cup	chopped fresh coriander	50 mL
2 tbsp	vegetable oil	25 mL
2 tbsp	lime juice	25 mL
Pinch	salt	Pinch
Pinch	freshly ground black pepper	Pinch

1. In a large bowl, mix together all the ingredients. Let sit for about 1 hour to develop flavors before serving.

NUTRITIONAL ANALYSIS (PER ¼ CUP/50 ML)

Energy	Protein	Carbohydrate	Fat	Fiber	Calcium	Iron	Sodium
30 kcal	0.4 g	2 g	2 g	1 g	5 mg	0.1 mg	17 mg

Kitchen Tips

To peel chickpeas, squeeze them gently and the thin skin will slide off. This will give your hummus a smoother texture. But if you're short of time, leave the skins on.

Tahini is sesame seed paste. It can be found in Middle Eastern grocery stores and in most large supermarkets.

Hummus (Chickpea Dip)

3 tbsp	tahini	45 mL
2 tbsp	cold water	25 mL
	Juice of 1 lemon	
1	can (19 oz/540 mL) chickpeas, peeled (see tip)	1
1	clove garlic, minced	1

1. In a small bowl, combine tahini with cold water, stirring until tahini turns white. Transfer paste to food processor along with chickpeas; blend until mixed. Add lemon juice and garlic; purée to desired consistency, adding more water as necessary. Serve with pita bread.

NUTRITIONAL ANALYSIS (PER 1 TBSP/15 ML)

Energy	Protein	Carbohydrate	Fat	Fiber	Calcium	Iron	Sodium
37 kcal	2 g	5 g	1 g	1 g	16 mg	0.5 mg	3 mg

Everybody likes to dip. And the smoky-sweet taste of roasted red peppers in this sour-cream-based dip is irresistible. Torn pieces of pita bread, bread sticks and fresh vegetables make excellent dippers.

Kitchen Tip

If you have time, roast your own peppers under a broiler or on a barbecue grill, then remove skin and seeds. This is especially worthwhile when peppers are in season. Roasted peppers can be frozen for later use.

Red Pepper Dip

½ cup	drained bottled roasted red peppers (see tip)	125 mL
¼ cup	sour cream	50 mL
2 tbsp	mayonnaise	25 mL
1 tsp	lemon juice	5 mL
½ tsp	ground oregano	2 mL
Pinch	granulated sugar	Pinch
Pinch	salt	Pinch

1. In a food processor or blender, combine red peppers, sour cream, mayonnaise and lemon juice; purée until smooth. Stir in oregano, sugar and salt. Spoon into a container with a tight-fitting lid. Refrigerate until ready to serve.

NUTRITIONAL ANALYSIS (PER 1 TBSP/15 ML)

Energy	Protein	Carbohydrate	Fat	Fiber	Calcium	Iron	Sodium
16 kcal	0.2 g	1 g	1 g	0.1 g	6 mg	0.1 mg	36 mg

This new take on a vegetable dip is sufficiently different that it makes a nice alternative to hummus. We have found that it is especially flavorful when served at room temperature or slightly warmed. And, of course, it doubles easily!

Warm Lentil Dip

½ cup	red lentils, rinsed and drained	125 mL
1½ cups	reduced-sodium vegetable or chicken broth	375 mL
1	small clove garlic, sliced	1
2 tsp	olive oil	10 mL
1 tsp	freshly squeezed lemon juice	5 mL
¼ tsp	dry mustard	1 mL
Pinch	salt	Pinch
Pinch	freshly ground black pepper	Pinch

1. In a saucepan, combine lentils, broth and garlic. Bring to a boil over high heat. Reduce heat to low, cover and cook for 10 minutes or until lentils are tender (do not overcook). Drain immediately.
2. In a food processor or blender, process drained lentils, oil, lemon juice, mustard, salt and pepper until mixture is smooth.
3. Serve immediately or transfer to an airtight container and store in the refrigerator for up to 5 days.

NUTRITIONAL ANALYSIS (PER 1 TBSP/15 ML)

Energy	Protein	Carbohydrate	Fat	Fiber	Calcium	Iron	Sodium
21 kcal	1.4 g	2.9 g	0.6 g	0.5 g	3.8 mg	0.4 mg	110 mg

Makes 4 fruit pops

This frozen yogurt snack is brimming with nutrition.

Food Safety Tip

Honey should only be given to children who are over 1 year of age. For younger children, replace honey in this recipe with granulated sugar.

Frozen Fruit Pops

1 cup	sliced strawberries or cubed cantaloupe	250 mL
½ cup	plain yogurt	125 mL
2 tbsp	instant skim milk powder	25 mL
2 tbsp	liquid honey (see tip)	25 mL
½ cup	evaporated milk	125 mL

1. In a food processor or blender, combine fruit, yogurt, milk powder and honey; process until smooth. Blend in milk.

2. Spoon mixture into small molds or paper cups. Freeze until pops are almost solid; insert a plastic spoon or tongue depressor into the center of each mold. Return to freezer. When frozen, store in a sealed plastic bag until ready to serve.

NUTRITIONAL ANALYSIS (PER FRUIT POP)

Energy	Protein	Carbohydrate	Fat	Fiber	Calcium	Iron	Sodium
96 kcal	5 g	16 g	2 g	1 g	189 mg	0.3 mg	74 mg

Makes 2½ cups (625 mL)

Children of all ages love frozen fruit pops. It's best to let younger babies enjoy this mixture off a spoon. Older children can eat a frozen pop as long as they are able to manage the stick.

Banana Pops

1 cup	plain or vanilla-flavored yogurt	250 mL
½ cup	orange juice	125 mL
1	banana, cut into chunks	1

1. In a food processor or blender, process yogurt, orange juice and banana until smooth.

2. Pour into ice pop molds or small dishes and freeze until firm, at least 2 hours. Store in the freezer for up to 1 month.

NUTRITIONAL ANALYSIS (PER ½ CUP/125 ML)

Energy	Protein	Carbohydrate	Fat	Fiber	Calcium	Iron	Sodium
64 kcal	3 g	12 g	1 g	0.5 g	95 mg	0.1 mg	36 mg

12 to 18 months

Makes 2½ cups (625 mL)

Here's a simplified "nuts and bolts" snack that children love. (They especially enjoy feeding themselves with the small, easily handled pieces.) It's quick to make and provides more food energy than the cereal alone.

Cereal Snack

1 tbsp	margarine or butter	15 mL
1½ cups	Cheerios-type oat cereal	375 mL
½ cup	pretzels, broken	125 mL
½ cup	finely chopped raisins	125 mL

1. In a large nonstick skillet, melt margarine over medium-low heat. Add cereal and cook, stirring constantly, for 5 minutes. Remove from heat and let cool. Stir in pretzels and raisins. Store in an airtight container.

NUTRITIONAL ANALYSIS (PER ¼ CUP/50 ML)

Energy	Protein	Carbohydrate	Fat	Fiber	Calcium	Iron	Sodium
48 kcal	1 g	10 g	2 g	1 g	11 mg	1 mg	58 mg

12 to 18 months

Makes 24 cookies

Kitchen Tip

These basic sugar cookies are quick and easy to make using ingredients that are always on hand. Keep an eye on them, since they can burn very quickly.

French Biscuits

Preheat oven to 375°F (190°C)
Baking sheet, ungreased

⅔ cup	butter or margarine	150 mL
⅔ cup	all-purpose flour	150 mL
⅓ cup	granulated sugar	75 mL

1. In a large bowl, with an electric mixer, blend together butter, flour and sugar. Drop small dollops onto baking sheet. Bake in preheated oven for 7 to 10 minutes or until golden brown.

NUTRITIONAL ANALYSIS (PER COOKIE)

Energy	Protein	Carbohydrate	Fat	Fiber	Calcium	Iron	Sodium
67 kcal	0.4 g	5 g	5 g	0.1 g	2 mg	0.2 mg	36 mg

Breadsticks are easy to hold, making them ideal for young children who are learning to feed themselves. Adults enjoy them, too, as an accompaniment to soup or chili.

Kitchen Tip

Keep unbaked bread sticks in the freezer, ready to pull out and bake at a moment's notice. Or bake them all at once for a crowd.

Herbed Breadsticks

Preheat oven to 425°F (220°C)
Nonstick baking sheet

1	long thin baguette	1
1/4 cup	butter or margarine, softened	25 mL
2 tsp	chopped fresh parsley	10 mL
1/4 tsp	ground dried basil	1 mL
1	small clove garlic, crushed (optional)	1

1. Cut baguette crosswise into quarters. Cut each quarter lengthwise into quarters to form 16 bread sticks.

2. In a small bowl, combine butter, parsley, basil and garlic, if using. Spread mixture thinly over cut sides of bread sticks. Place sticks in a single layer on baking sheet.

3. Bake in preheated oven for 10 minutes or until lightly toasted. Serve immediately, allowing child's portion to cool enough for safe and easy handling.

NUTRITIONAL ANALYSIS (PER BREADSTICK)							
Energy	Protein	Carbohydrate	Fat	Fiber	Calcium	Iron	Sodium
57 kcal	2 g	9 g	2 g	0.4 g	9 mg	0.5 mg	110 mg

Makes one 12-slice loaf

Five-grain cereal adds texture, flavor and great nutrients to this quick bread. Serve for dessert with a piece of fresh fruit.

Kitchen Tips

Five-grain cereal can be found in the bulk-food section of many supermarkets or in health food stores. If you can't find any, use Red River cereal, which is a 3-grain cereal of cracked wheat, cracked rye and flax.

Use dried fruit such as apricots, raisins, dates, prunes or pineapple.

Cut loaf into individual slices, wrap well and freeze until needed.

Five-Grain Loaf

Preheat oven to 350°F (180°C)
9- by 5-inch (2 L) loaf pan, greased

1 cup	5-grain cereal (see tip)	250 mL
1½ cups	buttermilk	375 mL
1	egg	1
¼ cup	packed brown sugar	50 mL
¼ cup	vegetable oil	50 mL
2 cups	all-purpose flour	500 mL
¼ cup	chopped dried fruit (see tip)	50 mL
1 tsp	baking powder	5 mL
1 tsp	baking soda	5 mL
1 tsp	ground cinnamon	5 mL
¼ tsp	salt	1 mL

1. In a small bowl, combine cereal and buttermilk. Let stand for 5 minutes. Add egg, brown sugar and oil; mix well.

2. In a large bowl, combine flour, fruit, baking powder, baking soda, cinnamon and salt. Add cereal mixture to flour mixture. Stir just until dry ingredients are moistened.

3. Spoon batter into prepared loaf pan. Bake in preheated oven for 45 minutes or until a cake taster inserted in center comes out clean. Let cool on a wire rack before cutting into slices.

NUTRITIONAL ANALYSIS (PER SLICE)

Energy	Protein	Carbohydrate	Fat	Fiber	Calcium	Iron	Sodium
167 kcal	4 g	27 g	5 g	1 g	63 mg	1 mg	216 mg

This loaf is really a quick bread — leavened with baking powder and soda rather than yeast. You can also think of it as a large muffin made in a loaf pan. Apples give it a delightfully fresh taste and moist texture that appeals to all ages.

Apple Loaf

Preheat oven to 350°F (180°C)
9- by 5-inch (2 L) loaf pan, greased

⅓ cup	butter or margarine	75 mL
½ cup	lightly packed brown sugar	125 mL
1	egg	1
1 tsp	vanilla extract	5 mL
1 tsp	grated orange zest	5 mL
2 cups	all-purpose flour	500 mL
1 tsp	baking powder	5 mL
1 tsp	ground cinnamon	5 mL
½ tsp	baking soda	2 mL
½ tsp	salt	2 mL
⅓ cup	freshly squeezed orange juice	75 mL
1 cup	finely chopped peeled apple (about 1 large)	250 mL

1. In a large bowl, with an electric mixer, cream butter until light and fluffy. Gradually add brown sugar, egg, vanilla and orange zest; beat until smooth.

2. In another bowl, sift together flour, baking powder, cinnamon, baking soda and salt. Add dry ingredients to creamed mixture alternately with orange juice; stir after each addition. Fold in apples.

3. Spoon batter into prepared loaf pan. Bake in preheated oven for 50 minutes or until a tester inserted in the center comes out clean.

NUTRITIONAL ANALYSIS (PER SLICE)

Energy	Protein	Carbohydrate	Fat	Fiber	Calcium	Iron	Sodium
133 kcal	2 g	22 g	4 g	1 g	23 mg	1 mg	145 mg

Makes one 16-slice loaf

This quick bread is especially tasty, with a moistness that appeals to everyone. Slices freeze well when a snack is required. Thaw frozen slices at room temperature or in the microwave, on a plate lined with paper towels, on Medium (50%).

Oat Pumpkin Loaf

Preheat oven to 350°F (180°C)
9- by 5-inch (2 L) loaf pan, greased

1 cup	buttermilk	250 mL
1 cup	large-flake old-fashioned rolled oats	250 mL
1 cup	whole wheat flour	250 mL
⅔ cup	lightly packed brown sugar	150 mL
1 tsp	baking powder	5 mL
1 tsp	baking soda	5 mL
½ tsp	ground nutmeg	2 mL
½ tsp	ground cinnamon	2 mL
½ tsp	ground ginger	2 mL
1 cup	unsweetened canned pumpkin purée (not pie filling)	250 mL
¼ cup	canola oil	50 mL
1	egg, beaten	1
½ tsp	vanilla extract	2 mL

1. In a bowl, stir buttermilk into rolled oats; let stand for 30 minutes.

2. In another bowl, combine flour, brown sugar, baking powder, baking soda, nutmeg, cinnamon and ginger.

3. Stir pumpkin, oil, egg and vanilla into buttermilk mixture. Add to dry ingredients and stir just until combined.

4. Spoon batter into prepared pan. Bake in preheated oven for 45 minutes or until a cake tester inserted in center comes out clean. Let cool in pan on a wire rack for 10 minutes, then remove to rack to cool completely.

NUTRITIONAL ANALYSIS (PER SLICE)

Energy	Protein	Carbohydrate	Fat	Fiber	Calcium	Iron	Sodium
143 kcal	4 g	23 g	4 g	3 g	50 mg	1 mg	125 mg

Makes one 16-slice cake

This cake makes a nice change from cookies and milk at snack time. Kids love it!

Kitchen Tip

If using a nonstick pan, there's no need to grease the cake pan.

Variation

If you like, you can add a streusel topping to this cake. In a bowl, combine 1/4 cup (50 mL) packed brown sugar, 2 tbsp (25 mL) all-purpose flour and 1 to 2 tsp (5 to 10 mL) ground cinnamon. Work in 1 tbsp (15 mL) butter or margarine to make a crumbly topping. Sprinkle over batter before baking.

Snacking Cake

Preheat oven to 375°F (190°C)
8- or 9-inch (20 or 23 cm) round cake pan, greased and floured

1 1/3 cups	whole wheat flour	325 mL
2 1/2 tsp	baking powder	12 mL
1/2 cup	granulated sugar	125 mL
1/2 tsp	salt	2 mL
1/4 cup	vegetable oil	50 mL
1	egg, beaten	1
1/2 tsp	vanilla extract	2 mL
3/4 cup	2% milk	175 mL

1. In a bowl, combine flour, baking powder, sugar and salt. Make a well or depression in the center.
2. In a small bowl, combine oil, egg, vanilla and milk. Pour into well in dry ingredients; mix just until blended. Pour into prepared cake pan.
3. Bake in preheated oven for 30 to 35 minutes or until a toothpick inserted in the center comes out clean.

NUTRITIONAL ANALYSIS (PER SLICE)

Energy	Protein	Carbohydrate	Fat	Fiber	Calcium	Iron	Sodium
114 kcal	2 g	18 g	4 g	1 g	42 mg	1 mg	61 mg

Makes 12 muffins

Muffins make a quick and easy snack for on-the-go toddlers and their mommies. These fruit-filled muffins are a healthier alternative to many "cake" type muffins, because the applesauce keeps them moist while eliminating the need for a lot of oil. They are also a source of dietary fiber.

Kitchen Tips

This recipe also makes 48 mini muffins. Reduce baking time to 8 minutes.

Muffins freeze well and make great snacks or treats for play dates with other children and their families.

Apple Raisin Muffins

Preheat oven to 375°F (190°C)
12-cup muffin tin, greased or paper-lined

1 cup	all-purpose flour	250 mL
1 tsp	baking soda	5 mL
1 tsp	baking powder	5 mL
½ tsp	ground cinnamon	2 mL
½ cup	lightly packed brown sugar	125 mL
½ cup	unsweetened applesauce	125 mL
¼ cup	vegetable oil	50 mL
1	egg	1
1 tsp	vanilla extract	5 mL
¾ cup	diced peeled apples	175 mL
½ cup	raisins, chopped	125 mL

1. In a large bowl, combine flour, baking soda, baking powder and cinnamon.
2. In another bowl, combine brown sugar, applesauce, oil, egg and vanilla. Stir until mixed well. Add to dry ingredients and stir until just combined. Stir in apples and raisins.
3. Spoon batter into prepared muffin cups. Bake for 20 minutes or until a toothpick inserted in the center of a muffin comes out clean. Let cool in pan on a wire rack for 10 minutes, then remove to rack to cool completely.

NUTRITIONAL ANALYSIS (PER MUFFIN)

Energy	Protein	Carbohydrate	Fat	Fiber	Calcium	Iron	Sodium
147 kcal	2 g	26 g	4 g	1 g	28 mg	1 mg	143 mg

Makes 36 cookies

Mashed bananas and rolled oats give body, taste, texture and nutritive value to these soft cookies. They are just the thing for a children's snack or to finish a family meal.

Variation

For a peanut-flavored version of these cookies — and where there is no danger of nut allergy — replace the butter or margarine with peanut butter.

Soft Cranberry Banana Cookies

Preheat oven to 350°F (180°C)
Baking sheets, greased

½ cup	finely chopped dried cranberries (optional)	125 mL
1	ripe medium banana, mashed	1
⅓ cup	butter or margarine (see tip)	75 mL
¼ cup	apple juice	50 mL
1	egg	1
½ tsp	vanilla extract	2 mL
1 cup	old-fashioned rolled oats	250 mL
½ cup	all-purpose flour	125 mL
¼ cup	packed brown sugar	50 mL
1 tsp	baking soda	5 mL

1. In a bowl, stir together cranberries (if using), banana, butter, apple juice, egg and vanilla; mix until smooth. Stir in rolled oats, flour, brown sugar and baking soda; blend well.

2. Drop by spoonfuls onto prepared baking pans; flatten with a fork. Bake in preheated oven for 10 minutes or until lightly browned. Let cool on a wire rack before storing in a tightly closed container.

NUTRITIONAL ANALYSIS (PER COOKIE)

Energy	Protein	Carbohydrate	Fat	Fiber	Calcium	Iron	Sodium
55 kcal	1 g	8 g	2 g	1 g	5 mg	0.4 mg	50 mg

Makes 45 cookies

Apple Oatmeal Cookies

Preheat oven to 375°F (190°C)
Baking sheets, greased

1 cup	whole wheat flour	250 mL
1¼ tsp	ground cinnamon	6 mL
½ tsp	salt	2 mL
¼ tsp	baking soda	1 mL
¼ tsp	ground nutmeg	1 mL
¾ cup	margarine	175 mL
¾ cup	lightly packed brown sugar	175 mL
1	egg	1
¼ cup	milk	50 mL
1½ tsp	vanilla extract	7 mL
3 cups	old-fashioned rolled oats	750 mL
1 cup	finely chopped peeled apple (about 1 large)	250 mL
1 cup	finely chopped raisins (optional)	250 mL

1. In a large bowl, combine flour, cinnamon, salt, baking soda and nutmeg.

2. In another large bowl, with an electric mixer, combine margarine, brown sugar, egg, milk and vanilla; cream together until smooth. Add flour mixture with mixer on low speed, just until blended. Stir in oats, apple and raisins, if using.

3. Drop dough by spoonfuls onto prepared baking sheets. Bake for 12 minutes or until golden brown.

NUTRITIONAL ANALYSIS (PER COOKIE)

Energy	Protein	Carbohydrate	Fat	Fiber	Calcium	Iron	Sodium
97 kcal	2 g	13 g	4 g	2 g	14 mg	1 mg	71 mg

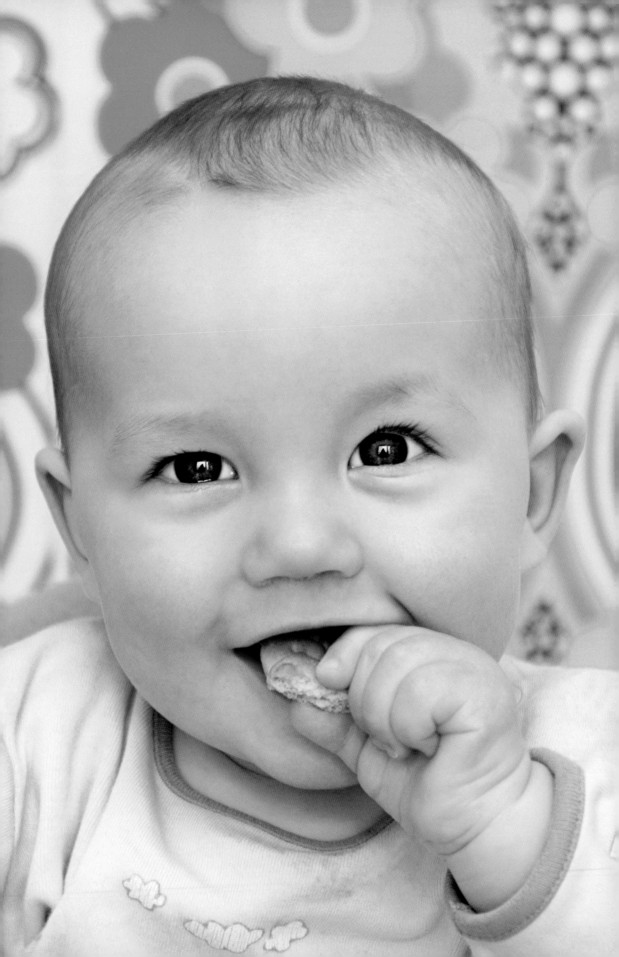

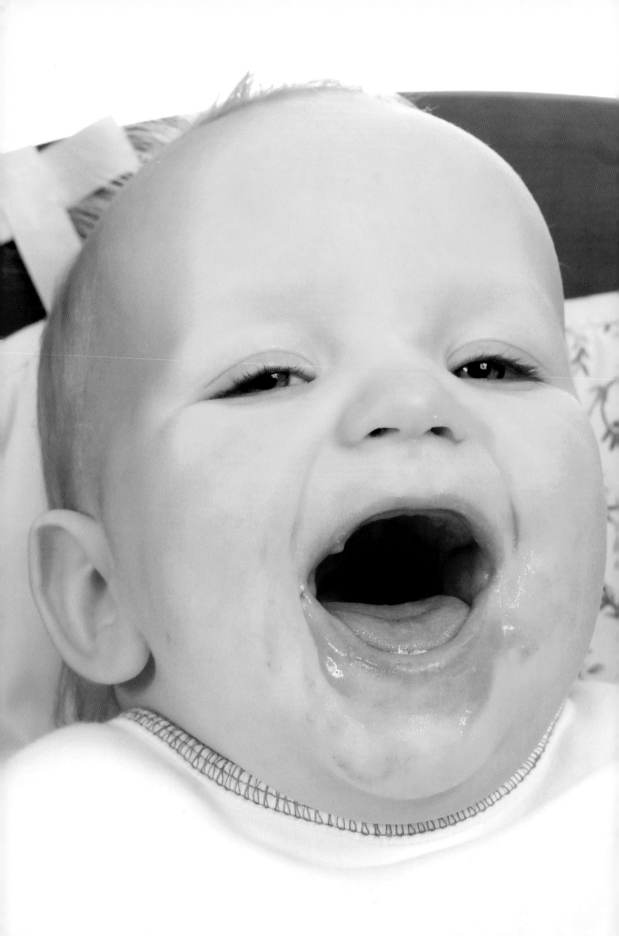

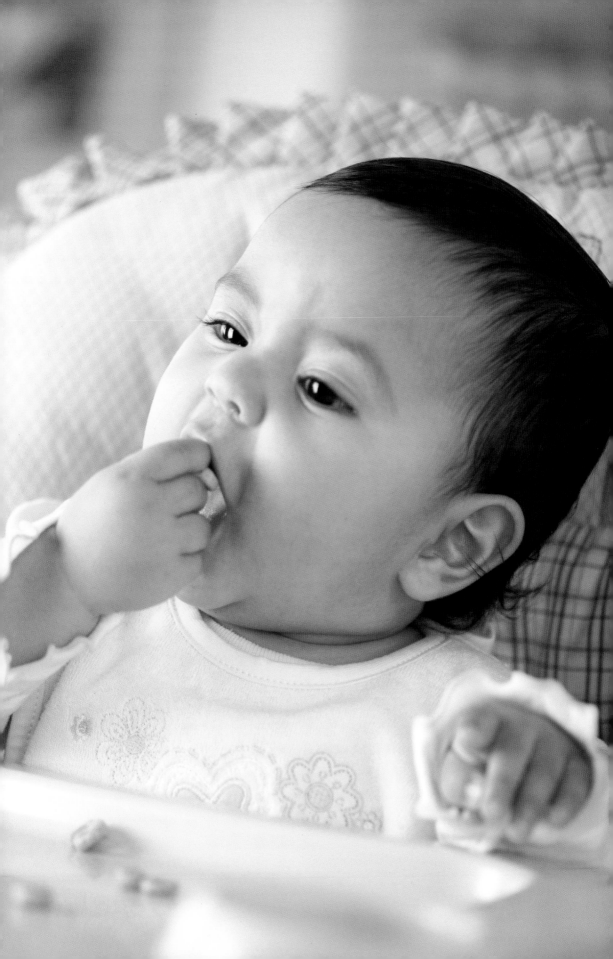

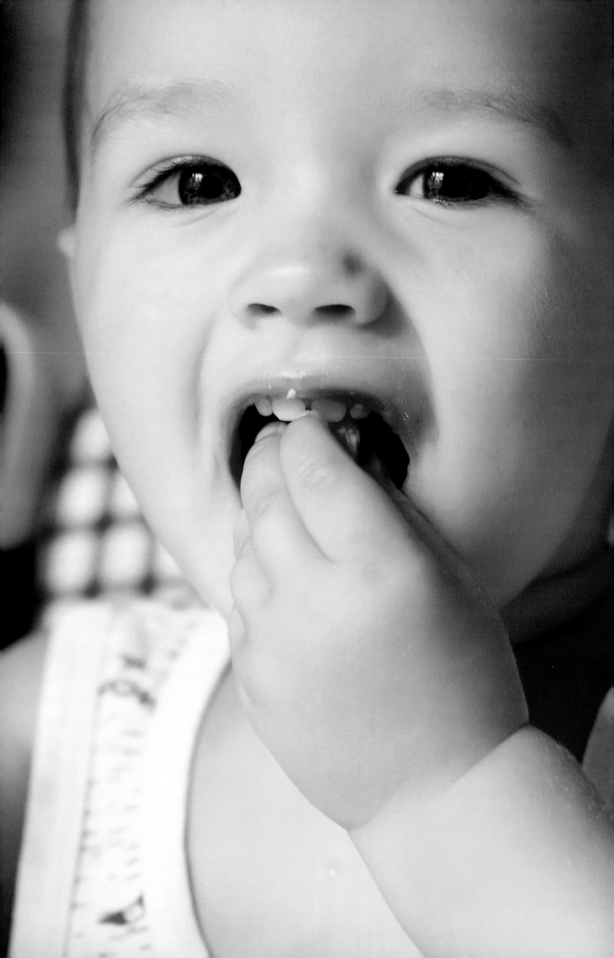

Iron-deficiency anemia is the most common nutritional deficiency in the U.S. and Canada. These cookies have a secret ingredient — infant rice cereal — which gives them a little boost of iron.

Iron-Boosted Oatmeal and Raisin Cookies

Preheat oven to 375°F (190°C)
Large baking sheet, ungreased

½ cup	butter or margarine, softened	125 mL
½ cup	lightly packed brown sugar	125 mL
½ cup	all-purpose flour	125 mL
1 cup	quick-cooking rolled oats	250 mL
½ cup	instant infant rice cereal	125 mL
½ tsp	baking soda	2 mL
½ tsp	baking powder	2 mL
½ tsp	salt	2 mL
1 tsp	vanilla	5 mL
½ cup	raisins, chopped	125 mL

1. In a large bowl, using an electric mixer, cream together butter and brown sugar. Add flour, oats, rice cereal, baking soda, baking powder, salt and vanilla. Mix well. Fold in raisins.

2. Drop dough by tablespoonfuls (15 mL) on baking sheet, at least 2 inches (5 cm) apart, and flatten with a fork. Bake for 10 minutes or until golden brown. Let cool on baking sheet for 5 minutes, then transfer to wire racks to cool completely.

NUTRITIONAL ANALYSIS (PER COOKIE)							
Energy	Protein	Carbohydrate	Fat	Fiber	Calcium	Iron	Sodium
77 kcal	1 g	11 g	3 g	1 g	14 mg	1 mg	66 mg

Oat and Rice Crisp Cookies

Makes 30 cookies

Serve these small cookies (just right for little hands) with a piece of fresh fruit at snacking time. Rolled oats add a nutritional variation on the more common rice cereal cookie.

Preheat oven to 350°F (180°C)
Nonstick baking sheets

¼ cup	vegetable oil	50 mL
½ cup	packed brown sugar	125 mL
1	egg	1
2 tbsp	corn syrup	25 mL
½ tsp	vanilla extract	2 mL
1 cup	all-purpose flour	250 mL
¼ cup	skim milk powder	50 mL
¼ tsp	salt	1 mL
¼ tsp	baking soda	1 mL
¾ cup	old-fashioned rolled oats	175 mL
½ cup	crisp rice cereal	125 mL

1. In a large bowl, with an electric mixer, combine oil, brown sugar, egg, corn syrup and vanilla; beat until light and fluffy.

2. In another bowl, combine flour, skim milk powder, salt and baking soda. Gradually stir into creamed mixture; mix well.

3. Stir in rolled oats and cereal. Drop dough, by spoonfuls, 2 inches (5 cm) apart on baking sheets. Bake in preheated oven for 10 minutes or until cookies are golden brown. Let cool on wire rack before storing in an airtight container.

NUTRITIONAL ANALYSIS (PER COOKIE)							
Energy	Protein	Carbohydrate	Fat	Fiber	Calcium	Iron	Sodium
70 kcal	2 g	11 g	2 g	0.5 g	17 mg	1 mg	37 mg

Makes 36 cookies

These drop cookies have an old-fashioned taste that will remind you of your grandmother's sugar cookies. The difference is the carrots, which give the cookies colorful eye appeal and vitamin A. These cookies are sized just right for little hands.

Kitchen Tip

These cookies freeze well.

Carrot Cookies

Preheat oven to 400°F (200°C)
Baking sheets, ungreased

½ cup	butter or margarine, softened	125 mL
½ cup	packed brown sugar	125 mL
1	egg	1
1 cup	finely shredded carrots (about 2 medium)	250 mL
1½ cups	all-purpose flour	375 mL
1 cup	whole wheat flour	250 mL
1 tsp	ground cinnamon	5 mL
1 tsp	baking powder	5 mL
½ tsp	ground nutmeg	2 mL
½ tsp	salt	2 mL

1. In a large bowl, with an electric mixer, cream together butter and sugar until light and fluffy. Beat in egg and carrots.

2. In another bowl, combine flours, cinnamon, baking powder, nutmeg and salt. Gradually stir into creamed mixture, blending well after each addition.

3. Shape cookies into small balls, place on baking sheets and press down with a moistened fork. Bake in preheated oven for 15 minutes or until cookies are golden and crisp. Let cool on wire racks.

NUTRITIONAL ANALYSIS (PER COOKIE)							
Energy	Protein	Carbohydrate	Fat	Fiber	Calcium	Iron	Sodium
73 kcal	1 g	10 g	3 g	1 g	12 mg	0.5 mg	61 mg

Makes 1½ cups (375 mL)

Children are especially fond of avocados — perhaps because of their mushy consistency, as well as their great tropical flavor.

Kitchen Tips

Avocado discolors quickly, so make this dip only a short time before serving. Brush cut side of unused avocado with lemon juice, cover with plastic wrap and refrigerate. (Even with this treatment, however, the avocado will become browned; this can be cut off before use.)

Buy ripe avocados that yield to gentle palm pressure and are unblemished and heavy for their size.

Avocado Dip

1	ripe medium avocado, peeled (see tip)	1
2 tsp	lemon juice	10 mL
¼ cup	finely chopped onion	50 mL
¼ tsp	salt	1 mL
Pinch	freshly ground black pepper	Pinch
¼ cup	sour cream	50 mL
	Crisp corn tortillas	

1. In a bowl, with a fork, mash avocado until smooth. Stir in lemon juice, onion, salt and pepper. Cover and refrigerate for 30 minutes.
2. Gently stir sour cream into avocado mixture. Spoon into a serving bowl, surround with tortilla chips and serve.

NUTRITIONAL ANALYSIS (PER 1 TBSP/15 ML)

Energy	Protein	Carbohydrate	Fat	Fiber	Calcium	Iron	Sodium
17 kcal	0.2 g	1 g	2 g	1 g	4 mg	0.1 mg	21 mg

Makes 1¼ cups (300 mL)

Children seem to enjoy food they can get right into, and dips fit the bill, although both child and high chair will need a good wash-up afterwards! Raw veggies are a good dipper.

Variations

If your child is adventurous, by all means add some chili or curry powder, or try fresh or dried dill.

Cheese and Carrot Dip

½ cup	finely shredded carrots	125 mL
½ cup	finely shredded Cheddar cheese	125 mL
⅓ cup	mayonnaise	75 mL
2 tbsp	finely chopped raisins	25 mL
1 tsp	freshly squeezed lemon juice	5 mL

1. In a bowl, combine carrots, cheese, mayonnaise, raisins and lemon juice. Stir until blended.
2. Serve immediately or transfer to an airtight container and store in the refrigerator for up to 3 days.

NUTRITIONAL ANALYSIS (PER 2 TBSP/25 ML)

Energy	Protein	Carbohydrate	Fat	Fiber	Calcium	Iron	Sodium
62 kcal	2 g	4 g	4 g	0.2 g	48 mg	0.1 mg	96 mg

*Serve as a snack-time spread
for crackers, toast or apple
slices.*

Kitchen Tips

If your child is ready to eat
apple skin, there is no need to
peel the apples. Naturally,
there is more fiber in the
unpeeled apple.

Prepare only as many apple
slices as are needed for the
snack. The spread may be
kept refrigerated for another
use for up to 3 days. Spoon
into several small containers,
then remove just one
container at a time.

To prevent browning, apple
slices may be dipped into a
lemon-water mixture, using
1 part freshly squeezed lemon
juice to 3 parts water.

Creamy Apple Cheese Spread

4 oz	cream cheese, softened	125 g
½ cup	shredded mild Cheddar cheese	125 mL
2 tbsp	mayonnaise	25 mL
2 tsp	freshly squeezed lemon juice	10 mL
Pinch	dry mustard	Pinch
3	apples	3

1. In a bowl, using an electric mixer, beat cream cheese until smooth. Beat in Cheddar cheese, mayonnaise, lemon juice and mustard until creamy.

2. Peel and grate 1 apple; stir into cheese mixture. Cover and refrigerate for about 2 hours.

3. Remove from refrigerator and let stand at room temperature for 15 minutes, until mixture is softened to spreading consistency.

4. Core and peel remaining apples (see tip). Cut into thin slices. Dip each slice into a water and lemon juice mixture (see tip) to prevent browning. Spread apple slices with cheese mixture.

NUTRITIONAL ANALYSIS (PER 2 TBSP/25 ML)							
Energy	Protein	Carbohydrate	Fat	Fiber	Calcium	Iron	Sodium
159 kcal	4 g	10 g	12 g	1 g	92 mg	0.4 mg	152 mg

Makes 32 chips

In this recipe, corn or flour tortillas (or pitas) become tasty crisp morsels for between-meal bites. Make them in sizes that little fingers can handle.

Flavored Snacking Chips

Preheat oven to 425°F (220°C)
Baking sheet

4	corn or flour tortillas or pita bread halves	4
¼ cup	vegetable oil	50 mL
½ tsp	garlic powder or onion powder	2 mL
½ tsp	herb blend	2 mL

1. Lightly brush corn or flour tortillas or pita halves with oil. Sprinkle with garlic powder and herbs. Cut each with scissors into 8 wedge-shaped pieces. Arrange in a single layer on baking sheet. Bake for 8 minutes or until crisp and golden brown. Let cool before storing in a tightly sealed container.

NUTRITIONAL ANALYSIS (PER 4 CHIPS)							
Energy	Protein	Carbohydrate	Fat	Fiber	Calcium	Iron	Sodium
28 kcal	1.5 g	2.5 g	2 g	0.3 g	1 mg	0.1 mg	23 mg

Makes 10 cups (2.5 L)

Snack Mix

¼ cup	vegetable oil	50 mL
6 cups	Chex-type cereal	1.5 L
8 oz	mini crackers (such as Ritz)	250 g
1	package (1 oz/28 g) ranch-style salad dressing mix (powder)	1
2 to 3 tbsp	dried dill	25 to 45 mL

1. In a small bowl, heat oil in microwave for 45 to 60 seconds, until warm.

2. In a large bag, combine cereal, crackers, ranch powder and dill. Sprinkle with oil and shake. Store in an airtight container.

NUTRITIONAL ANALYSIS (PER ¼ CUP/50 ML)							
Energy	Protein	Carbohydrate	Fat	Fiber	Calcium	Iron	Sodium
78 kcal	2 g	11 g	3 g	1 g	18 mg	2 mg	127 mg

Makes 20 baby servings, or 4 adult servings

Delicious when served warm with vanilla ice cream.

Kitchen Tips

If peaches are difficult to peel, plunge into boiling water for 1 minute.

If you wish, replace peaches with additional apples.

Apple Peach Crisp and Oats

Preheat oven to 375°F (190°C)
8-inch (2 L) casserole dish

7	medium apples, peeled and sliced	7
3	medium peaches, peeled and sliced	3
1 tbsp	lemon juice	15 mL
⅔ cup	all-purpose flour	150 mL
⅔ cup	quick-cooking rolled oats	150 mL
⅓ cup	packed brown sugar	75 mL
½ tsp	ground cinnamon	2 mL
¼ cup	butter or margarine, melted	50 mL

1. Place apple and peach slices on bottom of casserole dish. Sprinkle with lemon juice; toss to coat thoroughly.

2. In a bowl, combine flour, oats, brown sugar and cinnamon. Pour melted butter over. Mix together to make a crumbly mixture. Sprinkle mixture evenly over fruit.

3. Bake in preheated oven for 45 minutes or until fruit is softened and crumbly topping is crisp.

NUTRITIONAL ANALYSIS (PER BABY SERVING)

Energy	Protein	Carbohydrate	Fat	Fiber	Calcium	Iron	Sodium
83 kcal	2 g	16 g	2 g	1 g	9 mg	0.5 mg	16 mg

Makes 48 cookies

Kids love these cookies, as do adults. Best of all, they're simple and quick to bake.

Kitchen Tip

If desired, you can add 1 cup (250 mL) raisins with the dry ingredients.

Great Oatmeal Cookies

Preheat oven to 350°F (180°C)
Baking sheet, greased

1 cup	butter or margarine, softened	250 mL
¾ cup	brown sugar	175 mL
1	egg	1
½ tsp	vanilla extract	2 mL
1½ cups	all-purpose flour	375 mL
½ tsp	salt	2 mL
1 tsp	baking soda	5 mL
2 cups	old-fashioned rolled oats	500 mL

1. In a bowl, with an electric mixer, combine butter, brown sugar, egg and vanilla. Beat until smooth.

2. In another bowl, combine flour, salt, baking soda and oats. Add to butter mixture; mix well.

3. Spoon out about 1 tbsp (15 mL) dough and shape into a round ball. Place on prepared baking sheet. Flatten with a moistened fork. Bake in preheated oven for about 12 minutes or until lightly browned.

NUTRITIONAL ANALYSIS (PER COOKIE)

Energy	Protein	Carbohydrate	Fat	Fiber	Calcium	Iron	Sodium
93 kcal	2 g	11 g	5 g	1 g	9 mg	1 mg	79 mg

Best Chocolate Chip and Oatmeal Cookies

Preheat oven to 375°F (190°C)
Baking sheet, greased

1 cup	old-fashioned rolled oats	250 mL
1 cup	all-purpose flour	250 mL
¼ tsp	salt	1 mL
½ tsp	baking powder	2 mL
½ tsp	baking soda	2 mL
½ cup	butter or margarine, softened	125 mL
1 cup	packed brown sugar	250 mL
1	egg	1
½ tsp	vanilla extract	2 mL
1½ cups	semisweet chocolate chips	375 mL

1. In a large bowl, combine oats, flour, salt, baking powder and baking soda. Set aside.

2. In another large bowl, with an electric mixer, combine butter, brown sugar, egg and vanilla; beat until smooth. Add flour mixture; mix well. Fold in chocolate chips.

3. Spoon batter onto prepared baking sheet, making 1-inch (2.5 cm) round balls. Bake in preheated oven for 8 to 10 minutes or until just browned.

NUTRITIONAL ANALYSIS (PER COOKIE)							
Energy	Protein	Carbohydrate	Fat	Fiber	Calcium	Iron	Sodium
142 kcal	2 g	20 g	7 g	1 g	17 mg	1 mg	67 mg

Old-Fashioned Chocolate Chip Cookies

Preheat oven to 350°F (180°C)
Baking sheet, ungreased

⅓ cup	shortening	75 mL
⅓ cup	butter or margarine, softened	75 mL
½ cup	granulated sugar	125 mL
½ cup	brown sugar	125 mL
1	egg	1
1 tsp	vanilla extract	5 mL
1½ cups	all-purpose flour	375 mL
½ tsp	salt	2 mL
½ tsp	baking soda	2 mL
¾ cup	chocolate chips	175 mL

1. In a large bowl, with an electric mixer, cream together shortening and butter. Add granulated sugar, brown sugar, egg and vanilla. Mix until smooth. Stir in flour, salt and baking soda. Fold in chocolate chips.
2. Drop dough by spoonfuls onto baking sheet. Bake in preheated oven for 8 to 12 minutes or until browned.

NUTRITIONAL ANALYSIS (PER COOKIE)							
Energy	Protein	Carbohydrate	Fat	Fiber	Calcium	Iron	Sodium
94 kcal	1 g	12 g	5 g	0.4 g	6 mg	0.4 mg	56 mg

Makes 40 cookies

These wholesome whole wheat cookies are a good way to use up those overripe bananas you have tossed into the freezer.

Whole Wheat Banana Spice Cookies

Preheat oven to 375°F (190°C)
Baking sheets, greased

2 cups	whole wheat flour	500 mL
1 tsp	baking soda	5 mL
½ tsp	ground cinnamon	2 mL
¾ cup	lightly packed brown sugar	175 mL
½ cup	margarine or butter, softened	125 mL
1	egg	1
2	ripe bananas, mashed	2
¼ cup	chopped raisins	50 mL

1. In a bowl, combine flour, baking soda and cinnamon.

2. In another bowl, cream brown sugar, margarine and egg until fluffy. Stir in bananas and raisins. Stir in dry ingredients.

3. Drop batter by spoonfuls, 2 inches (5 cm) apart, on prepared baking sheets. Bake in preheated oven for 12 minutes or until set. Let cool on baking sheets for 10 minutes before removing to wire racks to cool completely.

NUTRITIONAL ANALYSIS (PER COOKIE)							
Energy	Protein	Carbohydrate	Fat	Fiber	Calcium	Iron	Sodium
68 kcal	1 g	10 g	3 g	1 g	8 mg	0.4 mg	68 mg

Makes 48 cookies

Old-Fashioned Gingersnaps

Preheat oven to 350°F (180°C)
Baking sheet, ungreased

3 cups	all-purpose flour	750 mL
2 tsp	baking soda	10 mL
1 tsp	ground ginger	5 mL
1 tsp	ground cinnamon	5 mL
$\frac{1}{2}$ tsp	salt	2 mL
$\frac{1}{2}$ tsp	ground cloves	2 mL
$\frac{3}{4}$ cup	margarine	175 mL
$\frac{1}{2}$ cup	packed brown sugar	125 mL
1	egg	1
$\frac{1}{2}$ cup	molasses	125 mL
$\frac{1}{2}$ cup	granulated sugar	125 mL

1. In a bowl, sift flour together with baking soda, ginger, cinnamon, salt and cloves.

2. In a large bowl, with an electric mixer, beat margarine until creamy. Gradually add brown sugar. Beat in egg and molasses. Stir in flour mixture and mix well. Wrap dough in plastic wrap or waxed paper; refrigerate for about 1 hour or until firm enough to handle.

3. Shape dough into $1\frac{1}{2}$-inch (4 cm) balls and roll in sugar. Place balls on baking sheet, 2 inches (5 cm) apart. Bake in preheated oven for 8 to 10 minutes or until browned. Let cool on wire racks.

NUTRITIONAL ANALYSIS (PER COOKIE)

Energy	Protein	Carbohydrate	Fat	Fiber	Calcium	Iron	Sodium
85 kcal	1 g	14 g	3 g	0.3 g	13 mg	1 mg	115 mg

Desserts

Makes 5 cups (1.25 L)

For this recipe, we used vanilla soymilk, but the pudding can be made with chocolate if you prefer. The spices can be tied in a cheesecloth bag, but if you don't have cheesecloth, you can just add them directly to the pudding and remove them once it's cooked.

Kitchen Tip

If you do not have whole cinnamon, cloves and cardamom, they can be replaced with ground spices. Use about ¼ tsp (1 mL) of each.

Vanilla Soymilk Rice Pudding

¾ cup	short-grain rice (such as Arborio)	175 mL
2	cardamom pods (see tip)	2
2	whole cloves	2
1	3-inch (7.5 cm) cinnamon stick	1
2 cups	vanilla-flavored soymilk	500 mL
⅓ cup	granulated sugar	75 mL
1	egg	1
1 tsp	vanilla extract	5 mL

1. In a large bowl, cover rice with cold water. Stir until water becomes cloudy; drain. Repeat until water is no longer cloudy.
2. Place rice in a saucepan and add 2 cups (500 mL) cold water; bring to a boil over medium-high heat. Cover, reduce heat to low and cook for 15 minutes or until liquid is absorbed. Remove from heat and stir in cardamom, cloves and cinnamon. Let stand, covered, for 10 minutes.
3. Stir soymilk and sugar into rice; bring to a boil over high heat. Reduce heat to low and cook, uncovered, for 15 minutes, stirring constantly. Discard spices.
4. In a bowl, beat a small amount of hot rice mixture into egg; stir into saucepan and cook, stirring constantly, for 3 minutes or until slightly thickened. Remove from heat and stir in vanilla. Serve warm.

NUTRITIONAL ANALYSIS (PER ½ CUP/125 ML)

Energy	Protein	Carbohydrate	Fat	Fiber	Calcium	Iron	Sodium
79 kcal	3 g	13.5 g	1.5 g	0.5 g	68 mg	0.7 mg	31 mg

Makes 1 cup (250 mL)

This delicious combo of fruits is high in vitamin C and fiber.

Strawberry-Kiwi Medley

1 cup	strawberries	250 mL
2	kiwifruit	2

1. In a food processor or blender, purée strawberries and kiwis until smooth.

NUTRITIONAL ANALYSIS (PER ¼ CUP/50 ML)

Energy	Protein	Carbohydrate	Fat	Fiber	Calcium	Iron	Sodium
40 kcal	1 g	9 g	0.4 g	2 g	21 mg	0.3 mg	2 mg

Makes 1 cup (250 mL)

This dessert is easily made in the microwave oven in one-quarter of the time required by conventional baking. It is readily handled by young eaters just learning to manage a spoon.

Kitchen Tips

Use regular or 2% evaporated milk.

For even cooking, prepare in individual cups.

Serving Suggestion

For adults, sprinkle top of each dessert with 1 tsp (5 mL) brown sugar. Arrange cups on a baking pan; place under preheated broiler. Broil until sugar is melted and browned. Fresh fruit makes a nice garnish. (The crisp sugar topping is not suitable for children.)

Microwave Crème Brûlée

Four ⅓-cup (75 mL) microwave-safe custard cups

1	can (6 oz/160 mL) evaporated milk	1
⅓ cup	granulated sugar	75 mL
2	eggs	2
1 tsp	vanilla extract	5 mL

1. In a small microwave-safe bowl, combine milk and granulated sugar. Microwave at High for 1 minute or until hot. Stir to dissolve sugar.

2. In a second bowl, combine eggs and vanilla; beat until well mixed. Stir in hot milk mixture; pour into custard cups. Arrange cups in a circle in microwave oven; microwave at Medium for 2 minutes or until each cup shows signs of bubbling. (Do not overcook; desserts should still be slightly liquid, but will thicken on standing.) Let cool at room temperature. Chill until time to serve.

NUTRITIONAL ANALYSIS (PER ¼ CUP/50 ML)

Energy	Protein	Carbohydrate	Fat	Fiber	Calcium	Iron	Sodium
138 kcal	6 g	20 g	3 g	–	131 mg	0.4 mg	78 mg

Makes 2½ cups (625 mL)

Serving Suggestion

Pour this cream over fresh fruit for dessert or serve plain on its own. You can also use whole milk in place of the evaporated milk.

Variation

Raspberry Vanilla Parfait: Dissolve ½ package (3 oz/ 85 g) of raspberry gelatin in ¼ cup (50 mL) boiling water. Top it up to 1 cup (250 mL) with cold water. Let cool. When the gelatin has almost set, layer the vanilla cream with the raspberry gelatin in parfait glasses. Refrigerate until set.

Vanilla Cream

¾ cup	evaporated 2% milk	175 mL
1¾ cups	water	425 mL
¼ cup	cornstarch	50 mL
¼ cup	granulated sugar	50 mL
¼ tsp	vanilla extract	1 mL

1. In a saucepan, combine evaporated milk and water. Bring to a boil, stirring constantly. Remove from heat.
2. In a small bowl, combine cornstarch and sugar with 1 tbsp (15 mL) of the milk mixture. Stir back into milk in saucepan. Return to a boil and cook, stirring constantly, for 3 to 4 minutes or until thick. Add vanilla. Let cool before serving.

NUTRITIONAL ANALYSIS (PER ¼ CUP/50 ML)

Energy	Protein	Carbohydrate	Fat	Fiber	Calcium	Iron	Sodium
44 kcal	1 g	9 g	0.4 g	–	53 mg	–	22 mg

Makes 2 cups (500 mL)

Variation

To make this a chocolate pudding, add 3 tbsp (45 mL) unsweetened cocoa powder to dry ingredients.

Vanilla Pudding

2 cups	2% milk, divided	500 mL
3 tbsp	cornstarch	45 mL
⅓ cup	granulated sugar	75 mL
¼ tsp	salt	1 mL
½ tsp	vanilla extract	2 mL

1. In the top of a double boiler, heat 1¾ cups (425 mL) of the milk over medium heat.
2. In a saucepan, blend cornstarch, sugar, salt and remaining ¼ cup (50 mL) milk. Gradually stir in heated milk from the double boiler; cook over medium heat, stirring constantly, until the mixture boils. Continue cooking for 1 minute. Remove saucepan from heat and stir in vanilla. Let cool before serving.

NUTRITIONAL ANALYSIS (PER ¼ CUP/50 ML)

Energy	Protein	Carbohydrate	Fat	Fiber	Calcium	Iron	Sodium
74 kcal	2 g	14 g	1 g	–	76 mg	–	86 mg

Makes 3 cups (750 mL)

Apple Pudding

Preheat oven to 375°F (190°C)
9-inch (23 cm) pie pan

4	medium baking apples, peeled, cored and sliced	4
1/3 cup	water	75 mL
1/3 cup	butter or margarine	75 mL
1/3 cup	granulated sugar	75 mL
2	eggs	2
1 cup	all-purpose flour	250 mL
1 1/2 tsp	baking powder	7 mL
1/4 tsp	salt	1 mL

1. Place apples in pan with the water. Bake in preheated oven for 10 minutes.

2. In a large bowl, with an electric mixer, cream together butter and sugar. Gradually beat in eggs. Stir in flour, sifted with baking powder and salt. Spread mixture over hot apples; bake for another 35 to 40 minutes.

NUTRITIONAL ANALYSIS (PER 1/4 CUP/50 ML)

Energy	Protein	Carbohydrate	Fat	Fiber	Calcium	Iron	Sodium
138 kcal	2 g	19 g	6 g	1 g	26 mg	1 mg	122 mg

Makes 6 servings

Apples, cinnamon and nutmeg elevate humble bread pudding to make this very special dessert. You can enhance it even more by adding a serving of Lemon or Vanilla Custard Sauce (see recipes, pages 318 and 319). Its soft texture is ideal for wee ones still lacking a full set of teeth.

Kitchen Tip

Instead of apples, try other fruit in season, such as strawberries, raspberries, pears or peaches.

Apple Bread Pudding

Preheat oven to 350°F (180°C)
6-cup (1.5 L) square baking dish

2 cups	2% milk	500 mL
⅓ cup	packed brown sugar	75 mL
½ tsp	ground cinnamon	2 mL
½ tsp	ground nutmeg	2 mL
2	eggs	2
1 tsp	vanilla extract	5 mL
2 cups	bread cubes	500 mL
2 tbsp	butter or margarine	25 mL
1	large apple, peeled, cored and thinly sliced (see tip)	1

1. In a bowl, whisk together milk, brown sugar, cinnamon, nutmeg, eggs and vanilla. Stir in bread and let stand for 10 minutes.

2. Meanwhile, place butter in baking dish and heat in preheated oven until melted; swirl to cover bottom of dish. Pour in bread mixture. Top with apples, pushing slices down into bread mixture.

3. Bake in preheated oven for 40 minutes or until puffed and browned. Serve warm, ensuring that infant portions have cooled to a safe temperature.

NUTRITIONAL ANALYSIS (PER SERVING)							
Energy	Protein	Carbohydrate	Fat	Fiber	Calcium	Iron	Sodium
183 kcal	6 g	24 g	7 g	1 g	132 mg	1 mg	146 mg

Creamy Rice Pudding

Rice pudding has a long history of being one of the great "comfort" desserts. Traditionalists demand raisins in their rice pudding, but why not try cranberries for a change? Self-feeding little ones can easily cope with rice pudding. It sticks equally well to a spoon or to fingers.

Kitchen Tips

For all the creaminess that you expect from a great rice pudding, use Arborio rice for this recipe. But if you can't find any, conventional long-grain rice will do the job. Just stay away from instant rice — it doesn't work very well.

Add vanilla to this or any other dessert after it has been removed from the heat. If added before, the vanilla flavor will evaporate.

3 cups	2% milk	750 mL
½ cup	Arborio or long-grain rice (see tip)	125 mL
¼ cup	granulated sugar	50 mL
1	cinnamon stick	1
¼ tsp	freshly gated nutmeg	1 mL
¼ tsp	salt	1 mL
1 tsp	vanilla extract	5 mL
¼ cup	chopped raisins or dried cranberries	50 mL

1. In a heavy saucepan over medium-high heat, combine milk, rice, sugar, cinnamon stick, nutmeg and salt. Bring to a boil. Reduce heat to low and cook, uncovered and stirring frequently, for 25 minutes or until rice is tender and creamy.

2. Remove and discard cinnamon stick. Stir in vanilla and raisins; cover and let stand for 10 minutes. Spoon into serving dishes and serve warm.

NUTRITIONAL ANALYSIS (PER ¼ CUP/50 ML)							
Energy	Protein	Carbohydrate	Fat	Fiber	Calcium	Iron	Sodium
113 kcal	4 g	20 g	2 g	0.3 g	109 mg	0.3 mg	89 mg

Makes 5¼ cups (1.3 L)

This pudding is delicious served warm with whole or evaporated milk poured on top.

Baked Rice Pudding

Preheat oven to 375°F (190°C)
8-cup (2 L) casserole dish, greased

½ cup	chopped raisins	125 mL
4 cups	water	1 L
1 cup	rice	250 mL
½ cup	granulated sugar	125 mL
2	eggs, beaten	2
2 cups	2% milk	500 mL
1 tbsp	butter or margarine	15 mL
	Ground cinnamon	

1. In a small bowl, cover raisins with hot water and let soak.
2. In a saucepan, boil 4 cups (1 L) water. Add rice and cook for about 15 minutes. Drain.
3. Drain raisins. Add rice to prepared casserole dish, along with sugar, eggs and raisins; mix well. Pour milk over. Top with small pieces of butter. Bake, uncovered, in preheated oven for about 1 hour or until crust is golden. Sprinkle with cinnamon just before serving.

NUTRITIONAL ANALYSIS (PER ¼ CUP/50 ML)							
Energy	Protein	Carbohydrate	Fat	Fiber	Calcium	Iron	Sodium
89 kcal	2 g	16 g	2 g	0.3 g	40 mg	0.3 mg	22 mg

Makes 12 servings

Thanks to the bananas and applesauce, this flavorful cake is very moist, without added fat.

Spiced Banana Yogurt Cake

Preheat oven to 350°F (180°C)
13- by 9-inch (3 L) baking dish, greased

2 cups	cake and pastry flour	500 mL
2 tsp	baking powder	10 mL
1 tsp	baking soda	5 mL
½ tsp	ground cinnamon	2 mL
½ tsp	ground nutmeg	2 mL
2	eggs	2
½ cup	granulated sugar	125 mL
1 cup	mashed banana (about 2)	250 mL
½ cup	unsweetened applesauce	125 mL
⅔ cup	plain yogurt	150 mL

1. In a bowl, combine flour, baking powder, baking soda, cinnamon and nutmeg.

2. In a large bowl, whisk eggs until frothy. Gradually beat in sugar until very thick. Stir in banana and applesauce. Stir in dry ingredients alternately with yogurt, making three additions of dry and two of yogurt. Spread in prepared pan.

3. Bake in preheated oven for 30 minutes or until center is firm to the touch. Let cool completely in pan on a wire rack before cutting into squares.

NUTRITIONAL ANALYSIS (PER SERVING)							
Energy	Protein	Carbohydrate	Fat	Fiber	Calcium	Iron	Sodium
165 kcal	4 g	34 g	1 g	1 g	56 mg	1 mg	178 mg

Carrot Cupcakes

Kitchen Tip

Enjoy these cupcakes on their own or with a cream cheese frosting of your choice.

Preheat oven to 325°F (160°C)
Two 12-cup muffin tins, greased or paper-lined

2 cups	all-purpose flour	500 mL
2 cups	granulated sugar	500 mL
1 tsp	baking powder	5 mL
1 tsp	baking soda	5 mL
1 tsp	salt	5 mL
1 tsp	ground cinnamon	5 mL
3 cups	finely shredded carrots	750 mL
1 cup	vegetable oil	250 mL
4	eggs, slightly beaten	4

1. In a large bowl, combine flour, sugar, baking powder, baking soda, salt and cinnamon. Add shredded carrots, oil and eggs; beat until combined.

2. Pour batter into prepared cupcake tins and bake in preheated oven for 20 to 25 minutes or until toothpick inserted in center comes out clean. Let cool before serving.

NUTRITIONAL ANALYSIS (PER CUPCAKE)

Energy	Protein	Carbohydrate	Fat	Fiber	Calcium	Iron	Sodium
213 kcal	2 g	28 g	11 g	1 g	21 mg	1 mg	192 mg

Makes 6 servings

This tangy fruit crisp wins acclaim with everyone who tries it. Plus, it is a good way to start adding tofu to recipes!

Apple Cranberry Crisp

Preheat oven to 400°F (200°C)
6-cup (1.5 L) baking pan, greased

4 cups	sliced peeled apples (about 4 medium)	1 L
½ cup	fresh or frozen cranberries	125 mL
½ cup	frozen orange juice concentrate, thawed, divided	125 mL
¼ cup	granulated sugar, divided	50 mL
½ tsp	ground cinnamon	2 mL
½ cup	soft tofu	125 mL
½ cup	plain yogurt	125 mL
1 tbsp	whole wheat flour	15 mL
Topping		
2 tbsp	quick-cooking rolled oats	25 mL
2 tbsp	wheat germ	25 mL
2 tbsp	packed brown sugar	25 mL

1. In a bowl, combine apples, cranberries, 2 tbsp (25 mL) orange concentrate, 2 tbsp (25 mL) sugar and cinnamon. Spoon mixture into prepared pan.

2. In another bowl, beat together tofu, yogurt, flour, remaining orange concentrate and remaining sugar. Pour over apple mixture.

3. *Topping:* In a small bowl, combine rolled oats, wheat germ and brown sugar. Sprinkle evenly over tofu mixture.

4. Bake in preheated oven for 25 minutes or until apples are tender.

NUTRITIONAL ANALYSIS (PER SERVING)							
Energy	Protein	Carbohydrate	Fat	Fiber	Calcium	Iron	Sodium
131 kcal	3 g	30 g	1 g	2 g	28 mg	1 mg	6 mg

Spiced Semolina Pudding

Preheat oven to 400°F (200°C)
4-cup (1 L) casserole dish, greased

2½ cups	2% milk	625 mL
3 tbsp	semolina	45 mL
1 tsp	ground allspice	5 mL
⅓ cup	granulated sugar	75 mL
	Grated zest of ½ lemon	
2	eggs, separated	2
¼ cup	chopped currants	50 mL

1. In a saucepan over medium-high heat, combine milk, semolina and allspice. Bring to a boil and cook, stirring, until mixture thickens. Continue to cook for approximately 5 minutes. Remove saucepan from heat. Stir in sugar, zest, egg yolks and currants.
2. In a medium bowl, whisk egg whites until they are stiff; gently fold into pudding mixture.
3. Transfer mixture to prepared casserole dish and bake in preheated oven for about 20 minutes or until lightly browned.

NUTRITIONAL ANALYSIS (PER ¼ CUP/50 ML)							
Energy	Protein	Carbohydrate	Fat	Fiber	Calcium	Iron	Sodium
173 kcal	7 g	31 g	2 g	1 g	74 mg	2 mg	32 mg

A real comfort food, gingerbread appeals to young and old alike. The apple gives this gingerbread extra moisture and a fresh flavor.

Apple Gingerbread

Preheat oven to 350°F (180°C)
13- by 9-inch (3 L) metal baking pan, greased

1 cup	whole wheat flour	250 mL
1 cup	all-purpose flour	250 mL
¼ cup	granulated sugar	50 mL
2 tsp	baking powder	10 mL
1 tsp	baking soda	5 mL
1 tsp	ground ginger	5 mL
½ tsp	ground cinnamon	2 mL
½ tsp	ground nutmeg	2 mL
½ cup	butter or margarine, softened	125 mL
2	eggs	2
½ cup	light (fancy) molasses	125 mL
⅓ cup	2% milk	75 mL
1¾ cups	grated peeled apple (about 2 medium)	425 mL

1. In a bowl, combine whole wheat flour, all-purpose flour, sugar, baking powder, baking soda, ginger, cinnamon and nutmeg.
2. In a large bowl, cream butter until light and fluffy. Stir in eggs and molasses. Stir in dry ingredients alternately with milk, making three additions of dry and two of milk. Fold in apples. Spread into prepared baking pan.
3. Bake in preheated oven for 35 minutes or until a cake tester inserted in the center comes out clean. Cool in pan on a wire rack before cutting.

NUTRITIONAL ANALYSIS (PER SERVING)

Energy	Protein	Carbohydrate	Fat	Fiber	Calcium	Iron	Sodium
187 kcal	3 g	27 g	8 g	2 g	59 mg	1 mg	190 mg

Makes one 12-slice cake

This moist, delicious cake is a great way to use up overripe bananas.

Kitchen Tip

For a different flavor twist, try adding 1 cup (250 mL) chocolate chips.

Banana Cake

Preheat oven to 325°F (160°C)
9- by 5-inch (2 L) loaf pan

1 cup	butter or margarine, softened	250 mL
1¾ cups	granulated sugar	425 mL
4	eggs, beaten	4
2 tsp	vanilla extract	10 mL
3 cups	all-purpose flour	750 mL
2 tsp	baking powder	10 mL
2 tsp	baking soda	10 mL
½ tsp	salt	2 mL
½ tsp	ground allspice	2 mL
½ tsp	ground cinnamon	2 mL
5	ripe bananas	5

1. In a large bowl, with an electric mixer, cream together butter and sugar. Beat in eggs and vanilla.

2. In another bowl, combine flour, baking powder, baking soda, salt, allspice and cinnamon. Stir into egg mixture. Add bananas and mix thoroughly. Transfer mixture to loaf pan.

3. Bake in preheated oven for 30 minutes. Increase temperature to 350°F (180°C) and bake for another 30 minutes.

NUTRITIONAL ANALYSIS (PER ½ SLICE)							
Energy	Protein	Carbohydrate	Fat	Fiber	Calcium	Iron	Sodium
226 kcal	3 g	33 g	10 g	1 g	23 mg	1 mg	243 mg

Makes 6 servings

Children really love the lemon flavor of this old-fashioned dessert. It never seems to go out of fashion.

Kitchen Tip

Instead of a single baking dish, use 6 individual baking dishes and reduce baking time to 30 minutes.

Lemon Custard Pudding Cake

Preheat oven to 350°F (180°C)
8-cup (2 L) baking dish, lightly greased

⅓ cup	all-purpose flour	75 mL
⅓ cup	butter or margarine, melted	75 mL
1½ cups	granulated sugar, divided	375 mL
4	eggs, separated	4
1½ cups	2% milk	375 mL
	Grated zest of 1 lemon	
2 tbsp	lemon juice	25 mL

1. In a large bowl, combine flour, butter and 1 cup (250 mL) of the sugar. In a small bowl, beat egg yolks; add to flour mixture along with milk and zest. Mix well. Stir in lemon juice.

2. In another bowl, beat egg whites until stiff, but not dry. Gradually beat in remaining sugar until stiff peaks form. Fold into batter.

3. Pour batter into prepared baking dish. Place in a shallow pan of hot water and bake in preheated oven for 55 minutes or until lightly browned. Serve warm.

NUTRITIONAL ANALYSIS (PER SERVING)

Energy	Protein	Carbohydrate	Fat	Fiber	Calcium	Iron	Sodium
393 kcal	7 g	60 g	15 g	0.3 g	97 mg	1 mg	139 mg

Makes 18 cupcakes

Banana and sour cream combine to give these cupcakes delicious flavor and moisture that lasts for several days, and will please the youngest appetite. One child we know loves to eat two cupcakes at a time, one held in each fist. If you're lucky, you may be offered a taste!

Kitchen Tip

Since one of your muffin tins will be only half-filled, fill empty cups with water to prevent the muffin tin from warping in the oven.

Banana Sour Cream Cupcakes

Preheat oven to 350°F (180°C)
Two 12-cup muffin tins, nonstick or paper-lined

2 cups	cake and pastry flour	500 mL
2 tsp	baking powder	10 mL
1 tsp	baking soda	5 mL
¼ cup	butter or margarine, softened	50 mL
⅔ cup	granulated sugar	150 mL
2	eggs	2
1 cup	mashed bananas (about 2 small)	250 mL
⅔ cup	sour cream	150 mL
½ tsp	vanilla extract	2 mL

1. In a small bowl, combine flour, baking powder and soda. Set aside
2. In a large bowl, with an electric mixer, cream butter until light and fluffy. Gradually beat in sugar, eggs and banana; blend until batter is smooth. Add flour mixture a bit at a time, alternating with sour cream and vanilla, stirring after each addition.
3. Spoon batter into muffin tins, leaving 6 cups empty (see tip). Bake in preheated oven for 16 minutes or until firm to the touch.

NUTRITIONAL ANALYSIS (PER CUPCAKE)							
Energy	Protein	Carbohydrate	Fat	Fiber	Calcium	Iron	Sodium
134 kcal	2 g	22 g	4 g	0.5 g	30 mg	1 mg	132 mg

Makes 3 cups (750 mL)

The whole family will enjoy this flavorful compote of fall fruits and citrus. Inexpensive and easy to make, it keeps well in the refrigerator and can be frozen for longer storage.

Kitchen Tip

Use your favorite dried fruits, such as apricots, pears, banana chips, prunes, dates or figs.

Fall Fruit Compote

2	large apples or pears, peeled, cored and sliced	2
1	medium orange	1
1	lemon	1
4 oz	dried mixed fruit (see tip)	125 g
2 tbsp	packed brown sugar	25 mL
¾ cup	water	175 mL
1	cinnamon stick	1

1. Place apple slices in a saucepan. Remove large strips of zest from orange and lemon; add to apples. Peel orange, cut into chunks and add to apples. Squeeze lemon and measure 1 tbsp (15 mL) juice; add to apples along with dried fruit, sugar, water and cinnamon stick.

2. Bring mixture to a boil. Reduce heat to medium-low, cover and cook for 10 minutes or until fruit is tender. Remove orange and lemon strips, as well as cinnamon stick; discard. Let cool slightly. Serve at room temperature or cover and refrigerate for 4 hours or longer.

NUTRITIONAL ANALYSIS (PER ¼ CUP/50 ML)

Energy	Protein	Carbohydrate	Fat	Fiber	Calcium	Iron	Sodium
40 kcal	0.3 g	9 g	1 g	1 g	18 mg	0.4 mg	1 mg

Makes 1¼ cups (300 mL)

Make a dessert into something extra special with one of these sauces. Try them on Apple Bread Pudding (see recipe, page 306). They are also great on pancakes or over fresh fruit.

Kitchen Tip

Unused egg whites can be stored in the refrigerator for several days or frozen for several months.

Saucy Finishes

Vanilla Sauce

¼ cup	granulated sugar	50 mL
1 tbsp	all-purpose flour	15 mL
Pinch	salt	Pinch
1 cup	2% milk, divided	250 mL
1	egg yolk	1
1 tbsp	butter or margarine	15 mL
½ tsp	vanilla extract	2 mL

1. In a small saucepan, combine sugar, flour and salt. Add ½ cup (125 mL) of the milk; stir until mixture is smooth. Whisk in remaining milk. Bring to a boil. Reduce heat and simmer, stirring constantly, for 2 minutes.

2. In a small bowl, stir egg yolk with a fork. Stir in some of the hot milk mixture and return to saucepan; cook, stirring constantly, for 1 minute (be careful not to boil). Remove from heat. Stir in butter and vanilla. Serve immediately.

NUTRITIONAL ANALYSIS (PER 1 TBSP/15 ML)

Energy	Protein	Carbohydrate	Fat	Fiber	Calcium	Iron	Sodium
24 kcal	1 g	3 g	1 g	–	16 mg	0.1 mg	17 mg

Lemon Sauce

⅓ cup	granulated sugar	75 mL
2 tbsp	cornstarch	25 mL
1 tsp	grated lemon zest	5 mL
Pinch	salt	Pinch
1 cup	boiling water	250 mL
2 tbsp	butter or margarine	25 mL
2 tbsp	lemon juice	25 mL

1. In a small saucepan, combine sugar, cornstarch, lemon zest and salt. Gradually stir in boiling water. Cook over medium heat, stirring constantly, until sauce is clear and thickened. Remove from heat. Stir in butter and lemon juice. Serve immediately.

NUTRITIONAL ANALYSIS (PER 1 TBSP/15 ML)

Energy	Protein	Carbohydrate	Fat	Fiber	Calcium	Iron	Sodium
24 kcal	–	4 g	1 g	–	1 mg	–	15 mg

Makes 8 servings

Clafouti is a specialty of the Limousin region in central France. It features a thick egg batter which is poured over fresh fruit before baking. The result is sure to be a family favorite — and it is one of the easiest desserts you will ever make!

Fruit Clafouti Dessert

Preheat oven to 350°F (180°C)
Shallow 8-cup (2 L) baking dish, greased

2 tbsp	butter or margarine	25 mL
6 cups	sliced fruit (such as peeled peaches, pears or apples)	1.5 L
½ cup	2% milk	125 mL
⅓ cup	all-purpose flour	75 mL
⅓ cup	granulated sugar	75 mL
3	eggs	3
¼ tsp	baking powder	1 mL
1 tbsp	granulated sugar	15 mL
½ tsp	ground cinnamon	2 mL

1. In a large microwave-safe container, melt butter on High for 20 seconds. Stir in fruit; microwave for 4 minutes or until fruit is barely tender. Transfer to prepared baking dish.

2. In a food processor or blender, combine milk, flour, ⅓ cup (75 mL) sugar, eggs and baking powder; process until smooth. Pour over fruit mixture in baking dish, lifting slices with a fork to allow batter to run through. Sprinkle 1 tbsp (15 mL) sugar and cinnamon over top. Bake in preheated oven for 45 minutes or until knife inserted in center comes out clean. Serve warm.

NUTRITIONAL ANALYSIS (PER SERVING)							
Energy	Protein	Carbohydrate	Fat	Fiber	Calcium	Iron	Sodium
158 kcal	4 g	26 g	5 g	2 g	40 mg	0.6 mg	55 mg

Should your family prefer fruit other than strawberries, this recipe is also wonderful with peaches, raspberries, bananas or blueberries.

Yogurt Strawberry Freeze

8-inch (2 L) square pan

1 cup	crushed strawberries	250 mL
1 cup	plain or vanilla-flavored yogurt	250 mL
½ cup	granulated sugar, divided	125 mL
¼ cup	pasteurized egg whites	50 mL

1. In a bowl, combine crushed strawberries, yogurt and ⅓ cup (75 mL) sugar.

2. In another bowl, beat egg whites with remaining sugar until stiff peaks form. Fold into strawberry mixture. Spread evenly in pan. Cover pan and freeze until firm, at least 2 hours or for up to 1 week. Scoop out servings of an appropriate size for each family member.

NUTRITIONAL ANALYSIS (PER ½ CUP/125 ML)

Energy	Protein	Carbohydrate	Fat	Fiber	Calcium	Iron	Sodium
105 kcal	4 g	22 g	1 g	1 g	82 mg	0.1 mg	47 mg

Resources

Breastfeeding Information

Canadian Lactation Consultants
Association
www.clca-accl.ca

Hollister Ltd.
www.hollister.com
Breast pump manufacturer

Jack Newman
www.breastfeeding.com

La Leche League International
www.llli.org
www.lalecheleaguecanada.ca (Canada)
Provides breastfeeding support

Medela Inc.
www.medela.com
Breast pump manufacturer

Motherisk
www.motherisk.org
1-877-327-4636

Infant Formula Companies

Abbott Nutrition
www.abbottnutrition.com (U.S.)
www.abbottnutrition.ca (Canada)

Mead Johnson Nutritionals
www.meadjohnson.com

Nestle Nutrition
www.verybestbaby.com (U.S. only)
www.nestle-baby.ca (Canada)

Baby Food Companies

Beechnut
www.beechnut.com (U.S.)
www.beechnut.ca (Canada)

Gerber Baby Foods
www.gerber.com (U.S.)
www.gerbercanada.com (Canada)

Heinz Canada
www.heinzbaby.com

Professional Organizations

American Academy of Pediatrics
www.aap.org
*Professional association of American
pediatricians*

American College of Obstetricians and
Gynecologists
www.acog.org
*Professional association of American
obstetricians and gynecologists*

American Dietetic Association
www.eatright.org
*Professional association of dietitians in
the U.S.*

Canadian Dental Association
www.cda-adc.ca
Professional association of Canadian dentists

Canadian Paediatric Society
www.cps.ca
Professional association of Canadian pediatricians

Dietitians of Canada
www.dietitians.ca
Professional association of registered dietitians in Canada

Food Allergy and Anaphylaxis Network
www.foodallergy.org
Provides a communication link on allergy and anaphylaxis for affected children and adults and for caregivers

Public Health Agency of Canada
www.phac-aspc.gc.ca
Provides Internet access to credible health information

Society of Obstetricians and Gynecologists of Canada
www.sogc.medical.org
Professional association of Canadian obstetricians and gynecologists

Other

Canadian Food Inspection Agency
www.inspection.gc.ca

Eating Well with Canada's Food Guide
www.hc-sc.gc.ca/fn-an/food-guide-aliment/index_e.html

Environmental Protection Agency (U.S.)
www.epa.gov

The Food Pyramid (U.S.)
www.nal.usda.gov/fnic/Fpyr/pyramid.gif

Health Canada
www.hc-sc.gc.ca

Hospital for Sick Children
www.sickkids.ca
Toronto's world-renowned pediatric hospital

March of Dimes
www.marchofdimes.com
Provides pregnancy and newborn health education

Specialty Food Shop
www.sickkids.on.ca/specialtyfoodshop/
Associated with the Hospital for Sick Children; allergen-free products available for purchase; dietitians available to answer questions

United States Food and Drug Administration
www.cfsan.fda.gov

World Health Organization
www.who.int

References

American Academy of Pediatrics — Committee on Nutrition. Policy Statement. Prevention of pediatric overweight and obesity. Pediatr 2003;112(2):424–30.

American Heart Association. Dietary recommendations for children and adolescents: A guide for practitioners. Pediatr 2006;117(2):544–59.

Auestad N, et al. Growth and development in term infants fed long-chain polyunsaturated fatty acids: A double-masked, randomized, parallel, prospective, multivariate study. Pediatr 2001;108:372–81.

Bazzano LA. The high cost of not consuming fruits and vegetables. JADA 2006;106:1364–68.

Blumberg S. Infant feeding: Can we spice it up a bit? JADA 2006;106:504–5.

Brenna JT, et al. Docosahexaenoic and arachidonic acid concentrations in human breast milk worldwide. Am J Clin Nutr 2007;85:1457–64.

Calvo MS, et al. Vitamin D fortification in the United States and Canada: Current status and data needs. Am J Clin Nutr 2004;80(Suppl):1710S–16S.

Carruth BR, et al. Prevalence of picky eaters among infants and toddlers and their caregivers' decisions about offering a new food. JADA 2004;104:s57–64.

Cotterman K. Reverse pressure softening: A simple tool to prepare areola for easier latching during engorgement. J Human Lactation 2004;20:227–37.

Dell S, To T. Breastfeeding and asthma in young children: Findings from a population-based study. Arch Pediatr Adolesc Med 2001;155:1261–65.

de Onis M, et al. Comparison of the WHO child growth standards and the CDC 2000 growth charts. J Nutr 2007;137:144–48.

de Onis M, Onyango AW. The Centers for Disease Control and Prevention 2000 growth charts and the growth of breastfed infants. Acta Paediatr 2003;92:413–19.

Domellof M, et al. Iron absorption in breast-fed infants: Effects of age, iron status, iron supplements, and complementary foods. Am J Clin Nutr 2002;76:198–204.

Eberhardt MV, et al. Antioxidant activity of fresh apples. Nature 2000;405:903–4.

Ekstrom A, Nissen E. A mother's feelings for her infant are strengthened by excellent breastfeeding counseling and continuity of care. Pediatrics 2006;118:e309–14.

Fewtrell MS, et al. Optimal duration of exclusive breastfeeding: What is the evidence to support current recommendations? Am J Clin Nutr 2007;85(Suppl):635S–38S.

Finkelstein JN, Johnston CJ. Enhanced sensitivity of the postnatal lung to environmental insults and oxidant stress. Pediatrics 2004;113:1092–96.

Fiocchi A, et al. Food allergy and the introduction of solid foods to infants: A consensus document. Adverse Reactions to Foods Committee, American College of Allergy, Asthma and Immunology 2006;97:10–20.

Forastiere F, et al. Consumption of fresh fruit rich in vitamin C and wheezing symptoms in children. Thorax 2000;55:283–88.

Forestell CA, Mennella JA. Early determinants of fruit and vegetable acceptance. Pediatr 2007;120:1247–54.

Fox MK, et al. Sources of energy and nutrients in the diets of infants and toddlers. JADA 2006;106:S28–42.

Friedman NJ, Zeiger RS. The role of breast-feeding in the development of allergies and asthma. J Allergy Clin Immunol 2005;115:1238–48.

Gale CR, et al. Critical periods of brain growth and cognitive function in children. Brain 2004;127:321–29.

Garriguet D. Sodium consumption at all ages. Health Reports 2007;18(2):47–52. Statistics Canada Catalogue 82-003.

Gillman MW, et al. Family dinner and diet quality among older children and adolescents. Arch Fam Med 2000;9:235–40.

Greer FR, et al. Effects of early nutritional interventions on the development of atopic disease in infants and children: The role of maternal dietary restriction, breastfeeding, timing of introduction of complementary foods and hydrolyzed formulas. Pediatr 2008;121:183–91.

Guenther PM, et al. Most Americans eat much less than recommended amounts of fruits and vegetables. JADA 2006;106:1371–79.

Hanson LA. Breastfeeding provides passive and likely long-lasting active immunity. Ann Allergy Asthma Immunol 1998;81:523–33.

Hawkins SS, et al. Maternal employment and breast-feeding initiation: Findings from the millennium cohort study. Pediatr Perinatal Epi 2007;21:242–47.

Hibbeln JR, et al. Maternal seafood consumption in pregnancy and neurodevelopmental outcomes in childhood (ALSPAC study): An observational cohort study. Lancet 2007;369:578–85.

Hollis BW, Wagner CL. Assessment of dietary vitamin D requirements during pregnancy and lactation. Am J Clin Nutr 2004;79:717–26.

Iacono G, et al. Gastrointestinal symptoms in infancy: A population-based prospective study. Dig Liver Dis 2005;37:432–38.

Jensen CL. Effects of n-3 fatty acids during pregnancy and lactation. Am J Clin Nutr 2006;83:1452S–57S.

Kramer MA, Kakuma R. Maternal dietary antigen avoidance during pregnancy or lactation, or both, for preventing or treating atopic disease in the child. Cochrane Database Syst Rev 2006;3:CD000133.

Kramer MS, et al. Feeding effects on growth during infancy. J Pediatr 2004;145:600–605.

Krebs NF, Hambidge KM. Complementary feeding: Clinically relevant factors affecting timing and composition. Am J Clin Nutr 2007;85(Suppl): 639S–45S.

Labbok MH. Effects of breastfeeding on the mother. Pediatr Clin North Am 2001;48:143–58.

Lee WWR. An overview of pediatric obesity. Pediatr Diabetes 2007;8(Suppl 9):76–87.

Loening-Baucke V. Prevalence, symptoms and outcome of constipation in infants and toddlers. J Pediatr 2005;146:359–63.

Lozoff B, et al. Double burden of iron deficiency in infancy and low socioeconomic status. A longitudinal analysis of cognitive test scores to age 19 years. Arch Pediatr Adolesc Med 2006;160:1108–13.

Lozoff B, et al. Behavioral and developmental effects of preventing iron-deficiency anemia in healthy full-term infants. Pediatr 2003;112: 846–54.

Marlett JA, et al. Position of the American Dietetic Association: Health implications of dietary fiber. JADA 2002;102:993–1000.

Martin R, et al. Human milk is a source of lactic acid bacteria for the infant gut. J Pediatr 2003;143:754–58.

Martin RM, et al. Breast-feeding and childhood cancer: A systematic review with metaanalysis. Int J Cancer 2005;117:1020–31.

McCann D, et al. Food additives and hyperactive behaviour in 3-year-old and 8/9-year-old children in the community: A randomized, double-blinded, placebo-controlled trial. Lancet 2007;370:1560–67.

Mennella JA, et al. Flavor programming during infancy. Pediatrics 2004;113:840–45.

Mennella JA, et al. Prenatal and postnatal flavor learning by human infants. Pediatrics 2001;107:1–6.

Mozaffarian D, et al. Trans fatty acids and cardiovascular disease. NEJM 2006;354:1601–13.

Nainar SM, Hohummed S. Diet counseling during the infant oral health visit. Pediatr Dent 2004;26:459–62.

O'Connor DL, et al. Growth and development in preterm infants fed long-chain polyunsaturated fatty acids: A prospective, randomized controlled trial. Pediatr 2001;108:359–71.

Oddy WH. Breastfeeding protects against illness and infection in infants and children: A review of the evidence. Breastfeed Rev 2001;9:11–18.

Ogden CL, et al. Obesity among adults in the United States — no change since 2003–2004. NCHS data brief no 1. Hyattsville, MD: National Center for Health Statistics. 2007.

Oski FA. Iron deficiency in infancy and childhood. NEJM 1993;329:190–93.

Porter J. Treating sore, possibly infected nipples. J Human Lactation 2006;20:221–22.

Position of the American Dietetics Association and Dietitians of Canada: Dietary fatty acids. JADA 2007;107:1599–1611.

Position of the American Dietetic Association and Dietitians of Canada: Nutrition and women's health. JADA 2004;104:984–1001.

Quigley MA, et al. Breastfeeding and hospitalization for diarrheal and respiratory infection in the United Kingdom Millennium Cohort Study. Pediatrics 2007;119:e837–42.

Schneider JM, et al. Anemia, iron deficiency, and iron deficiency anemia in 12–36-mo-old children from low-income families. Am J Clin Nutr 2005;82:1269–75.

Sherwood KL, et al. One-third of pregnant and lactating women may not be meeting their folate requirements from diet alone based on mandated levels of folic acid fortification. J Nutr 2006;136:2820–26.

Snethen JA, et al. Childhood obesity: The infancy connection. Journal of Obstetric, Gynecologic & Neonatal Nursing 2007;36:501–10.

Stricker T, Braegger CP. Cholesterol intake, biosynthesis of cholesterol and plasma lipids in infants. Effects of early cholesterol intake on cholesterol biosynthesis and plasma lipids among infants until 18 months of age. J Pediatr Gastroenterol Nutr 2006;42:591.

Thorley V. Latch and the fear response: Overcoming an obstacle to successful breastfeeding. Breastfeeding Rev 2005;13:9–11.

Videon TM, Manning CK. Influences on adolescent eating patterns: The importance of family meals. J Adolesc Health 2003;32(5):365–73.

Wall CR, et al. Milk versus medicine for the treatment of iron deficiency anaemia in hospitalized infants. Arch Dis Child 2005;90:1033–38.

Williams CL. Dietary fiber in childhood. J Pediatr 2006;149:S121–30.

Zutavern A, et al. Timing of solid food introduction in relation to eczema, asthma, allergic rhinitis, and food and inhalant sensitization at the age of 6 years: Results from the prospective birth cohort study LISA. Pediatr 2008;121:e44–52.

Library and Archives Canada Cataloguing in Publication

Kalnins, Daina
  Better baby food : your essential guide to nutrition, feeding & cooking for all babies & toddlers / Daina Kalnins, Joanne Saab. — 2nd ed.

Includes index.
ISBN-13: 978-0-7788-0195-5
ISBN-10: 0-7788-0195-0

1. Cookery (Baby foods). 2. Infants—Nutrition. I. Saab, Joanne. II. Title.

TX740.K34 2008   641.5'622   C2008-902467-2

Index